Routledge Revivals

Sufferers and Healers

Lucinda McCray Beier's remarkable book, first published in 1987, enters the world of illness in seventeenth-century England, exploring what it was like to be either a sufferer or a healer. A wide spectrum of healers existed, ranging between the housewife, with her simple herbal preparations, local cunning-folk and bonestters, travelling healers, and formally accredited surgeons and physicians. Basing her study upon personal accounts written by sufferers and healers, Beier examines the range of healers and therapies available, describes the disorders people suffered from, and indicates the various ways sufferers dealt with their ailments. She includes several case-studies of healers and sufferers, and looks in detail at the ways in which women's identities and duties were associated with childbirth, illness and healing. This title will be of interest to students of history.

Sufferers and Healers

The Experience of Illness in Seventeenth-Century England

Lucinda McCray Beier

Routledge
Taylor & Francis Group
Routledge Revivals

First published in 1987
by Routledge & Kegan Paul Ltd

This edition first published in 2015 by Routledge
2 Park Square, Milton Park, Abingdon, Oxon, OX14 4RN
and by Routledge
711 Third Avenue, New York, NY 10017

Routledge is an imprint of the Taylor & Francis Group, an informa business

A Library of Congress record exists under LC control number: 87020771

ISBN 13: 978-1-138-18263-9 (hbk)
ISBN 13: 978-1-315-64621-3 (ebk)

SUFFERERS & HEALERS

The experience of illness in Seventeenth-Century England

LUCINDA McCRAY BEIER

ROUTLEDGE & KEGAN PAUL
LONDON AND NEW YORK

First published in 1987 by
Routledge & Kegan Paul Ltd
11 New Fetter Lane, London EC4P 4EE

Published in the USA by
Routledge & Kegan Paul Inc.
in association with Methuen Inc.
29 West 35th Street, New York, NY 10001

Set in Bembo
by Columns of Reading
and printed in Great Britain
by Richard Clay Ltd.,
Bungay, Suffolk

Library of Congress Cataloging in Publication Data
Beier, Lucinda McCray.
Sufferers and healers.
Bibliography: p.
Includes index.
1. Physician and patient – England – History – 17th century. 2. Medicine – England – History – 17th century.
I. Title.
R727.3.B43 1987 610'.941 87–20771
ISBN 0–7102–1053–1

British Library CIP Data also available
ISBN 0–7102–1053–1

To Lee, with gratitude and love.

CONTENTS

N.B. In quotations from original sources, spelling and punctuation have been modernised and abbreviations and suspensions have been extended. Dates are given in new style, the year beginning on 1 January.

ACKNOWLEDGMENTS

No book can be attributed to its author alone. This is especially true of first books, even truer of the books resulting from Ph.D. theses. If I were to thank all of those who influenced the conception, preparation and execution of this work, this brief note would be longer than the book itself. Thus, I must be economical.

First of all, thanks are due to my parents, Robert and Janet McCray, who encouraged my earliest interest in history and medicine. I also wish to thank my first history teachers, foremost among them Professor A. R. Hogue of Indiana University. Later inspiration, support and criticism came from the history faculty at the University of Illinois at Urbana, especially from Professor Walter Arnstein and Dr Caroline Hibbard. My thesis would never have been finished without the help of my supervisor at the University of Lancaster, Dr Roger Smith. My external examiners, Dr Paul Slack and Dr Roy Porter, have rendered assistance above and beyond the call of duty. I am grateful to Dr David Hamilton for his careful reading of Chapter 3. I would also like to thank the Cambridge University Press for allowing me to reprint material on the Josselins' experience contained in my essay 'In sickness and in health: a seventeenth-century family's experience' (in *Patients and Practitioners*, ed. Roy Porter, Cambridge University Press, 1985).

I am especially grateful to the Interlibrary Loan department at the University of Lancaster and the staffs of the Library of the Wellcome Institute for the History of Medicine and the British Library. I also wish to thank the Royal Society, without whose grant I would have been unable to complete my research. Andrew Wheatcroft, my editor at Routledge & Kegan Paul, has provided practical and moral support throughout the process of converting thesis to book, proving that the clichéd enmity between publishing staff and writers need have no basis in fact.

Finally, I must thank my family. My sons, Robert Joseph, Jesse, Jacob and Zachary, were all born during the years spent researching and writing this book. They have tolerated the haphazard housekeeping resulting from 'mummy's work' without complaint and with much good humour. To my husband, Lee, I owe a debt which can never be repaid. His practical aid, imaginative criticism and expert advice have helped turn a vague fantasy into a reality. The faults in this book are my own; much of the good in it is his.

1

INTRODUCTION

Along with death, taxes and the poor, illness, injury, childbirth and old age are always with us. These human universals are, and have always been, intrinsically interesting, permeating day-to-day conversation, providing comedy and tragedy in entertainment, and forming the subject matter of research in a multitude of disciplines.

Today we are obsessed by various aspects of health and illness. We exercise and diet according to infinitely mutable theories. Endlessly we debate the moral and ethical issues of abortion, contraception and euthanasia. We criticise, exploit and are addicted to our medical services, expecting far more than we can ever receive. We live in fear of diseases such as cancer, multiple sclerosis and AIDS, enraged because they are beyond our control.

Our vulnerability, fear and anger are not new. These also are common aspects of the human condition, products, like other pieces of mental baggage, of the Western tradition which has never become reconciled to the existence of evil and mortality. Some things do not change. Suffering and death come to us all.

However, the twentieth century has produced a major change in our expectations. We expect our children to be born alive and perfect. We expect health and a sense of well-being. We expect to live for at least the biblical three score and ten years. We expect our healers, like trained auto mechanics, to be able to fix damaged parts of us with a minimum of fuss and discomfort, putting us back on the road in peak running condition. We are losing the concept of natural death, that ancient loop-hole which comforted and exonerated survivors in ages past. These days death, regardless of age or circumstances, is usually somebody's fault.

Our inflated expectations have resulted, in part, from a combination of public health measures and developments in medical science. Perhaps understandably, in the past century medical historians have concentrated upon tracing the progress of medical science and eulogising the great doctors whose discoveries contributed to that progress. Scholars such as Charles Singer, Erwin Ackerknecht and Lester King produced general studies which concentrated on the development of rational, scientific medicine.[1] Biographers like Kenneth Dewhurst and Geoffrey Keynes described the lives and discoveries of those practitioners who contributed to that development.[2] These historians and others like them internalised the values and prejudices of the twentieth-century medical community. For them, the learned and licensed medical practitioners of the past might have been mistaken, but were always altruistic; unlearned and unlicensed healers were quacks, deliberately taking advantage of a vulnerable lay population; 'modern medicine' represented a victory of reason over superstition, knowledge over ignorance, life over death. This Whig interpretation of the history of medicine protects the medical status quo by creating and articulating the myth of uninterrupted medical heroism and inevitable progress. Our doctors inherit the mantle of their sainted ancestors.

Until fairly recently traditional medical history satisfied the needs of both the medical profession and the general public. The medical profession as we know it is a recent phenomenon. The pedigree provided for it by medical historians contributed to a necessary *esprit de corps* and allowed for a gradual inflation of its demands for respect and rewards. The general public, relieved from the age-old tyranny of infection and encouraged by a rise in living standards, gave its gratitude to the doctors who were the most visible agents of the improvements it perceived. Miracle medicine and miracle surgery heralded the dawn of a new age. People wanted to believe in 'modern medicine' because this belief offered an irresistible combination of confidence in the future and relief from personal responsibility for the health and illnesses of themselves and their loved ones.

Predictably the second half of the twentieth century has witnessed a re-examination of medicine and the provision of medical care. Developments in medical science have outrun the cultural context within which they operate. People are not sure about how to use the opportunities now available to them. By the same token, despite its enormous capabilities, medicine still cannot provide a guarantee of health and happiness for all. Disappointed consumers, like naïve children, blame the medical profession for its all-too-human frailties. Furthermore, there is the feeling that lay-people, in their enthusiasm for the medical revolution, have given too much responsibility and power to doctors. Childbirth has become an arena where mothers struggle for good birth experiences, while medical professionals fight for safety and domination. Patient–doctor relationships are examined for evidence of control strategies on the part of the doctors, passivity and lack of satisfaction on the part of patients. In the Age of the Expert, lay-people grow increasingly uncomfortable about their own powerlessness.

Like the profession with which it is associated, the history of medicine is undergoing a process of reassessment and change. Traditional historians, concerned with mapping the advance of medical science, implicitly treated patients as irrelevant, except as the vehicles or beneficiaries of medical discoveries. Doctors were expected and seen to be totally in control of the experience of illness. However, it is impossible to relate illness and medicine to its social context without recognising the significance of the sufferer's feelings, attitudes and behaviour. Thus, medical historians increasingly study the experiences of both healers and sufferers, examining the social impact of epidemics, gathering information about the provision of medical care, and re-examining the development of medical occupations.[3]

The social history of medicine might more correctly be called the social history of suffering because it combines the study of medical theories, treatments and practitioners with the study of the disorders people underwent and the ways they experienced and dealt with those disorders. Because it is a young field, it has the advantage for the historian of being relatively uncharted territory. It has the complementary disadvantage of providing few standard authorities either to build upon or to disagree with. Like general social history, it borrows analytical techniques from anthropology and sociology, attempting to place medical events, along with the participants in those events, in their appropriate cultural and social contexts.

This book examines the experience of ill-health in seventeenth-century England. It is essentially a one-question study: what did people of that time do when they became ill, were injured, or had babies? Neither the approaches to this question nor the conclusions reached are simple. One must first examine the conditions surrounding the experience of suffering, then allow for the great diversity in individual responses to these conditions. This book will describe the ailments seventeenth-century English people had and the many ways they dealt with these ailments. It will also describe the enormous variety of healers available in the period. In addition, it will investigate popular attitudes regarding illness and medical practitioners. Although the diversity of medical ideas and behaviour will be emphasised, several case studies of individual healers and sufferers will be included. These will allow us to experience vicariously what seventeenth-century illness and therapy could be like in a way general discussion cannot. One study cannot hope to provide a definitive view of seventeenth-century illness experience. Limits must be imposed. This book will not give a demographic or epidemiological view of seventeenth-century diseases. It will not attempt to describe contemporary living conditions or suggest any cause-effect relationship between these conditions and the disorders people suffered from. It also will not attempt indepth analysis of the relationship between medical theories and therapies.

Because of the nature of the questions asked and the source materials consulted, arguments and conclusions will be impressionistic rather than quantitative. The question of how representative these conclusions can be is justifiable. However, this study will argue that few generalisations about human experience can successfully be made. Despite common living conditions and the options generally available for handling illness, injury and childbirth, the individual's experience is ultimately unique. It depends on numerous factors, such as individual character, religious orientation, geographical location, social class, economic status, pain threshold and personal 'medical history', in combinations which prove quite resistant to attempts at generalisation. One can describe what individuals suffered and what they did about their problems. The more similar the accounts available, the more possible tentative generalisations become.

With the above reservations always in mind, some arguments will be made. In seventeenth-century England the most commonly used kinds of medical therapy were self-treatment and treatment rendered by lay-people – relations, friends and neighbours. Women acted as amateur healers, regardless of their social status. Medical information was widely disseminated in the population. Although certain types of medical knowledge, such as learned medicine, based on academic training, and popular medicine, based on oral tradition, can be identified, there is no clear demarcation between these types. Rather, there was a spectrum of medical knowledge shared by the population as a whole. Licensed physicians sometimes used popular therapies; lay-people were acquainted with learned medical theories and prescribed officially endorsed remedies for themselves and their friends.

Further, it will be argued that despite the efforts and aspirations of occupational organisations, there was no medical profession in seventeenth-century England. Providers of medical services, licensed and unlicensed, competed in an open market where the consumer remained largely in charge of his or her own care. Licensed medical practitioners had a monopoly over neither practice nor medical knowledge. Thus, although they and their unlicensed competitors might make claims of expertise, there was no consensus in the general population that licensed healers were the sole authorities in medical matters. The creation of a profession requires such a consensus.

Seventeenth-century sufferers' experience of illness and medicine was very different from that of their twentieth-century descendants. The modern inflation of expectations has been mentioned above. In the early modern period, whatever their hopes, people did not actually expect healers and medicines to cure them. Furthermore, as we shall see, they did not expect medicine-taking to make them feel better; most of the time, medicine made people feel very ill.

In addition, seventeenth-century illnesses, births and deaths were very social, in contrast to the privacy required by twentieth-century conventions. All of these events took place at home, witnessed by crowds of family members, friends and neighbours, as well as healers. All women were expected to prescribe for and nurse relatives, friends and neighbours. A married woman who had not been invited to the childbirth of someone closely connected to her might justifiably feel slighted. Visiting the sick was a religious and social duty performed by both sexes. Routine responsibility for and witnessing of birth, illness and death brought seventeenth-century people closer to the events of their own mortality than are those living in the twentieth century.

Source materials for this book are of six major types. The secondary literature dealing with both the general social history and the medical history of seventeenth-century England has been widely drawn upon. Indeed, the debts owed by this study for aid in articulating questions, finding resource materials and formulating conclusions are too great to be accurately enumerated. Keith Thomas's *Religion and the Decline of Magic* and Lawrence Stone's *The Family, Sex and Marriage in England 1500–1800* provided an enormous amount of background information and bibliographical help.[4] Although many of the arguments and conclusions of these seminal works may be challenged, their wide-ranging scholarship, imaginative approaches and superb readability were inspirational. Alan Macfarlane's *Witchcraft in Tudor and Stuart England: A Regional and Comparative Study*, along with Thomas's work, suggested ways in which anthropological perspectives could be brought to bear upon historical questions. It also added to the information gleaned from Thomas's book concerning unlearned and unlicensed healers.[5] A collection of essays edited by Charles Webster on *Health, Medicine and Mortality in the Sixteenth Century* suggested numerous ways of approaching that subject in the following century.[6] Michael MacDonald's pioneering study *Mystical Bedlam: Madness, Anxiety and Healing in Seventeenth-Century England* offered one method of using a healer's casebook as the primary source material for a discussion of seventeenth-century illness.[7] And Paul Slack's *The Impact of Plague in Tudor and Stuart England* illuminated ways in which disease can be viewed in its social context.[8] Unfortunately, I have been unable to cite Harold J. Cook's useful *The Decline of the Old Medical Regime in Stuart London*, which appeared after this book was completed.[9]

Such secondary reading served as the conceptual foundation upon which the information gleaned from primary sources was built. Casebooks kept by seventeenth-century medical practitioners give insight into the therapeutic routines and clienteles of healers. Diaries and correspondence of lay-people provide information about the disorders people suffered from, the treatments they used and the healers they consulted. These private papers also reveal general religious and theoretical orientations which are useful in explaining the medical behaviour of their writers. As historical sources they have obvious limitations. Writers of such documents are usually of upper or middling social origins. How representative can their records be of general experience? Firstly, it should be observed that the illness experience of even upper-class sufferers is rarely studied. As part of the wider picture, forming one end of the spectrum of observation and therapeutical attention, this experience offers a necessary perspective from which to view contemporary illness and medicine. Secondly, half a loaf is better than none at all; the historian must make the best possible use of whatever documents exist. Thirdly, although the writers of medical and surgical casebooks were of middling and upper status, many of their patients were not. Thus, casebooks allow inferences to be made about the general experience of medical and surgical care. Finally, sources originating with the social elite can be balanced by those having more direct links with a broader cross-section of the population.

The London Bills of Mortality and selected parish records have been consulted for evidence about causes of death. While the diseases people died from are not necessarily the same as those people lived with, they do act as a partial guide to the seventeenth-century medical 'scene'. For instance, the large number of plague deaths in the period helps to explain the general fear of plague felt even by people who lived far from the places usually threatened by epidemics.

Seventeenth-century popular literature and vernacular medical literature have been examined for information about attitudes concerning disease, healers and patients. This large body of writing tells a confused and sometimes contradictory tale. However, its complex character is useful in itself, underlining the general impression of complexity and diversity in matters relating to illness and medicine given by the other source materials.

This book is an exploratory study. It joins the small but growing body of work dealing with the sufferer's experience.[10] Rather than providing a complete picture of suffering and healing in seventeenth-century England, it hopes to suggest a number of directions for further research.

History is all about continuity and change. Historians have traditionally seen the seventeenth century as a watershed in the development of English medicine. Significant changes took place during the period. William Harvey discovered the circulation of the blood. Thomas Sydenham, the great clinician, advocated a return to empirical observation in the practice of medicine. The apothecaries stepped out of their medieval role as the servants of licensed physicians, increasingly becoming general practitioners in their own right. Man-midwives grew in number and power, giving promise of their eventual takeover of the practice of 'obstetrics' in the subsequent two centuries. Metallic 'Paracelsian' remedies increased in popularity, rivalling traditional herbal medicines. The spa became well established, offering a combination of fashionable social life and medicinal waters which would not decline in popularity until the late nineteenth century.

More examples could be given. However, for the individual sufferer, the early seventeenth century appears to have been much the same as the late seventeenth century. Remedies came in and out of fashion, but therapeutic evacuation was a constant. The medical marketplace was staffed by the same population of vendors at the beginning as at the end of the period. Although the plague disappeared after 1666, other seventeenth-century diseases remained to be suffered, feared and treated well after the new century began. Thus, this study concentrates on continuity rather than change, leaving the discussion of medical innovation to those not primarily concerned with the sufferer's point of view.

2

THE MEDICAL MARKETPLACE

In order to describe the seventeenth-century medical marketplace, we must first divest ourselves of the assumption that the licensed medical practitioner belonged to a recognised profession. Professor Geoffrey Holmes defines professional status as follows:

> a profession is a calling or vocation, exclusive . . . of occupations 'purely commercial, mechanical, agricultural or the like'; and . . . what gives it its distinctive social stamp is the fact that, through education and a career-oriented training, a particular body of specialised knowledge is acquired and is then applied to the service . . . of others.[1]

Only seventeenth-century physicians could have claimed to fulfil the requirements of such a definition. And even the physicians' claims were suspect. Their numbers were very small.[2] Relatively few sufferers ever became their patients. Even the patients of physicians were not in uniform agreement about the physicians' service motivations.[3] And the physicians themselves were quite vocally insecure about their status, complaining about their many competitors and about the insufficient respect they received from lay-men.

Other medical occupations had no pretensions to such 'professional' status in the seventeenth century. Healers such as surgeons, apothecaries, midwives, empirics and cunning-folk sold their services quite openly. Their training, usually by some form of apprenticeship, was similar to that employed by other trades and crafts.

Margaret Pelling describes the approaches of traditional historians to the analysis of the medical occupations for the period before 1800 as follows:

> Some of these emphasised the literary qualifications of a minority; some, to point a contrast, stressed earlier credulity or eccentricity;

> others entered into controversy over the craft origins of surgeons and apothecaries. Analysts have followed these leads without embarking on a freer discussion of the earlier period in terms outside those period-specific concepts used to describe the modern professions. This has had three main effects. First, by far the larger part of medical activity remains undescribed. Secondly, there is a disguising of the elements of continuity before and after 1800. Thirdly, there is a persistent underestimate of the connections between medicine and other economic and social activities.[4]

While the period after 1700 is outside the scope of this study and enterprises other than healing engaged in by medical practitioners will not be explored, an attempt will be made to describe as much of seventeenth-century medical activity as possible, and to place that activity in the context of the general social life of the period.

In order to do this, the links between seventeenth-century healers and the twentieth-century medical profession will be forgotten. The healers whose activities will be described will be seen, rather, as inhabiting a medical marketplace where services were advertised and sold to those sufferers who cared to shop. As this study can derive no benefit from attempting to make a qualitative distinction between medical and other occupations, no such distinction will be made. The society physician, in his red robe and full wig, may as easily be compared to the prosperous London merchant as to the bishop. Whether or not he was professional is unimportant; use of that label may well obscure more than it clarifies.

The following chapter will describe the many types of seventeenth-century healers. It will go on to examine healers' attitudes about themselves, other healers and the lay-population. Finally, it will turn to the question of healers' aspirations and public responses to them.

I LICENSED HEALERS

The truly licensed healers of seventeenth-century England were the physicians, surgeons and midwives. Physicians were licensed by bishops, universities and the Royal College of Physicians of London. They also sometimes became members of provincial medical guilds.[5] Surgeons were licensed by bishops and universities. They were also admitted to practise by the London Company of Barbersurgeons and provincial surgeons' companies or craft guilds. Midwives were licensed by bishops.[6]

Apothecaries, although they were technically neither healers nor licensed, will be included in the category of licensed healers. In London their position was legitimised by the Worshipful Society of Apothecaries (founded in 1617). They were alternately protected and persecuted by the physicians, depending upon whether they were perceived by their superior colleagues as loyal servants or renegade competitors. And, although their official function was merely to prepare medications, they often gave medical advice to those who patronised their shops.[7]

Theoretically the functions of these practitioners were very different. Physicians, although empowered by law to practise surgery and make up medications, were mainly expected to diagnose internal maladies and prescribe internal remedies. Partly because of their humanist training, partly because of their high social status, they were expected to be authorities, delegating most of the physical aspects of treatment to surgeons, apothecaries, nurses and servants. Surgeons were entrusted with injuries and the outward manifestations of disease. They set fractured bones, lanced infected swellings, dealt with obstructions such as bladder stones and treated skin rashes. They also treated venereal diseases and helped in difficult childbirths. They were expected to use only 'outward' remedies, leaving internal medicine to the physicians. Apothecaries, as indicated above, were expected to be experts in medical ingredients. Their function was to prepare remedies according to the directions given by physicians and surgeons.

Again theoretically, apothecaries and surgeons were expected to act under the direction of the learned physicians. The theory is well stated by Francis Herring, an early seventeenth-century Fellow of the Royal College of Physicians:

> So that the Physician, as a great Commander, hath as subordinate to him cooks for Diet, the surgeons for manual Operation, the Apothecaries for confecting and preparing medicines. You see then how goodly large and ample patrimony Physick hath, and that all her store and skill, consisteth not in compounding and mingling of a medicine. If that were all, then all our skillful chirurgeons and apothecaries . . . should be absolute and complete physicians. . . . And yet how far the cunningest of them are, from being able to give counsel in physic, both themselves will . . . freely acknowledge.[8]

Physicians had the highest social and economic status among all seventeenth-century medical practitioners. Their training was long and academic. They were expected to be able to read, write and speak in Latin and classical Greek. They were also expected to be familiar with a small library of classical and medieval medical works.[9] They obtained this education at university, attending Oxford or Cambridge and sometimes continuing their training at a continental university, such as Padua, Montpellier or Basel.

Several options were open to seventeenth-century medical students. For example, after 1570 Cambridge students became qualified physicians in one of two ways. Some obtained the MB by spending six years in residence, attending medical lectures, viewing dissections and participating in disputations in the schools, and acquired the MD five years later. Others took an MA, requiring seven years in residence, and then obtained a university medical licence which was both less expensive and easier to get than the MB.[10] English medical students who completed their educations at continental universities often returned to incorporate their degrees at one of the English universities, thus qualifying for membership of the Royal College of Physicians.

Not all of those who practised 'physic' in seventeenth-century England bothered to obtain English university degrees or licences. Some held bishops' licences which simply involved examination by the bishop of the diocese (or, in London, the Dean of St Paul's) and a panel of four physicians.[11] Many holders of foreign medical degrees practised both within and outside immigrant communities without bothering to obtain English accreditation.[12] All of the above practitioners, however, considered themselves learned and opposed the multitude of unlearned practitioners, be they surgeons, apothecaries, midwives, or part of the multitude of 'smiths, weavers and women' who prescribed internal remedies in spite of all legal and organisational attempts to stop them.[13]

Not all of those licensed to practise medicine were full-time physicians. Many, like the Buckinghamshire astrological physician, Richard Napier, were also clergymen.[14] The minister's duty to visit and comfort the sick made a combination of roles quite natural. The academic skills required for studying theology and medicine were similar. A suggestion has even been made that during times of religious turmoil, 'clerics prudently studied medicine as a safeguard'.[15] The Royal College of Physicians objected to the granting of licences to scholars who ultimately became clergymen.[16] However, this practice continued throughout the seventeenth century. The relationship between medicine and theology was a two-way street. While vicars sometimes were licensed physicians, physicians, such as the late sixteenth-century author, Timothy Bright, abandoned medicine for the church.[17]

At the top of the medical elite was the Royal College of Physicians of London (RCP), founded in 1518. From the beginning its members had a monopoly over the practice of medicine within the City of London and a seven-mile radius around the metropolis. After 1523 its monopoly was extended to include the whole country in an attempt to take the licensing of physicians out of the hands of the bishops and make it the responsibility of the RCP. Despite an unsuccessful attempt at regulating provincial practice by using 'Visitors', the RCP never developed the administrative machinery necessary to enforce its power outside London.[18] The RCP had the power to fine, imprison and bar from practice any person they found to be violating its monopoly. Numerous efforts were made to enforce this monopoly.[19] However, membership of the RCP was exclusive. At no time in the seventeenth century did it recognise more than forty Fellows. The membership of the RCP was so small and the numbers of those illegally prescribing internal medicines so large that attempts at enforcement were doomed to failure.

Furthermore, although the RCP's monopoly had been awarded in the first place to protect the populace from the depredations of the unlearned and unskilled, it frequently attacked practitioners such as Thomas Bonham, holder of a Cambridge MD, and John Banister, a learned surgeon, writer and translator.[20] Such actions make a nonsense of the RCP's claims of altruism and suggest questions about the reasons for its exclusivity, despite the obvious demand for medical services in London. The RCP appears to have been defeated by its own desire to protect its increasingly old-fashioned allegiance to lengthy classical education and its somewhat dubious claims regarding the gentility of physicians. By enlarging its membership and lowering the fees physicians charged, the RCP could most likely have made real the monopoly it claimed by law. However, to do so might have cheapened the physician in both his own estimation and in the eyes of the general public. For the RCP, such a result would have made the effort futile.

Surgeons were the most numerous of all licensed seventeenth-century healers.[21] Although the English universities licensed surgeons, most received their training by apprenticeship. They then could apply for bishops' licences, which were granted upon successful examination by the bishop and four expert

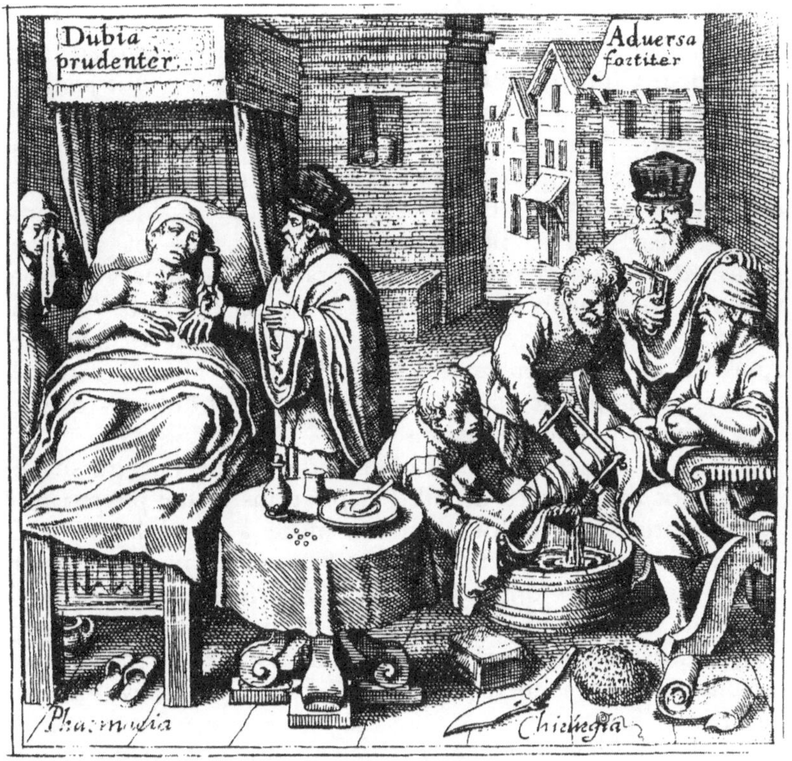

Engraving illustrating the duties of seventeenth-century apothecaries and surgeons. (Matthaeus Merian, *c.* 1646, Wellcome Library)

surgeons.[22] They could, alternatively, practise under the protection of one of the many craft organisations regulating surgeons which operated in towns and cities throughout the country.[23] In London the Barbersurgeons' Company, founded in 1540, was the largest of all the City Companies, numbering 293 members in 1641, of whom approximately half were surgeons.[24]

Surgeons were not expected to be multilingual or learned to the same degree as the physicians. However, they were expected to be literate in English and to have a sound basic understanding of such subjects as anatomy. Within the occupation there was an enormous diversity in training and social status, ranging from the learned surgeons, such as the sixteenth-century luminary William Clowes, to the local barbersurgeon who cut hair and drew teeth, in addition to performing surgical operations. The surgical elite pressed for higher standards. In 1564 the 'Master Surgeon' Thomas Gale lamented that 'every person good and bad, learned and unlearned, Chirurgeon or no Chirurgeon, do without penalty and correction of laws . . . take on them the practice of Chirurgerie'.[25] In order to remedy the situation, numerous handbooks for surgeons were published in English.[26] However, the craft organisations were most important in maintaining standards. The Barbersurgeons' Company of London punished its own members for malpractice and supervised the treatment of patients thought to be in danger of death.[27] It also prosecuted those who undertook surgical cases without the approval of the Company.[28] In addition, it housed surgical lectures and public dissections, thus contributing to the education of London surgeons.

Although surgeons shared neither the relatively high social status, nor the upward mobility aspirations of the physicians, the potential existed for them to make a good living and socialise with well-to-do people. Samuel Pepys numbered several surgeons among his friends. By performing a necessary function and providing relief from pain and handicap, the surgeons demonstrated their utility far more easily than could the physicians. It is therefore not remarkable that they were so numerous.[29]

For the apothecaries, the seventeenth was a very important century. Having formed their Worshipful Society in 1617 with the aid of the Royal College of Physicians, the apothecaries, both within and outside London, proceeded to spend the rest of the century challenging their erstwhile patrons for the right to practise internal medicine.[30] Their shops served both as outlets for merchandise and as consulting-rooms.

Like the surgeons, apothecaries were trained by apprenticeship. They were literate and, because of the demands made upon them by physicians, knew more than a little Latin. They were expected to be familiar with an enormous variety of medical ingredients, vegetable, animal and mineral, and were entrusted with the task of compounding the complicated recipes dear to the hearts of seventeenth-century physicians and patients. In addition to their familiarity with these ingredients, they were expected to understand the humoral qualities of the ingredients they used. Partly to standardise the remedies available and partly to help apothecaries in their work, the Royal College of Physicians published the first London *Pharmacopoeia* in Latin in 1618. This, in addition to the physicians' official duty to inspect apothecaries' shops, was expected to help the physicians control the apothecaries.

The apothecaries benefited from the general seventeenth-century greed for medicines. They also were able to capitalise on two important trends in the drug trade. English exploration and colonial expansion sent a steady stream of exotic foreign substances home throughout the century. Remedies such as tobacco, guaiacum and, late in the century, 'Jesuit's bark' increased apothecaries' incomes. Perhaps more important were the non-herbal Paracelsian remedies, such as mercury, antimony and vitriol, which were becoming popular by the beginning of the century. Shunned at first by the conservative 'Galenical' physicians, apothecaries and their Paracelsian colleagues, the chemists, prepared and sold these medicines alongside the surgeons.

Although the physicians tried to control the apothecaries, both by prosecuting individuals for practising medicine and by encouraging physicians to make their own remedies, the apothecaries were ultimately victorious.[31] For one thing, there were many more apothecaries than there were physicians. For another, what happened in apothecaries' shops was a private matter between the apothecary and the client. It was difficult for a physician to prove that an apothecary had been prescribing unless the apothecary wished to be found out.[32] By the end of the century, apothecaries were routinely acting as general practitioners, particularly in provincial areas.[33]

Last under the heading of officially recognised medical personnel, the midwives were uneasy companions of their more learned male colleagues. Although, like physicians and surgeons, they were licensed by the bishops, the licensing of midwives had more to do with their moral character than with their skill.

From the middle ages until the late sixteenth century at least, midwives were obliged to baptise infants who seemed likely to die before the sacrament could be administered by a priest.[34] Clergymen were expected to instruct midwives in the orthodox baptismal formula.

In addition, the midwife served a legal function, acting, along with the other women present, as a witness of the birth and an informal inquisitor of the labouring woman. A sixteenth-century midwife's licence makes her duties clear:

> ITEM you shall neither cause nor suffer any woman to name or put other father to the child, but only him that is the very father indeed thereof. ITEM you shall not suffer any woman to p'tend feign surmise herself to be delivered of a child which is not indeed neither to claim any other woman's child for her own. ITEM that

> ye shall never consent agree give or keep counsel that any woman be delivered secretly of that she goeth with but that in the presence of two or three honest women and that there be two or three lights always ready.[35]

It was obviously in the interests of both church and state that midwives be honest, loyal and spiritually orthodox.

Midwives were, of course, employed to deliver babies. They were summoned early in labour and stayed with their clients until the baby was born. In addition, like sick-nurses, they often performed household tasks during labour and sometimes after delivery.[36] Midwifery training was generally informal, although, according to the seventeenth-century man-midwife, Percival Willughby, 'The young midwives at London be trained seven years first under the old midwives, before they be allowed to practise for themselves'.[37] For the most part, the midwife was trained through her own experience and her observation of many births. Since not only she, but also a number of other neighbour women were present during the birth process, all had the opportunity to add to the local stock of information on the subject.[38] The midwife also served as an authority on matters of women's diseases and sexual relations.

Until the eighteenth century midwives delivered almost all of the babies born in England. Only occasionally were surgeons summoned to difficult births. In these cases the infant was usually delivered in pieces, and the woman endangered as well. Beginning in the sixteenth century, however, male healers began to show an interest in midwifery techniques, which was reflected in a gradually increasing body of literature published on the subject.[39] A few seventeenth-century practitioners became man-midwives. One of these, Peter Chamberlen, is traditionally credited with the invention of the midwifery forceps. However, the instrument was jealously guarded as a family monopoly by generations of Chamberlen *accoucheurs*. Not until it was reinvented by Edmund Chapman in 1733 did it come into general use.[40]

Surgeons accused midwives of ignorance. Indeed, midwives themselves were aware of their own need for reliable training. In 1616 several London midwives, with the help of Peter Chamberlen, petitioned the King and Parliament for the incorporation of a midwives' company which would be responsible for the training and licensing of midwives.[41] However, the formation of such a company was blocked by the Royal College of Physicians on the following grounds:

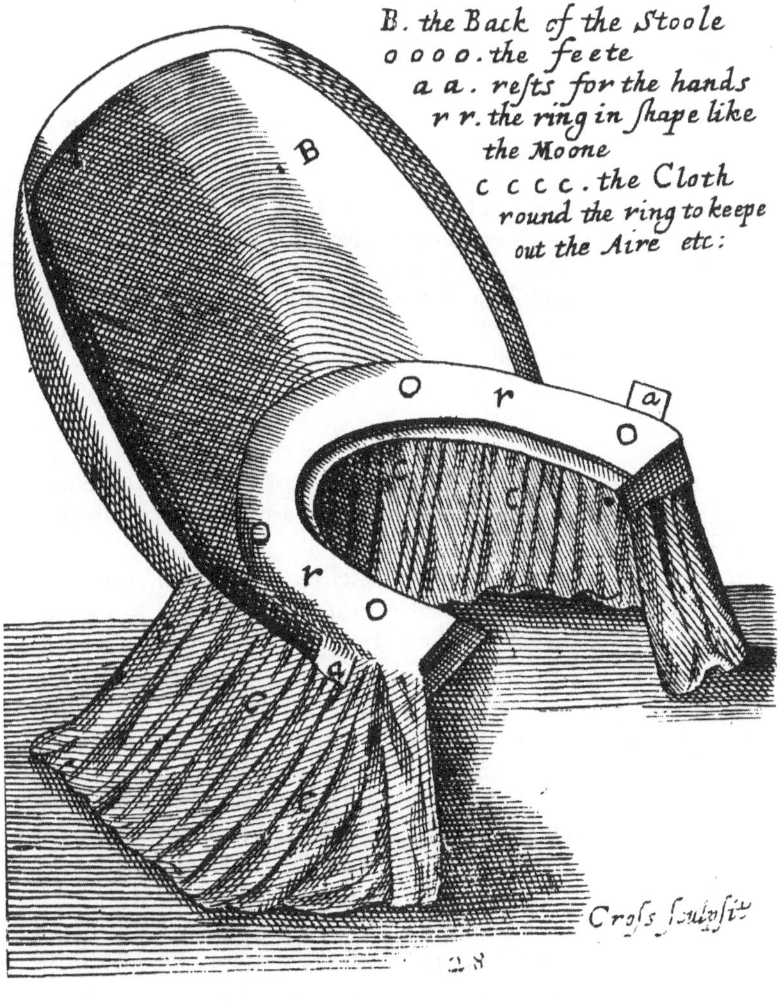

A birthing chair recommended by a seventeenth-century author of a book on midwifery. (J. Wolveridge, *Speculum Matricis*, London, 1671.)

> Nevertheless they [the RCP] think it neither necessary nor convenient that they [the midwives] should be made a Corporation to govern within themselves, a thing not exampled in any Commonwealth.[42]

Two more efforts were made to incorporate midwives. In 1634 another Peter Chamberlen (son of the first mentioned of that name) proposed a scheme for the training and licensing of midwives. Unfortunately he wanted to control the programme himself. His proposal was opposed by the midwives Mrs Hester Shaw and Mrs Whipp as follows:

> That through the molestation of a Dr. Chamberlen by appointing them [the midwives] to meet at his house once every month without authority, and with intention, as they suppose to bring about a project of his to have the sole licensing of them or approving of all such as shall hereafter be licensed out of an opinion of himself, and his own ability in the art of midwifery, implying a necessity of using him and no other both in those cases and in all other occasions that shall happen to women with child, presuming that he shall not repair unto such women as are distressed whose midwives have refused to conform themselves to him.[43]

They went on to accuse Chamberlen of extreme violence in his use of instruments. Chamberlen's attempt to monopolise midwifery in London failed.

In 1687 the midwife Elizabeth Cellier petitioned James II for 'the Foundation of a Royal Hospital and raising a Revenue of five or six thousand pounds a year by, and for the Maintenance of a Corporation of skilful midwives, and such Foundlings or exposed children, as shall be admitted therein'.[44] Her scheme was unsuccessful, partly because of her own notoriety (she was a convert to Catholicism, accused of involvement in the obscure Meal-Tub Plot), and partly, perhaps, because the monarch had other things on his mind. Not until 1902 were the midwives successful in obtaining their own corporation, including adequate training facilities and licensing rights.

Midwives may be viewed as being more similar to unlearned unlicensed healers than they were to physicians, surgeons and apothecaries. Like their unlicensed brethren, they were attacked by licensed healers for ignorance and immorality. Worse, their occupation was traditionally linked with witchcraft. Visitation articles of 1559 included the question,

> Whether you know of any that do use charms, sorcery, enchantments, invocations, circles, witchcrafts, soothsayings, or any like crafts or imaginations invented by the Devil and specially in time of women's travail.[45]

Although by the eighteenth century midwives were no longer being accused of witchcraft, they retained the negative reputation publicised by their detractors. The eighteenth-century midwife, Margaret Stephen, wrote,

> Those who have found it in their interest to bring midwives into disrepute, have charged them with intemperance, and even obscenity. How the being a midwife should make women possess such vices is to me a mystery. I know no way of life in which a woman can be engaged, that is more calculated to fix sentiments of piety and morality upon the mind, nor have I ever been acquainted with any midwife who did not possess them.[46]

Despite such defenders, and despite the support of those who viewed as immoral the presence of man-midwives in the birth chamber, the stereotype, of which Dickens's Sairey Gamp was but one example, stuck to midwives.[47]

Rather than offering them training, the physicians and surgeons attempted to drive midwives and other unlearned healers from medical practice altogether. Their methods of attack and the probable reasons for their success will be discussed in greater detail below. Although licensed male practitioners were unable entirely to rid England of female midwives, they were able to take over the practice of 'obstetrics' among all but the poorest classes of patients, thus essentially eliminating their competition.

II UNLICENSED HEALERS

> Forasmuch as the science and cunning of Physick and surgery (to the perfect knowledge whereof be requisite both great learning and ripe experience) is daily within the Realm exercised by a great multitude of ignorant persons, of whom the greater part have no manner of insight in the same, nor in any other kind of learning: Some also can no letters on the Book, so far forth that common Artificers, as smiths, weavers, and women boldly and accustomably take upon them great cures, and things of great difficulty: in the which they partly use sorcery and Witchcraft, partly apply such Medicines unto the disease as be very noxious, and nothing meet therefore; to the high displeasure of God, great infamy to the Faculty, and the grievous hurt, damage, and destruction of the King's liege people; most especially of them that cannot discern the uncunning from the cunning.
>
> *An Act for the Appointing of Physicians and Surgeons* (1512)[48]

The vast majority of people practising medicine in seventeenth-century England did so without the blessing of church, state or occupational organisation. It is difficult to obtain reliable information about either the activities or the numbers of these healers, because so much of what was written about them was written by their enemies. Nevertheless, it is certain that both urban and rural areas supported a host of unauthorised healers, some learned, most unlearned; some practising medicine as a full-time occupation, others dividing their attention between medicine and other trades; some engaging in general practice, others specialising in the treatment of a particular condition; some long-term members of a community, others itinerants who were subject to prosecution as vagrants in addition to their vulnerability to attack from licensed practitioners.[49]

Not all of these healers were the ignorant charlatans their competitors accused them of being. Some had received university training – a few holding foreign medical degrees.[50] A few were learned physicians or surgeons who, for one reason or another, had fallen foul of the medical organisations.[51] The group which provoked the most serious and sustained attacks from the supporters of learned licensed medicine, however, was the large number of empirics, who maintained that in medical practice experience was more important than theory and, thus, that the extensive book-learning of physicians was unnecessary. One popular sixteenth-century empirical writer, Leonardo Fioravanti, stated his position as follows:

> there is no science in the world wherewith a man may do good if therewith be no practice or experience, as a man may say. The which experience is master of all things, as it is plainly seen.[52]

That his common-sense approach to healing appealed to many simply made the attacks on empirics more vicious.

It is interesting to note that Fioravanti's scepticism regarding medical theory was echoed by the great clinician, Thomas Sydenham, a century later. In an unpublished treatise on dysentery, written in 1669, he wrote

> This way of cure will not be thought less expeditious and certain then [sic] courses usually prescribed are both tedious and dangerous, when the world valuing learning for that only therein which is necessary for the good of human life shall think as well of him that taught to cure diseases as those that taught to discourse learnedly about them.[53]

Although Sydenham himself came under attack for both his anti-intellectual views and his unorthodox methods, his general attitude was prophetic. Empiricism, or, at least, an empirical 'style', would characterise medical research and practice long after empirics themselves had been driven from the field.

None the less, for seventeenth-century orthodox physicians, their academic achievements were the basis for their claims of superiority and the right to a monopoly over medical care. The activities of those who openly professed a disregard for theory was both insulting to the *amour propre* of learned physicians and potentially injurious to their incomes.

The relatively large number of medical works produced by empirics and their sympathisers indicates that the medical establishment had cause for alarm.[54] Not only did these writers maintain that classical medical education was virtually useless, but also they wrote that the general public had the right to medical information which learned practitioners were deliberately keeping from them.

> How long would they [the physicians] have the people ignorant? Why grudge they physic to come forth in English? Would they have no man to know but only they? Or what made they themselves Merchants of our lives and deaths, that we should buy our health only of them, and at their prices?[55]

While some of the empirical writers demonstrate a tendency towards keeping as personal monopolies certain medical 'secrets', a practice their enemies often accused them of, most appear to have encouraged the popular penchant for self-medication.[56]

The term 'empiric' was a general one, intended by the enemies of unauthorised healers to have the same meaning as the word 'quack' has in modern parlance. Thus, the label stuck to a multitude of practitioners, some of whom were in general practice, and some of whom specialised in the treatment of particular disorders. Many specialists were quasi-respectable, so long as they did not poach on the territory of higher-status healers. The Barbersurgeons' Company of London awarded special licences to practitioners who specialised in bone-setting, scrofula, cutting for the stone and operating on ruptures, fistulae and cataracts.[57] Many such practitioners operated outside London as well – some living in towns and villages, some travelling from place to place.[58] Perhaps typical of these healers was the travelling shoemaker who showed up in Maidstone in the mid-sixteenth century, claiming to be able to heal sore eyes.[59]

It is difficult to generalise about the therapeutic methods of empirics, partly because they differed widely, one from another, partly because their methods are most often described by enemies, eager to discredit them. Empirics were accused of employing 'secret' remedies and of applying a single panacea

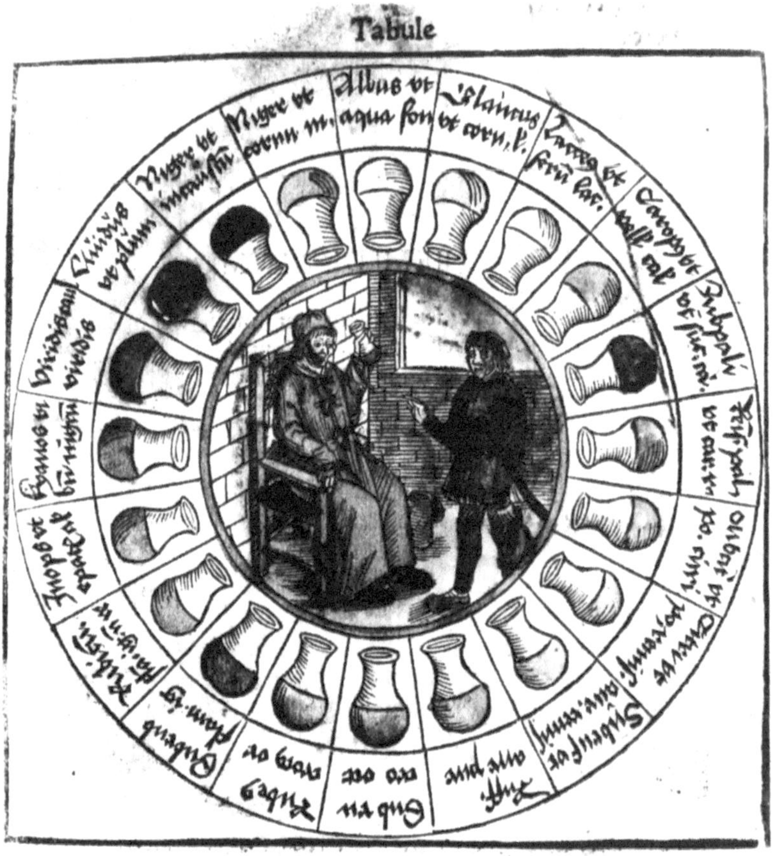

Woodcut of a sixteenth-century physician surrounded by a ring of urine flasks. Until the seventeenth century the distinctively-shaped urine flask was the major symbol of the service provided by physicians. Although diagnosis and treatment based upon the examination of a urine sample was increasingly frowned upon by learned physicians, many seventeenth-century healers and sufferers continued to use this technique.

to all disorders. However, licensed healers might with justice have been attacked for the same practices.

Certainly empirics borrowed techniques from higher-status colleagues. Two who specialised in the treatment of syphilis in mid-seventeenth-century London, 'one Bonorenige' and Kixton the Quack, used mercury preparations as did many licensed surgeons.[60] And a much-maligned group of healers, the so-called 'piss prophets', diagnosed and prescribed after examination of the patient's urine – a technique which had simply become out of date among most physicians by the mid-seventeenth century.

A revealing description of diagnosis from urine appeared in Thomas Brain's *The Piss-Prophet, or Certain Piss-Pot Lectures . . .*, published in 1637. Brain, a licensed physician, admitted that he had diagnosed pregnancy from examining urine samples, but wrote that he had known he was practising 'trickery' and had stopped using that method.[61] He claimed that his book had been written in order to give patients 'inside information' about how piss prophets operated, describing how a practitioner could tell a lot about the patient and the patient's condition by carefully observing the person who delivered the urine sample and questioning that person in so subtle a way that he or she would never realise that information had been divulged.

In spite of the scepticism of Brain and other physicians regarding the usefulness of the examination of urine samples, the practice continued for a long time, both among healers and among patients. The diarists Samuel Pepys and Ralph Josselin routinely examined their own urine during times of illness.[62]

A group of practitioners whose methods diverged more widely from those of licensed healers were the magical practitioners. A wide variety of such healers existed. At the top of the scale, in terms of both social status and expense, was the magical astrologer. His position, *vis-à-vis* learned physicians, the state and the church, was an uneasy one.

In the seventeenth century astrology was a respectable science, taught in the universities and frequently employed by physicians and apothecaries to help them gather herbs, prepare medicines and administer treatment at the most propitious times.[63] However, astrology's associations with 'art magic' were both recognised and practised. For Tudor and Stuart Englishmen, conscious of the presence and danger of witchcraft, high magic was simply a learned cousin of sorcery and demonianism. The physician John Cotta wrote

> As it is not obscure, that some men under the colour of astrology have practised magic and sorcery, so it is no less evident that many others under the pretense of advising and counselling in physick for curation or Prognostication of disease have likewise exercised the same devilish practice.[64]

Famous magical practitioners, such as Simon Forman and John Dee, testify both to the popularity of their services and the upper-class patronage such services could command.[65] Less notorious astrological physicians, such as Richard Napier, mentioned above, illustrate the respectability of such practices in some hands.[66] However, astrological physicians were in danger of being accused of sorcery. Simon Forman was accused of practising magic (which, indeed, he admitted doing), and was many times imprisoned for practising medicine without a licence.[67] Dr John Lambe, another magical practitioner patronised by the great, faced an even worse fate. After having been imprisoned and examined by the Royal College of Physicians for his unlicensed practice, Lambe was battered to death in the streets.[68]

Lower in status than the astrological physicians were the cunning-folk, wise-men and -women, white witches and wizards who, in addition to healing, found lost or stolen goods, identified thieves and witches, made love potions and foretold the future.[69] These practitioners treated a full spectrum of diseases in both animals and humans, ranging from readily diagnosable physical ailments to disorders caused by witchcraft. Their fees varied considerably, but compared favourably with the charges of other types of healers. Some charged only when the treatment was successful. Others would accept no money at all, but took their fees in foodstuffs.[70]

These healers mingled traditional medical knowledge, folk magic and prayer to produce their cures. They employed word charms which were either recited or written on pieces of paper and hung around the sufferer's neck.[71] They used other magical techniques, such as 'girdle-measuring' and transferring the illness from the sick person to themselves.[72] They also employed herbal preparations similar to those used by empirics and licensed medical practitioners.

Unlearned magical practitioners were open to attack on many fronts. They were prosecuted for unlicensed medical and surgical practice. They were also particularly vulnerable to the charge of witchcraft. For one thing, they were frequently employed to diagnose illnesses which had been caused by witchcraft, and could identify witches. For another, they claimed to be able to cure diseases caused by witchcraft. Such talents were dangerous, for, it was reasoned, magic was identified by magic. Although art magicians like Richard Napier argued in favour of angelic magic (Napier conjured up the Archangel Raphael), the consensus of opinion was that to traffic with the unseen world was either to invoke Satan or to act in obedience to him.[73] Thus, although the magical healer might use magical arts only for the benefit of mankind, he or she was as guilty of treating with the Devil as was the black witch.

Akin to such magical healers were those who healed by touch. Some, such as seventh sons – and particularly seventh sons of seventh sons – healed by virtue of their peculiar genealogical circumstances. Others, like modern faith healers, healed as a result of powers given them by God.[74] Most famous of the latter type of healer was Valentine Greatrakes, an Irish gentleman who began by healing his neighbours of the King's Evil (scrofula or struma – a tubercular inflammation of the glands of the neck) in 1662.[75] In 1665 Greatrakes found he could heal other diseases.[76] He gained a great reputation, first in Ireland, then in England, healing by stroking the patient.[77] Philosophers, scientists and physicians observed him at work, and testified to his cures.[78] Such intellectuals as Robert Boyle and Henry More believed in him.

Greatrakes took no payment for his work. Indeed, he cited this as the reason why he had not applied for an episcopal licence to practise medicine when he was examined at the Court of Lismore.

> Then the Judge asked me, where is your licence for practising, as all Physicians and Chirurgeons ought to have from the Ordinary of the Diocese? My answer was, that I knew no reason I had to take a licence, since I took no reward from any one, and that I knew no law of the Nation which prohibited any person from doing what good he could to his neighbours.[79]

Greatrakes claimed to have had

> no further design in the distribution of that talent which the all-healing God has entrusted him withal, than the honour of his maker, and the good of his poor fellow-creatures, whose Distempers (many of them) neither Art nor Physick probably could reach.[80]

His career as a healer ended abruptly in May 1666, when he failed to cure in a demonstration before Charles II and his court.[81]

This monarch must have been most interested in Greatrakes's claims, since he made similar ones himself. Beginning with Edward the Confessor, English monarchs had touched people suffering from the King's Evil.[82] This practice reached its height under the Stuarts. Charles II touched 90,798 people in the years 1660–4 and 1667–82.[83] Keith Thomas describes the ceremony as follows:

> At a special religious service conducted by leading Anglican clergy the monarch laid his hands upon each member of the long queue of sufferers. The patients approached one by one and knelt before the monarch, who lightly touched them on the face, while a chaplain read aloud the verse from St. Mark: 'They shall lay hands on the sick and they shall recover'. They then retired and came forward again so that the king might hang round their necks a gold coin strung from a white silk ribbon.[84]

The monarch did not guarantee a cure, and did not charge for his or her services. Patients resorted to the royal touch very much as they did to other medical and surgical aid. Mrs Elizabeth Barker was treated for scrofula for four years by the London surgeon, Joseph Binns, before being touched by Charles II.[85] Queen Anne was the last English monarch to touch for the King's Evil.[86]

Scrofula was not the only ailment monarchs cured. Until the reign of Elizabeth I, monarchs also ministered to sufferers from epilepsy and associated disorders, such as convulsions, rheumatism and muscle spasms. Applicants were given 'cramp rings' which the monarch had rubbed between his or her fingers in a special ceremony.[87] The rings had originally been made of the money offered by the king on Good Friday. This money was believed to have magical properties.[88] Upon the accession of Elizabeth I, the blessing of cramp rings was abandoned.

Of all the unlicensed healers discussed above, only the monarch was immune from prosecution for practising without a licence. Unauthorised healers did claim some protection under the law, however. In 1543 the so-called 'Quack's Charter' was enacted which empowered

> every person being the King's subject, having knowledge and experience of the nature of Herbs, Roots and Waters, or of the operation of the same, by speculation or practice within any part of the Realm of England, or within any other the King's Dominions, to practise, use and minister in and to any outward sore . . . , wound, apostemations, outward swelling or disease, any herb or herbs, ointments, baths, poultices and plasters, according to their cunning, experience and knowledge in any of the diseases, sores and maladies beforesaid, and all other like to the same, or drinks for the stone and strangury, or agues, without suit, berations, trouble, penalty or loss of their goods.[89]

The act was passed in order to enable poor people who could not pay surgeons' fees to obtain help.

There is no doubt that unlearned unlicensed healers were widely consulted in seventeenth-century England. Their licensed competitors and detractors, about whom more will be said below, were convinced that their numbers were growing. Although such allegations cannot be proven, recent scholarship has shown that unlicensed healers were widely distributed throughout the country and that sufferers did use their services. Alan Macfarlane writes, 'Nowhere in Essex was there a village more than ten miles from a known cunning man'.[90] And Margaret Pelling and Charles Webster estimate that some 250 unauthorised healers were practising in London between 1581 and 1600.[91] Their fees were, by and large, lower than those of licensed surgeons and apothecaries. And sometimes, as in the case of magical practitioners, they provided services not usually offered by their competitors.

Medical coverage in the seventeenth century is a difficult subject to tackle. Those who have undertaken it now agree that there were more medical practitioners available – both licensed and unlicensed – than has heretofore been thought. John Raach's pioneering study identified 814 known physicians practising in the period.[92] Of these, 635 matriculated at a university, 328 received a BA, 280 an MA and 246 an MD. Most of these physicians studied at English universities, but some 137 attended a continental university, 75 taking a foreign MD.[93] Concerning geographical distribution, Raach found the largest concentrations of physicians in the coastal counties, especially Kent, Sussex, Lincoln, Norfolk, Suffolk and Devon, as well as in the Home Counties.[94]

Needless to say, Raach's work only scratches the surface. He was interested only in 'reputable' physicians. Further, as R. S. Roberts points out, it remains to be demonstrated that the holders of medical degrees Raach included actually practised, some such people apparently appearing in the *Directory* simply on the strength of possessing a degree. 'This is particularly true of the seventy-odd physicians listed for the cities of Oxford and Cambridge, for such a figure is quite disproportionate to the population.'[95]

In addition, Raach was uninterested in the practices of surgeons and apothecaries, many of whom were in general practice. Some of these healers were formally licensed to practise, either by ecclesiastical authorities or by local occupational organisations. For instance, Margaret Pelling has identified 150 members of the Barbersurgeons' Company of Norwich (which included physicians) for the period 1550–1640.[96] Many locally recognised practitioners were never licensed, yet practised alongside their licensed colleagues without being challenged.

Still other practitioners changed their occupational 'tags' or combined the characteristics of several medical occupations in the course of their careers. For instance the inventory attached to the 1637 will of John Periam, 'physician' of Plymouth, indicated that he kept a shop with merchandise in it worth £20.[97] The use of the term 'Doctor', which became increasingly common toward the end of the seventeenth century, also confuses matters. Torrington Churchwardens referred to Dr Bradford and Dr Potter who were, respectively, a surgeon and an apothecary who was also called surgeon in other documents.[98]

Indeed, one can say only that the seventeenth-century medical marketplace was plentifully staffed. This is not to say that qualified practitioners were always available wherever and whenever they were needed. On 26 August 1601 Lady Margaret Hoby, who lived in a remote part of Yorkshire and practised medicine informally among her family and neighbours, reported

> this day in the afternoon I had had a child brought to see [me] that was born at Silpho, one Talliour son, who had no fundament [anus], and had no passage for excrements but at the mouth: I was earnestly entreated to cut the place to see if any passage could be made, but, although I cut deep and searched, there was none to be found.[99]

Lady Hoby had received no formal training in surgery. We must assume that the desperate parents of this unfortunate baby consulted her as a last resort. Either no trained surgeon was available to them, or the local surgeon had refused to perform an operation so likely to end in the patient's death. However, there were multitudes of healers offering a variety of medical and surgical wares throughout the country. The evidence indicates that prospective patients shopped around for the practitioners and therapies which best suited their needs, means and tastes.

Distinctions made among licensed practitioners and between licensed and unlicensed healers are by no means as clear as some would have us believe. Apothecaries and surgeons prescribed internal medicines. Physicians compounded and sold physic from their own shops, as did apothecaries.[100] Clients made no distinction between licensed and unlicensed healers. With the exception of the relatively few academically trained practitioners, training in all cases was composed of apprenticeship (formal or informal) and personal experience.

Furthermore, the practice of medicine and surgery was often combined with other trades. The connection between medicine and the ministry has been mentioned above. The relationship between the apothecaries and the grocers, although formally dissolved in London by the foundation of the Society of Apothecaries in 1617, still exists in the present day in the form of non-prescription drugs sold in food stores. The association between barbering and surgery was an ancient one. Indeed, barbers were still pulling teeth and letting blood well into the eighteenth century. Not until 1745 were London barbers and surgeons governed by separate companies.[101]

Barbersurgeons exercised many skills in addition to the obvious ones. With wax-chandlers they shared the task of embalming the dead. Other associated trades included music-making, the brewing and selling of drink, net-making and school-teaching.[102]

Midwives occasionally kept lodging houses where they cared for women before, during and immediately after delivery. They also sometimes served as cunning-women. Indeed, the association of midwifery with magic was a time-honoured one, as we have seen.[103] In addition, midwives had the unfortunate reputation of being bawds and abortionists. Thomas Heywood's *The Wise-woman of Hogsden*, a play published in 1638, has as its central character a woman who undertook many of these activities. She says of herself,

> Let me see how many Trades have I to live by: First, I am a Wise-woman and a Fortune-teller, and under that I deal in Physick and Fore-speaking, in Palmistry, and recovering of things lost. Next, I undertake to cure Mad folks. Then I keep Gentlewoman Lodgers, to furnish such Chambers as I let out by the night: Then I am provided for bringing young Wenches to bed: and for a need, you see I can play the Match-maker.[104]

In addition, there were a number of occupations traditionally associated with medicine and surgery. Housewives and gentlewomen were expected to be able to keep herb gardens, compound remedies and treat the illnesses and injuries of their families and neighbours. As the 1512 *Act for the Appointing of Physicians and Surgeons* indicates, smiths and weavers sometimes healed. The sixteenth-century surgeon, Lanfranc of Milan, wrote that

> Cutlers, Carters, Cobblers, Coopers, Coriars of Leather, Carpenters, and a great rabble of women . . . foresake their handicrafts, and for filthy lucre abuse physick and Chirurgerie.[105]

Lanfranc was certainly biased about the motivations of those who attempted to cure in addition to exercising their original trades. However, he was right about the diversity of tradesmen and women who practised medicine and surgery.

Thus, the task of classifying, counting or even identifying the healers practising in seventeenth-century England is a virtually impossible one. Instead of the relatively neat categories available to us today – consultant, general practitioner, chiropractor, homeopath – medical personnel of that time can be viewed as inhabiting a spectrum where all distinctions were blurred, ranging from the university-trained physician to the housewife, all of whom spent at least some of their time treating the sick.

A distinction has traditionally been made between 'folk' (or 'traditional' or 'popular') and 'learned' (or 'Western' or 'modern') medicine. This distinction is most useful in medical anthropology, where two discrete systems of medical theory and provisions are often seen in opposition. Thus, the anthropologist David Landy writes on 'Role Adaptation: Traditional Curers under the Impact of Western Medicine' and his colleague, Harold A. Gould, on 'Modern Medicine and Folk Cognition in Rural India'.[106]

The distinction between 'popular' and 'modern' medicine also is found in the works of medical historians, however. F. N. L. Poynter writes,

> Many of the most important problems which confront man today arise from the conflict between new ideas and traditional beliefs, whether these be religious, social or economic. . . . In two great societies of Asia, for example, China and India, there are two rival systems of medicine, the one traditional and popular, the other modern and scientific.[107]

The earlier popular medical historian, Howard M. Haggard, wrote, 'There are two philosophies of medicine: the primitive or superstitious, and the modern or rational. They are in complete opposition to one another.'[108]

In the hands of medical historians, the opposing categories of learned and popular medicine have been applied, respectively, to literary medicine, with its Greek, Roman, Arabic, scholastic and humanist associations, and to an oral tradition of superstition and herb-lore only sporadically mentioned in any sort of written record.[109] This categorisation is dangerous for several reasons. It is self-congratulatory, viewing the adherents and beneficiaries of 'modern' medicine as rational and civilised, while the users of 'traditional' medicines are at best old-fashioned, at worst uncivilised, furry little natives. It also supports the claims of the learned physicians of past ages to have been lonely protectors of enlightened knowledge in periods darkened by superstition and ignorance. And finally, it suggests a total polarity between those believing in learned medicine and those believing in popular medicine.

Although this polarity may have existed in some places at some times, even among so-called 'primitive' peoples in today's world the reality is far more complex. The anthropological evidence indicates that sufferers generally adapt the medical systems existing in their societies to their own needs.[110] This observation certainly applies to the medical choices made by seventeenth-century English sufferers. While it is possible to identify 'traditional' and 'classical' elements in seventeenth-century medicine, a polarisation between folk and learned medicine simply did not exist.[111] Licensed and unlicensed, educated and unlearned healers shared both theories and therapies among themselves.

Virtually all healers and sufferers subscribed to a humoral view of disease and therapy. Illness or injury caused an imbalance in the body's idiosyncratic humoral complexion which was rectified by evacuation. A traditional body of herbal and astrological lore was directed at maintaining or restoring the equilibrium of the sanguine, choleric, melancholic and phlegmatic humours.[112] The great arsenal of medical texts by such sages as Hippocrates, Galen and Avicenna was directed at the same goal. Even Paracelsus, who wished to cure by sympathy rather than antipathy, was basically humoral in his therapeutic orientation.[113]

Thus, from the sufferer's point of view, it mattered little whether the healer he or she consulted was a learned physician, an empiric or a wise-woman. Treatment was almost certain to include a purge or emetic. Blood-letting or sweating might be recommended. Both herbal and metallic remedies were classified, in part, by the evacuative result they were likely to achieve.

By the same token, both licensed and unlicensed healers used techniques which were related to magical lore. Both used the aetites or eagle stone to aid in difficult births.[114] Both sanctioned stroking an afflicted part with a dead hand and putting pigeons to the feet of a person thought to be in danger of death.[115]

As Keith Thomas points out, it is difficult to distinguish between the natural properties thought to be inherent in some substances and objects and magical practices sanctioned either by local tradition or by the Neoplatonist belief in occult influences and sympathies.[116] The example he cites is the notorious weapon salve, the use of which was advocated in a book by Sir Kenelm Digby which went into twenty-nine editions.[117] This salve was applied to the weapon rather than to the wound itself. Digby claimed that the resulting cure was obtained through natural rather than magical means. However, it is doubtful whether patients made this sort of sophisticated distinction in their understanding of sympathetic cures.

In place of the generally assumed polarity between folk and learned medical theories, then, there existed a collection of medical lore which was drawn upon by both healers and laypeople. This information existed partly in the oral tradition passed from generation to generation. It was also disseminated in a large and growing vernacular medical literature which was directed at both medical practitioners and the general reading public.[118]

This is not to say that specialised medical knowledge did not exist. Astrological healers used a literature and language inaccessible to other healers and lay-men. Wizards and witches had occult secrets, rituals and incantations which they used to heal. Paracelsians and iatrochemists utilised literature and techniques wellnigh incomprehensible to the uninitiated. Learned physicians had encyclopedic knowledge of texts in languages unknown to uneducated people. Such works often remained unpublished, circulating in manuscript.

In spite – or, perhaps, because – of these arcane specialisms, the general public remained interested and comparatively well-informed in medical topics. It cultivated a healthy scepticism regarding professors of medical authority. And it reserved the right to choose healers or resort to self-treatment regardless of the efforts made by licensed healers to control its behaviour.

III ATTEMPTS TO PROFESSIONALISE: THE CREATION OF THE MYTH

Although licensed medical practitioners had the support of both the state and the church, their achievements concerning the control of medical care and provision lagged far behind their aspirations. The public, like the horse in the old adage, could be led to the wholesome waters of authorised medicine and surgery, but it could not be forced to drink. Thus, motivated partly by a desire to raise medical standards and protect gullible patients, and partly by the wish to protect and increase their own practices, incomes and social status, licensed medical practitioners launched what might be described as an advertising campaign to sell their own point of view. It was a two-pronged campaign which sought, on the one hand, to create a favourable image for licensed healers and, on the other, to destroy the reputation and practices of unlicensed healers. As its main agencies it used the powers of its occupational organisations and the vernacular medical literature referred to above.

This study will not address itself to the numerous prosecutions launched against unlicensed practitioners by the Royal College of Physicians and the Barbersurgeons' Company of London. These prosecutions have been ably discussed by other scholars.[119] Rather, we will be concerned with the medical propaganda which appeared in print. This approach to the efforts of licensed healers to consolidate and improve their own position in the medical marketplace has not been taken before. The utility of the popular press for forming popular opinion was not neglected by sixteenth- and seventeenth-century medical writers. Because the medical writers of these two centuries said substantially the same things about themselves and their competitors, sixteenth-century works will be quoted as well as those belonging to the century principally under examination.

Foremost among medical propagandists were the physicians. This is easy to understand, for they had much to gain by victory. Their aspirations, including control over all of licensed medical practice, extinction of unlicensed practice, public recognition of their rights to a high income, and general acceptance of their claims to be gentlemen, were very high. Their status was already higher than that of the surgeons and apothecaries. However, their position was insecure. Despite their officially endorsed privileges, they found competitors on all sides. And their numbers were too small, their administrative machinery too weak, to enforce the powers they had been given by law. Since their competitors were unlikely simply to disappear at a wish or command, the physicians directed some of their efforts at the market for medical services – the patients themselves.

The physicians were joined in their efforts by a small

number of learned surgeons. These surgeons were concerned about the activities of unlearned but licensed surgeons as well as about the behaviour of unlicensed healers. Together the physicians and learned surgeons attempted to create a pedigree for their crafts and distrust of the medical and surgical outlaws who surrounded them.

The pedigree constructed by licensed learned physicians and surgeons drew upon two resources dear to the hearts of educated Englishmen – classical tradition and religion. As ancestors for themselves, the physicians recalled Aesculapius and Hippocrates. And the sixteenth-century surgeon, Thomas Vicary, wrote,

> For did not that worthy and famous captain of the Greeks, Agamemnon, love dearly and reward bountifully both Podalerius and Machaon, through whose cunning skill in surgery, thousands of worthy Greeks were saved alive and healed, who else had died and perished.[120]

Similar efforts were made by early man-midwives who claimed direct descent from Adam – the first *accoucheur.*[121]

Furthermore, the ministrations of learned physicians and surgeons were authorised by God. John Cotta argued,

> For as God hath created all things for the good of man, so hath he appointed the physician to fit and accommodate all things unto the necessity and need of man, and hath farther also deputed him to supply unto man even those things which nature herself ofttimes cannot.[122]

Having mustered to their side God and the ancients, the learned healers lamented that their occupation had recently fallen into disrepute. The surgeon Franciscus Arcaeus wrote in 1588,

> But oh good God, is it tolerable that the ancient glory and renown of chirurgerie should be so defaced? Or that such men as have spent all their time in it, should so injuriously be put from the benefit of the same.[123]

The physician Francis Herring complained that the noble Romans had paid their physicians much more than seventeenth-century patients were willing to. He felt the smaller fees showed a decline in the physician's status, 'to the stain and blush of our present age'.[124]

Learned healers believed that the divinely sanctioned

services they offered and their arduous training entitled them to a monopoly over medical care. The great sixteenth-century physician, Andrew Boorde, described the education of a physician as follows:

> every physician ought to know first learning, and then practice, that is to say, first to have Grammar to understand what he doth read in Latin. Then to have logic to discourse or define by argumentation the truth from the falsehood. . . . And then to have a rhetoric or an eloquent tongue. . . . And also to have geometry, to ponder and weigh the drugs or portions the which ought to be ministered. Arithmetic is necessary to be had concerning numeration: but above all things next to Grammar, a physician must have surely his Astronomy, to know how, when, and at what time every medicine ought to be ministered, and then finally to know natural philosophy, the which consisteth in the knowledge of natural things.[125]

Physicians were particularly eager to defend their use of classical languages. The great body of classical medical texts were available only in Latin and Greek. In the words of the physician E. D., the books published in English were 'very little and light'.[126] More to the point, the physician John Securis argued:

> If English books could make men cunning physicians, then pouchmakers, threshers, ploughmen and cobblers might be Physicians as well as the best if they could read.[127]

So pervasive was the respect for Latin and Greek that almost every vernacular work on a medical subject, whether it supported or attacked the position of learned practitioners, opened with an apology and justification for publishing in English. Many physicians apparently feared that English works on medical topics would open the field to the unlearned. About such fears, Peter Levins, Oxford MA and student in physic and surgery, wrote,

> Certainly, these kind of people cannot abide that good and laudable arts should be common to many, fearing that their name and practice should decay, or at the least should diminish.[128]

Those who published in English claimed that their aim was to benefit the unlearned who otherwise might come to harm for lack of medical knowledge. Furthermore, they argued, physicians of other nations, including such writers as

Hippocrates, Galen and Avicenna, had published in their native languages. Thomas Brugis, whose book was intended for lay household use, wrote,

> for a great number of people perish for want of means to procure the advice of a physician; when perhaps with a little instructions they might have cured themselves; but we are to consider the general good and commonwealth; for in Italy, France, and other countries, scarce any Physician but hath published some book in his mother tongue, and rather than in any other language.[129]

The very defensiveness of such writers demonstrates that general respect for the physicians' academic attainments was one of their strongest cards. Another important selling point was the great length of the physicians' training. One physician maintained that it took a lifetime to learn physic, and used this argument against Paracelsians and empirics:

> And therefore it is a great error in such men, that do dream that the art of physick may be easily attained unto: so that if they have gotten two or three chemical medicines, without any other grounds; they profess themselves to be great Doctors and cunning physicians.[130]

Diagnosis and treatment depended upon an in-depth examination of the individual sufferer's symptoms, his general physical state and humoral complexion, the time of year and the humoral cause of the disorder. Therapy included a specially ordered diet, properly composed medicines and well-monitored habits of exercise, sleep and dress. Unlearned practitioners were often accused of taking a simplistic approach to disease, offering a standard treatment rather than one dictated by the particular circumstances of a particular patient.

Because of their sophisticated education and skills, physicians demanded respect and obedience from their patients. Punishment for failure to heed the physicians' instructions was death. Furthermore, the relatives and friends surrounding the patient should also obey the physician. Criticisms abound of the loving women who countered doctor's orders. For example:

> And from hence it may be evinced the erroneous practice of many, of women especially, who think the sick hath never food enough; and for this purpose they never cease to urge them to eat, morning and evening, night and day, all is one, their too too officious love and kindness having neither rhyme nor reason, as

we say, produceth often this contrary effect, that, according to the vulgar saying, *They kill their friend with kindness.*[131]

In contrast to such unhelpful meddling, members of the sick person's household should behave as follows:

> if there be any Physician or surgeon, which is with any sick man, woman or child, let no man disquiet them that be in the house nor tell them what they should do, let every person be tendable about them. And let every man in the house please and serve the Physician and Surgeon honestly, and let them lack nothing, to the end that they may be the more diligent to do the thing they go about.[132]

Above all, patients must not treat themselves:

> let not patients turn medicine mongers, but containing themselves within their proper spheres of Prayer, Confidence and Regularity, refer each cure to the honest care of the Rational Artist.[133]

Although learned healers were concerned about patients' behaviour, they would not bite the hands they hoped would feed them by directing their anger and scorn at the general public. They chose to believe that disobedient and fickle patients were duped. They saved their big guns for unauthorised healers.

So general was the concern displayed by medical authors about the dangers posed to an unsuspecting public by unlearned, unlicensed and unscrupulous medical practitioners that even works which dealt with practical subjects – handbooks for apprentice surgeons, plague tracts and herbals, for example – found space in dedications or introductions to criticise such healers. These attacks served as both a central part of the argument in favour of legal limitation of the practice of medicine and as a method of encouraging licensed practitioners to help raise educational and service standards within their own occupations.

In addition to these virtually automatic endorsements of conventional sentiment, a number of works were published in the sixteenth and seventeenth centuries which were exclusively devoted to the attack on unlearned healers.[134] The authors of what might be called the anti-quack literature were all licensed physicians or surgeons. They claimed that their motivation for writing was a public-spirited desire to open the eyes of unwary patients to the dangers which threatened them and to raise the general standards of medical care. The works of the anti-quack writers represent the most extreme and extensive statements of the conventional viewpoint. They were directed at licensed practitioners and at the general reading public. They were intended to inform, to shock, to convince and to entertain. They resemble nothing more than very early examples of yellow journalism, complete with villains, heroes, victims and the plea for a public meting out of justice to all concerned.

Unauthorised healers were accused of many errors and crimes. Chief among these was ignorance. One early-seventeenth-century anti-quack author wrote:

> But our Empirics and Imposters, as they are too ignorant either to teach or to practice Physic . . . and too insolent, and too arrogant to learn of the Masters of that Faculty, or to be reduced into order: so are they most dangerous and pernicious unto the Weale public. . . . These Crocodiles, disguised with the vizard of feigned knowledge and masking under the specious titles of Physicians and Doctors, not attained in Schools, but imposed by the common people, do with their Absolonicall Salutations steal away the affections of the inconstant multitude, from the Learned Professors of that Faculty, and with their Ioablike Imbracings, stab to the heart their poor and silly patients, ere they be aware or once suspect such uncouth Treachery.[135]

The anti-quack writers worked themselves into a lather of righteous indignation over their enemies' disrespect for medical theory. While they usually admitted that experience and observation of disease was desirable, they maintained that such experience and observation could not be understood without theory, and that to cure a disease one must understand its almost invariably invisible cause.[136] The physician E. D. wrote in 1606:

> What though they can judge of the gout, the palsy and the dropsy? So can simple women do: but to judge rightly of the causes and differences of these diseases . . . , that requireth Art, which is not in any Empiric.[137]

The sixteenth-century writer, John Halle, illustrated the learned surgeon's regard for academic theory in his examination of the travelling shoemaker, mentioned above, who 'pretended to be very cunning in curing diseases of the eyes'.

> Then I asked him whether he were a surgeon, or a physician: And he answered, no, he was a shoemaker, but he could heal all manner of sore eyes.

> I asked him where he learned that: he said that was no matter. Well, said I, seeing that you can heal sore eyes, what is an eye? whereof is it made? of what members or parts is it composed? And he said he knew not.[138]

Halle also indignantly described the ignorance of one Valentine, who arrived in Maidstone in 1560 claiming to be able to cure all diseases, as follows:

> The truth was so: he had no learning in the world, nor could read English (and, as I suppose, knew not a letter, or a b from a battledore), as it was well proved, yet made he the people believe that he could speak Latin, Greek and Hebrew.[139]

This crime made Halle angrier than Valentine's use of magical methods or the fact that he had three wives living in three different towns.

The anti-quack writers warned of the dangers of powerful medicines in the hands of ignorant healers. John Cotta wrote, 'Worse are the bad after-consequences of ill-applied medicines, than diseases themselves'.[140] He also fulminated against the claims of some empirics that a single preparation could cure all diseases.[141]

Even worse, perhaps, than the remedies of unlearned practitioners of physic, were the attentions of unskilful surgeons. Thomas Gale, then Master of the Company of Barbersurgeons, wrote in 1564, in his preface to a general work on surgery,

> thou mayest easily judge that the rabble of these rude Empirics (and dross of the earth which when they cannot otherwise live chip straight ways into the art of Chirurgery) be no chirurgeons: but mankillers, murderers, and robbers of the people: such are some hosiers, tailors, fletchers, minstrels, souters, horseleeches, jugglers, witches, sorcerers, bawds, and a rabble of that sect: which would by laws be driven from so divine an art, the exercise of which for want of knowledge, bringeth sometime loss of member, sometime of life, and sometime both of limb and life.[142]

The anti-quack authors agreed that a basic understanding of medical theory was desirable for the surgeon, despite the fact that surgery was a mechanical operation. The sixteenth-century physician, John Securis, wrote:

> There be many surgeons in this our time, that practise surgery, more by blind experience than by any science, who in using many

things appertaining to their art, know almost the virtue and operation of nothing that they do use.[143]

The self-advertisement and boasting of unlearned practitioners irritated their learned competitors almost past bearing. Licensed physicians felt insecure about their own ability to produce cures. Hearing unauthorised healers vaunting their successes – and realising that prospective patients believed their claims – added insult to injury. The fact that 'quacks' did sometimes succeed where learned practitioners had failed did not help matters. The learned defended their position by claiming that success on the part of licensed healers was due to art, while apparent success on the part of unlicensed healers was due to chance.[144] The physician James Hart wrote in 1624:

> Neither let this suffice, that some of their proctors plead for them a number of happy and successful events; since that thus we may often magnify the most vile wizard, and most ignorant old wife in the country: this argument taken from issue and event being a mere Paralogism, a fallacy and deceit, taking that often for a true cause which is no cause indeed.[145]

Dr E. D. pointed out that patients often consulted licensed practitioners only in cases of extremity after all other sources of medical care had been tried. He wrote:

> Here, if the sick person dies, all the fault will be laid by those that favour these Empirics, upon the last Physician, that they cannot see but that more die under the hand of the learned physician than under others, that they have no good luck, because they often times die to whom they come.[146]

Although the anti-quack writers attacked all unlicensed (and some licensed) providers of medical care, they were particularly virulent in their treatment of five popular types of healer – piss prophets, itinerant practitioners, women who practised medicine, magical healers, and ministers who treated bodies as well as souls.

The attack on piss prophets reflects a change in conventional medical treatment in the course of the sixteenth and early seventeenth centuries. In the Middle Ages diagnosis based on examination of urine had been so common that the distinctively shaped urinal flask had been the physician's symbol. In the early sixteenth century a number of handbooks designed to teach medical practitioners and laymen how to diagnose from urine samples appeared, and apparently sold well, judging by the number of editions printed in the mid-1520s.[147] By the seventeenth century, although physicians still examined urine, the Royal College of Physicians frowned on the practice. It was recognised that the colour and consistency of a urine sample was not necessarily the best guide to the patient's condition. Conversation with the patient and observation of symptoms, combined with other techniques such as pulse-taking, were by that time considered better aids in diagnosis.[148] However, as indicated above, there remained practitioners who offered to diagnose illness and pregnancy, to foretell the sex of an unborn child, and to predict whether a patient would recover or die on the basis of a urine sample, often brought to them by someone other than the patient.

Thomas Brain's description of piss prophets has been discussed above.[149] His tone was light and amused. The same cannot be said about the anti-quack writers' attacks on piss prophets.[150] These authors never assumed that the piss prophet might really believe in his own methods; to them, he was always fully aware of his treachery, deliberately deluding his patients in order to rob them of their money. Petrus Forestus spoke for all of the anti-quack writers in 1623:

> This scum and off-scouring of people, without conscience and honesty, yet seeking by all craft and cunning as well to attain to some credit and reputation amongst the people, as to convey unto themselves some part of their wealth and riches and that under some fair counterfeit colour of skill in the Profession of Physic, being withall conscious to themselves of their own insufficiency, and ignorant of the signs, causes, and consequently of the right cure of disease, to the attaining of which the most learned Physicians bestow no small labour and pains, then have they recourse to the sanctuary of unlearned fools, to wit, the judgement or rather imposture by Urines.[151]

No better than the piss prophets were itinerant healers. The most lengthy account of their activities was written by the surgeon John Halle and published as an appendix to Halle's translation of Lanfranc of Milan's *A Most Excellent and Learned Work of Chirurgerie . . .* in 1565.[152] This work, entitled 'An Historical Expostulation also against the Beastly Abusers, both of Chirurgery and Physic in Our Time', is a detailed description of some travelling practitioners who showed up in Kent in the years between 1555 and 1562. Their 'crimes' ranged from ignorant herbalism to sorcery; their patients, usually warned by Halle of the dangers of consulting such healers, ended up unhappy, disappointed or dead. Halle was concerned that so many of the inhabitants of Maidstone consulted unlicensed healers, despite the presence of seven learned physicians and a number of licensed surgeons in the town. He strongly advocated learning in both physicians and surgeons, and also pointed out the virtue of a healer maintaining a stable residence:

> It cannot be without suspicion therefore, either of the lack of cunning, or of a deceivable false conscience, that a chirurgeon, or physician, shall refuse to fix himself constantly in some dwelling place, and to become a wandering fugitive, as there were and are, of whom I have written.[153]

The situation had obviously not changed by 1612. John Cotta wrote disparagingly of

> they who in towns and villages hang up their banners and triumphant flags in fields of broken arms, rotted legs, and half faces, and haply also timber for new, displaying at large before the ignorant multitude.[154]

He admitted that travel was desirable in a physician, 'not as any part of his essence, but as an ornament'.[155] However, he distinguished between the well-travelled learned physician and the itinerant healer, saying of the latter,

> It is usual with these men, moving their wandering and uncertain steps from place to place and from town to town, by fair deluding promises and pollicitations to draw the lives of simple credulous men, for their own gain, into their own hands; and after they have by their common desperate courses provoked and drawn forth unwilling death (when they see him coming) to run away, and to leave the miserable beguiled innocent in his angry jaws, to answer their rash and needless challenge.[156]

Unlearned male practitioners were bad enough; unlearned female healers incensed the anti-quack writers by their femaleness as well as their ignorance. All of these authors castigated a wide variety of women, from the loving but misguided wife or mother who refused to follow the physician's instructions, to the unskilful midwife, to the female charlatan, to the witch. These healers, like their male counterparts, were considered unfit to practise medicine because of their ignorance and dishonesty. However, the anti-quack writers took the argument one step further, maintaining that women were unfit to practise because of their sex.

We cannot but acknowledge and with honour mention the graces of womanhood, wherein by their property, they are right and true sovereigns of affection: but yet, seeing their authority in learned knowledge cannot be authentical, neither hath God and nature made them commissioners in the sessions of learned reason and understanding . . . it is rash cruelty in them even there to do well, where unto the not judiciously foreseeing, that well might have proved ill, and that ill is no less than death.[157]

Women who wished to practise medicine were faced with a no-win situation. If they practised without training, they were attacked for their ignorance. However, many educational resources, such as university educations, were closed to them. Although women could and did become barbersurgeons, full participation in the activities of occupational organisations was denied them, and they were not encouraged to seek apprenticeship.[158] In a world in which men were considered the rational, strong, creative half of humanity and women the irrational, weak, destructive half, it is not surprising that learned upper- and middle-class male medical practitioners were contemptuous of the female healers who had the temerity to compete with them.[159] However, it is ironic that male practitioners happily accepted medical recipes and devoted nursing care from the women of their acquaintance who had the good sense not to charge for their services.

The most common sort of female practitioner in sixteenth- and seventeenth-century England was undoubtedly the midwife. While midwives were attacked for ignorance and butchery, as were unlicensed healers, the evidence regarding such attacks is ambiguous. It is notable that in the earlier period, male writers on the subject of midwifery agreed that female midwives performed a great service. The surgeon Jacob Rueff wrote in 1637:

It is observable that in all ages of the world and throughout all countries in the world, that the help of grave and modest women (with us termed midwives) hath ever been useful for relief and succour of all the daughters of Eve, whom God hath appointed to bear children into this world.[160]

However, he felt that women were unlearned and should be educated by skilful physicians and surgeons.[161] Later in the century, the man-midwife Percival Willughby, although generally well disposed toward midwives, criticised them for ignorance and for being over eager in their efforts to help women deliver.

> I leave all women to their liberty to make choice of their Midwife, yet I will not be forward to persuade them to take such a midwife as will bind them, perforce, in their chairs against their wills, or, that will pull, stretch, or hale their bodies, or use any violence to enforce the womb in hopes of a speedier delivery.[162]

By the same token, he warned against midwives being too hasty about sending for 'a young chirurgeon', who might injure both mother and baby in his efforts to extract the child.[163] Willughby never treated patients before having been summoned by the midwife. And he had to abide by the constraints placed on his activities by female modesty. He recorded details of a case where the midwife in charge was his daughter.

> About seven a clock that night labour approached. At my daughter's request, unknown to the lady, I crept into the chamber upon my hands and knees, and returned, and it was not perceived by the lady.[164]

He completed his examination in a partially darkened room, with his patient entirely covered with her own and the bedclothes.

By the eighteenth century male *accoucheurs*, having gained in both confidence and popularity, were ready to drive midwives from the birth chamber altogether. The physician William Smellie created a pedigree for man-midwives, calling Hippocrates the Father of Midwifery, unearthing a worthy called Paulus Aegineta (a fourth-century Greek medical writer who claimed to have been an *accoucheur*), and denying the existence of such ancient female physicians as the semi-legendary Trotula.[165] He and other writers again accused midwives of ignorance, but refused to instruct midwives in the use of instruments, including the midwifery forceps which were introduced in the 1730s. They also exaggerated the dangers of childbirth, which encouraged those with sufficient means to consult more learned and higher-status male practitioners. Fashion also came to the aid of the man-midwives, ladies with upward mobility aspirations summoning them rather than lower-status females in times of need. Thus, despite the chorus objecting to the invasion of the birth chamber by male practitioners, by the end of the century men had virtually taken over the practice of midwifery among all but the lower classes in society.[166]

Although midwives were not usually included in the list of

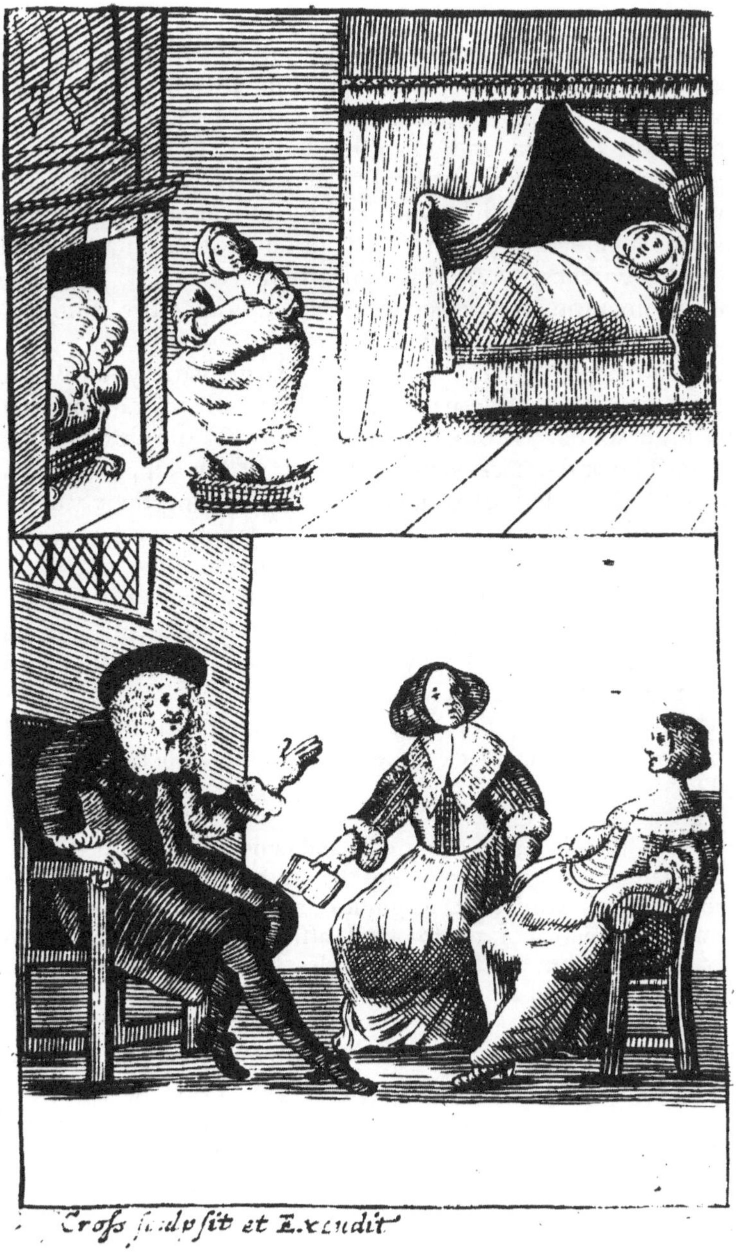

Man-midwives were consulted with increasing frequency by the beginning of the eighteenth century. However, pregnancy, birth and the care of infants remained in female hands among the majority of the population. (J. Wolveridge, *Speculum Matricis*, London, 1671, frontispiece.)

healers they chose to censure, the anti-quack writers devoted a good deal of venom to attacking another sort of healer who was likely to be female – the magical practitioner. Not all such healers were female. Indeed, the most notorious of them all, Dr Simon Forman and Dr John Lambe, for instance, were men. However, many magical healers were women. The mid-seventeenth-century licentiate in physic and surgery, Edward Poeton, included as the first item in a list of the characteristics of white witches, 'weak and unlearned women'.[167] Female or not, no unauthorised healer was viewed with more abhorrence than the magical practitioner.

As indicated above, there was a large variety of magical healers for prospective patients to choose from, ranging from the high-status astrological physician to the lowly white witch. The anti-quack writers, unsure of the support of other learned healers, left astrologers alone, confining their attention to the unlearned magic practised by cunning- and wise-folk, white witches and itinerant practitioners. This target was perfectly safe, for in their attack the anti-quack writers could rely on the combined support of organised medicine, the state and the church. In this way, these authors contributed to the escalation of the English witchcraze.

Magical healers, like other unlicensed practitioners, were condemned for their lack of learning. Oberndoerffer wrote in 1602,

> Others, that they may colourably and cunningly hide their gross ignorance, when they know not the cause of the Disease, refer it unto charms, witchcraft, magnifical incantations, and sorcery, vainly and with a brazen forehead, affirming that there is no way to help them but by characters, circles, figure-castings, exorcisms, conjurations, and other impious and godless means.[168]

In addition, despite the loyalty of many patients, the anti-quack writers felt such healers were evil. Forestus wrote,

> The devil likewise being a most cunning craftsmaster, makes choice of such unclean and wicked persons, receiving them into his service, to the end he may by their means more easily deceive and entrap others.[169]

The Essex clergyman George Gifford maintained that consultation of white witches endangered the patient's soul. He wrote,

> A man is sick, his sickness doth linger upon him, some do put

> into his head that he is bewitched, he is counselled to send unto a cunning woman, she says he is forespoken indeed, she prescribes what to use, there must be charms and sorcery used. The party finds ease, he is a glad man, he takes it that this is a common thing and well tried by experience, that many in great distress have been relieved by sending unto such wisemen or wisewomen. . . . Yet, now they cannot say that the Lord is their health and salvation, but their physician is the Devil.[170]

The anti-quack writers were obviously ambivalent about the talents of magical healers. They tended to believe that magic could heal. However, they were certain that such healers were both evil and dangerous. Cures produced by learned medical practitioners came from God: those produced by magical healers came from Satan.

Unfortunately the same could not be said about the medical activities of ministers. The anti-quack writers worried considerably about this source of competition. Ministers could not be accused of being either unlearned or evil. The worst the anti-quack writers could say about them was that it was unlikely that a clergyman could give proper attention to both the souls and the bodies of his parishioners. Cotta wrote of the

> Ecclesiastical persons, Vicars and Parsons, who now overflow this kingdom with this alienation of their own proper offices and duties and usurpation of others, making their holy calling a linsey wolsey, too narrow for their minds, and therefore making themselves room in others affairs, under pretence of love and mercy.[171]

Of course it was precisely the ministers' apparent usurpation of the practices – and financial rewards – of the physicians which made the anti-quack writers angry. They resented clergymen earning money by practising physic. Cotta himself admitted that he had no objection to ministers giving 'their medicinal advice with incorrupt hands free from implication of private gains'.[172] He wished only to attack ministers who set up 'in their houses apothecaries' shops' and travelled 'up and down to spoil the proper labour of his hire'.[173]

The complaint that their practices robbed licensed practitioners of both prospective patients and income was at the heart of all the anti-quack writers' attacks on unlicensed healers. It might be argued, of course, that learned physicians and surgeons were equally motivated by altruistic concern about the public welfare. However, the learned were, if anything, more upset by the successes than they were by the failures of their competitors. Success bred reputation which, in turn, bred an increase in clientele. One writer warned that if this situation were allowed to continue, 'verily it will greatly discourage men of learning hereafter to apply themselves to the study of physic'.[174] The remedy which the learned and licensed sought was new legislation to confine the practice of medicine to themselves, and increased help from the government in enforcing already existing legislation.[175]

Unlearned healers had their defenders. The renegade healer and author Nicholas Culpeper wrote,

> Who are they that cry out against Empericks? Who? The College of Physicians; And why do they do so? They kill Men for want of judgement; And who is the cause of this? Themselves forsooth; for if they taught men the true rules of Physick, is any Man so mad as to practise false ones?[176]

He accused physicians of keeping medical knowledge from the people in order to keep a financial monopoly over treatment. The midwife, Jane Sharp, went even further. She derided the physicians' academic approach to her craft. Although she advocated the training of midwives in anatomy and the mechanical operations they must perform, she wrote,

> It is not hard words that perform the work, as if none understood the Art that cannot understand Greek. Words are but the shell that we ofttimes break our teeth with them to come at the kernel. . . . It is commendable for men to employ their spare time in some things of deeper speculation than is required of the female sex: but the art of midwifery chiefly concerns us, which even the best learned man will grant, yielding something of their own to us when they are forced to borrow from us the very name they practise by, and to call themselves man-midwives.[177]

A sixteenth-century writer ridiculed academic education, which he felt prepared the physician for practice as much as reading books on navigation prepared a man to be a sea captain.[178] However, the principal defenders of unlearned and unlicensed healers were the loyal patients themselves who voted with both their feet and their purses.

Patients consulted unlicensed healers partly because they generally charged less than did licensed practitioners. This fact was recognised by the physician E. D., who wrote that patients consulted unlearned healers 'and magnify them above the learned Physician . . . because they can employ them for less reward'.[179] One obvious solution to the problem would have been for licensed practitioners to reduce their fees. However, learned healers valued both their high incomes and their relatively high social status. They knew as well as any modern social scientist that status was, to a certain extent, a reflection of how much clients were willing to pay them. Physicians and surgeons could not reduce their fees without reducing their worth in the public eye.

Unable to provide their services cheaply, unable to prove that they were the only healers able to cure diseases and heal wounds, licensed practitioners were forced to rely upon social and political clout and the powers of the pen in their competition with unlicensed practitioners. Both weapons eventually proved effective. However, the battle was a long one and had by no means been won by the end of the seventeenth century. Further, the eventual incarnation of the structure of professional medicine, which placed the consultant surgeon at the top of the hierarchy, drastically reduced the classical academic components in the physician's education in favour of empirical observation, and created of the apothecary the general practitioner, would have pleased neither the anti-quack writers nor their opponents.

Authorities on the subject of professionalisation concentrate on the activities of occupational organisations. They are most interested in the efforts of such organisations to control the services members provide and to govern themselves without outside interference.[180] While the growth of occupational organisations and their support by the state were important to the development of a medical profession in Britain, these elements were not the only necessary ones. Despite the fact that for most of the seventeenth century the medical and surgical monopolies had already been in existence for a hundred years or more, sick or injured people could not be forced to consult licensed physicians and surgeons. Nor could they be coerced into deserting unlicensed healers. The sociologist Eliot Freidson admits this fact, but does not shed much light upon the mechanisms by which people were encouraged to change their loyalties and their behaviour.[181]

The answer to this question lies outside the scope of this study. However, it is obvious that some explanation of lay public compliance with the goals of members of occupational groups aspiring to 'professionalise' should be included in professionalisation theory. If we cannot answer the question here, perhaps we can pose it fully. Why did people eventually accept physicians and surgeons at their own valuations? Surely the answer cannot be that the general public was impressed by a demonstrable superiority of licensed medical services over unlicensed ones. The record of medical success, usually kept by interested parties, was too confused to yield any sort of conclusive evidence about the value of various practitioners. General claims of success were balanced by general attacks for failure.

Is it not possible that the advertising campaign fought by licensed healers, partly in the form of the anti-quack literature, helped convince people that licensed medicine was the only true and safe medicine? The attack on quacks combined with the appeal to sufferers to protect themselves and their loved ones from the fearsome depradations of disease and injury by consulting healers who, if not perfect, were still the best available, must have seemed wellnigh irresistible to some. Certainly something occurred to shift popular opinion from the ambivalence it displayed throughout the seventeenth century.

This chapter has concentrated on the attitudes and behaviour of those staffing the teeming seventeenth-century medical marketplace. It has drawn little, however, on the evidence which exists about the day-to-day practices of individual healers. It is difficult to generalise about the activities of medical and surgical practitioners in the period. Their behaviour depended on where they practised, the expectations of their patients, the disorders they treated and their own social, economic and educational backgrounds. For instance, it is as easy to find an example of a seventeenth-century physician using magical methods as it is to find another physician who used no magic at all. None the less, examination and comparison of several of the surviving medical and surgical casebooks of the period will illuminate some of the methods and experiences of seventeenth-century healers and their patients. Thus, the next two chapters will consider in turn the casebook of a London surgeon and those kept by three provincial physicians. While these discussions will not provide an overall picture of seventeenth-century surgery and medicine, they will indicate the possibilities of conventional therapeutics in that period and will also explore the historical uses of such casebooks.

3

A LONDON SURGEON'S CAREER: JOSEPH BINNS

Although this study is chiefly concerned with the experiences and choices of seventeenth-century patients, it would be incomplete without reference to the records left by those who spent their occupational lives with people in their roles as patients – the medical practitioners. Numerous medical and surgical casebooks have survived the last three centuries. Although often neglected by medical historians, one, like that of the early-seventeenth-century physician Richard Napier, occasionally surfaces, providing scholars with the opportunity of examining the day-to-day activities of a medical practitioner.[1] Such casebooks yield information about a wide variety of subjects, ranging from the disorders treated and the therapy provided to the names, social status, addresses and (occasionally) personal idiosyncrasies of the patients. Casebooks vary, both in the kind of information recorded and in their value to historians. Some are simply lists of patients treated or prescriptions dispensed. Some are account books. A few are made up of detailed descriptions of each case the practitioner undertook.[2] Such a casebook is the one kept by the London surgeon Joseph Binns in the years between 1633 and 1663.[3]

It is difficult to find out much about Joseph Binns. In his own time he was respectable, but unremarkable. Histories of the Barbersurgeons' Company and St Bartholomew's Hospital, to which he was attached, mention his name. Two copies of his will are housed in the Public Record Office. His casebook, bound with other medical manuscripts in the Sloane manuscript collection, is the richest source of information about him, yet it reveals nothing about his personal or social life. However, this very anonymity gives the casebook some value. Unlike the records left by such medical luminaries as Sir Theodore Turquet de Mayerne or Sir Edmund King, Binns's casebook gives us an insight into the work of an 'ordinary' practitioner (if such a thing can be said to exist).[4]

Joseph Binns was born in Derbyshire. He was made free of

the Company of Barbersurgeons by apprenticeship to the London surgeon Joseph Fenton on 28 March 1637, and thought so highly of Fenton that he named his eldest son Fenton Binns. Binns was elected as one of the three surgeons to St Bartholomew's Hospital on 12 November 1647. He was paid £30 a year by the hospital and occupied his position there until his death on 18 May 1664. In addition to his work at St Bartholomew's, Binns had an active private practice. He finished his career as a warden of the Barbersurgeons' Company in 1662 and 1663.[5]

Joseph Binns married Mary Holland whose father, Master Richard Holland, was named as one of the executors of Binns's will.[6] The wedding probably took place in the late 1640s, when Binns was a well-established surgeon. At the time of Binns's death he had at least three living children, none of whom had reached the age of 21. During his working life Binns leased a house on Butchers Hall Lane in the parish of Christchurch. Numerous relatives of Joseph and Mary Binns are mentioned in both the casebook and the wills. Many of them appear to have lived close enough to Binns to consult him in times of sickness. Binns was survived by a sister, Jane Risson. He also left bequests to two aunts, five brothers-in-law and their wives, three cousins and four godchildren. Other relatives mentioned in the casebook apparently died before Binns did.

At the time of his death, Binns was in an enviably solid financial position. He was receiving income from properties in Berkshire, Oxfordshire and Middlesex. In 1664 he had loaned an Oxfordshire gentleman, Sir Bulstrode Whitelocke, £800, and a Middlesex property-owner £500. He left his eldest son Fenton £100 in cash, and his daughter Mary £125 set out in East India Company shares. He left £5 apiece to the poor of the parish of Christchurch and the Barbersurgeons' Company. He left £10 apiece to his executors. His will provides for mourning clothes for his two executors, the minister who was to preach his funeral sermon, his wife and children, his sister and brother-in-law, and his servants. In addition, he bequeathed between 10*s*. and 40*s*. apiece to seventeen friends and relations, to be used to purchase rings.[7]

Binns had wide contacts within the London medical establishment. His cousin and executor, Joseph Colston, was a physician. Binns's casebook mentions approximately forty names of physicians and surgeons with whom he had dealings with one kind or another. Some, like the surgeon John Woodall and the physician Charles Scarborough, are well known to medical historians. Most have been as totally forgotten as Binns himself. Binns apparently had a regular arrangement with at least one physician, Dr John Bathurst, whose patients he treated at the physician's house.

Joseph Binns was a dedicated surgeon. His casebook records his patience in the face of conditions which stubbornly refused to heal, and his flexibility regarding therapy. Unlike some healers, he was not so wedded to a pet theory or nostrum that he could not change treatments when the situation so required. He was not 'knife-happy'; out of approximately 671 cases, many of which concerned badly infected extremities, Binns recorded performing only three amputations.[8] He clearly loved his craft, and hoped that his sons would become surgeons. His will provided dressing cases and silver instruments for the first two of his sons to follow in their father's footsteps.[9]

His eldest son Fenton did indeed become a surgeon. In December 1690 Fenton was accused by the Royal College of Physicians of prescribing internal medicines. The Court of the Barbersurgeons' Company ordered that if Fenton Binns were arrested, he should be defended at the cost of the Company.[10]

Like other licensed medical practitioners, Joseph Binns displayed some contempt for unlearned unlicensed healers. According to the casebook, patients in Binns's practice who had consulted such healers before consulting Binns were the lucky ones; they got better. Those consulting unlicensed healers after Binns treated them died. In a case of breast cancer which Binns had been treating for a month, the patient moved to Shoreditch to be near 'one Poleman a Chemist who makes no doubt but to cure her, for he hath cured those that have been 10 times worse'. Poleman exhibited the characteristics thought usual of an empiric; not only did he promise a cure he could not produce, but also he used a 'secret preparation out of antimony and mercury fixed so he can command it at pleasure'. The patient died ten days after her move. Binns did not claim that if the patient had remained under his care she would have lived. He merely ridiculed the chemist for his ignorance and attempts to defraud his patients.[11]

More remarkable than his disparaging remarks about some unlicensed practitioners is his failure to criticise others. He was most likely to give a single value-free statement about any other healer the patient had consulted, whether licensed or unlicensed. For instance, a patient whom Binns treated for syphilis had earlier had 'his pains eased by the use of a cataplasm from one Bonorenige'.[12]

However, he felt free to criticise even licensed members of his own craft. In one case he expressed disapproval of the surgeon Edward Moollins for behaviour similar to that of Poleman the chemist. Both Moollins and Binns were working on the case of a lawyer who had mouth cancer. Binns left the case because 'Ed Moollins pretended he could do him good (though he said to me he did not desire to deal with it for no good could be done in it) but did not for he died in 14 days after'.[13]

Binns also had unpleasant contact with another member of the Moollins family, Will.

> 6 June 1643 7 o'clock at night on the backside of the Red Lion in Holborne one Samuel Ward, an old Gardener near 80 years of age, asking an alms of one Sergeant Major Jenkins, he refused to give, the old man replied some words, Jenkins drew his sword and thrust him into the belly . . . with a broad sword. I put my finger as I conceive into the cavity, the wound went somewhat upward toward the Liver. He had a puncture behind close to the left shoulder, bruised about the head and arm, dressed him up to stay blood, next morn his pulse high and he hot . . . 4th day, some digestion & they [sic] friends of Jenkins desired that Will: Moollins might join with me he goes with them next day (without me) and reports the patient afore the Justice to be past danger, so Major Jenkins was discharged out of prison upon bail. Next day Moollins dresses the patient without me, and leaves word that I must meddle no further.[14]

This case notwithstanding, Binns apparently got on reasonably well with both his colleagues and the opposition. He was occasionally called upon to consult on other practitioners' cases. In at least 30 out of the 671 cases recorded, Binns acted as a consultant rather than as the initial or the sole healer involved. This figure appears small unless it is recognised that the seventeenth-century pattern of treatment and consultation was very different from the one in operation today. Patients chose healers according to their symptoms, their pocketbooks and their opinions about the merits of various types of practitioners. Thus, surgeons competed with each other for the opportunity to treat the self-selected group of patients who chose to consult surgeons. Their incomes and reputations were based on the size of their practices, the social status of their patients and reports of their success in curing. Consultations were resorted to either in very unusual or difficult cases where the practitioner in charge wanted to make sure he was doing everything possible for the patient, or in cases where the patient had a high social status. In addition, a consultation involving senior members of the Barbersurgeons' Company was required in cases where the patient seemed likely to die. Failure to present such cases to the Master and Wardens of the Company could result in either a fine or the loss of the right to practise surgery.[15] Consultants of choice were those who could give expert advice and, at the same time, be relied upon not to try to steal the patient. Binns's colleagues must have both respected his skill and trusted his honour to have consulted with him as often as they did.

Joseph Binns's casebook mentioned approximately 671 patients. This number is necessarily approximate because some casenotes are incomplete, some illegible and some duplicates. Out of the total, only 616 are detailed enough to make any sort of analysis possible. Binns's casebook reveals a good deal about his patients. In addition to the descriptions of their illnesses and the therapeutic regimens they underwent, there is information about their social class origins, sex, addresses and the duration of their treatment by Binns. Such information is useful, both in attempting to sketch a fairly complete picture of the career of a mid-seventeenth-century London surgeon, and in trying to reconstruct the experience of being a seventeenth-century patient.

The traditional view of medical historians has been that in the sixteenth and seventeenth centuries few licensed medical practitioners existed, and that those few served the needs only of members of the upper classes who could afford them. This assumption has been successfully challenged in the work of Margaret Pelling, who has found that the numerous seventeenth-century London barbersurgeons lived in all parts of the metropolis, catering to all social classes.[16]

Binns's casebook supports these findings. Again, the numerical breakdown can only be approximate. Unless a title or occupation was specified, social class could be determined only on the basis of a mode of address (Mrs Jones seeming higher in the social register than Goodwife White or Jack Barker), or by other information about the patient given in a casenote. For instance, hospital patients were invariably poor. Hospitals were, after all, founded as charitable institutions. People with means were expected to pay for their own medical care.

Binns's casebook indicates that some 29 of his patients were upper class, 181 middle class, 50 artisans, 71 servants and 74 simply lower class (their occupations being unidentified). The social class of 266 of his patients is unknown; 300 patients were men and 220 were women [see Table 3.1].

Table 3.1 *Social Position and Sex of Joseph Binns's Patients*

	Upper	Middling	Artisan	Servant	Lower	Unknown
Female	7	64	12	34	33	70
Male	22	117	38	37	41	141
Unknown						55

However approximate these numbers may be, they indicate clearly that Binns treated members of all social classes. Perhaps his most famous patient was Archbishop Laud, whom Binns treated for a scurvy rash on his leg in 1644, during Laud's imprisonment in the Tower.[17] However, Binns's patients were predominantly middle class and below, finding the money to pay for his services because he seemed the most appropriate of the variety of healers available to deal with their problems.

Of Binns's patients, 249 were Londoners, and of these, 41 were in St Bartholomew's Hospital. Thirty patients came from outside London. Some of these had obviously met with an accident while visiting London.[18] Others had made a special trip to the metropolis in order to obtain expert medical or surgical help.[19] Of the many patients whose addresses are unidentified, most probably lived in London. Binns's practice was largely local [see Table 3.2]. Although information is sparse, it seems that he visited those patients he treated for any length of time, rather than expecting them to visit him. He very often visited a patient once or twice a day.

Table 3.2 *Geographical Origins of Joseph Binns's Patients*

London	208
St Bartholomew's Hospital	41
Outside London	30

Table 3.3 *Duration of Binns's Treatment*

One week to one month	211
One month to six months	164
Six months to one year	28
One year or more	13

Not all of Binns's patients required long-term care; 184 of them consulted him during a period of less than a week, many simply obtaining a prescription or two. Most, however, needed personal treatment. Binns treated 211 patients for between one week and one month, 164 patients for between one and six months, 28 patients for between six months and one year, and 13 patients for over a year [see Table 3.3].

As the descriptions of disorders and therapies given below will indicate, seventeenth-century illnesses and injuries lasted a long time and required a good deal of day-to-day supervision by the surgeon in charge [see Table 3.4]. Prescriptions and dressings were altered depending on the patient's response to the treatment given. Such decisions could be made only by the healer consulted. The responsibility for the outcome of the treatment was his or hers. If a patient became dissatisfied, he or she was free to consult another healer. By the same token, if the patient or the patient's 'friends' refused to follow the healer's instructions, the healer was at liberty to refuse further treatment.[20]

Table 3.4 *Frequency of Binns's Visits*

One consultation	81
One to five visits	99
More than five visits	227
Daily visits at any time	111

Table 3.5 *Joseph Binns's Cases*

Disorder	Female	Male	Unknown
Gonorrhoea		27	
Syphilis	29	74	2
Ague	4	3	
Pain in side	1		
Nausea		1	
Insomnia		1	
Stopping of urine		3	
Preventative medicine	1	1	
General illness		1	
Back pain	1	2	
Spitting blood	1	1	
Cough	1	1	
Fits like fits of the mother	2		
Asthma	1		
Scurvy	1	1	
New fever		1	
Looseness	2	2	
Cachexia	4		
Catarrh	1		
Colic		1	
Headache	3	2	
Stomachache	3	1	
Clanula	1		
Sore throat	5	1	
Epilepsy		1	
Burns	3	3	
Dog bite		2	1
Human bite		3	
Head wound	12	9	1
Gored by a bull		1	
Viper bite		1	
Sprained ankle		1	1
Fractures	18	24	2
Dislocation	2	12	
Gunshot wound		9	
Stab wound	1	11	
Wounds (misc.)	3	14	1
Knee wound		1	
Cut throat		2	
Wrist wound		1	
Bruises	4	8	
Sprains	3	1	
Leg wound		1	
Apostem	26	37	3

Table 3.5 *continued*

Disorder	Female	Male	Unknown
Hernia		10	
Hernia Aquosa		8	
Fistula	6	15	
Anal Fistula		4	
Ulcers	3	2	1
Ulcer on hand	1		
Ulcer and tumour in tongue	1	2	
Mouth ulcer	1		1
Ulcer on arm		1	
Ulcer on leg	6	1	
Ulcer on lip		1	
Ulcer on chin		1	
Ulcer on face		1	
Tumours	5	14	3
Tumour on arm		2	
Tumour on back		1	
Tumour on forehead		1	
Wen in armpit	1		
Corns		1	
Polyps in nose	1		
Swellings on back		1	
Scorbutical swelling	1		
Swollen legs	2	2	
Itch		2	
Skin rash	4		
Shingles	1		
Scald head	1		
Wry neck		1	
Scrofula	4	1	
Plague bubo			1
Gangrene	1	2	1
Hydrocephaly			3
Carious bones	2	4	
Amputation		1	
Haemorrhoids	1	1	
Nose problem		1	
Swollen testicle		1	
Arthritis		1	
Leg ailment			1
Aneurism		2	
Displaced artery	1		
Pain in leg	1	1	
Problem with gums	1	4	1
Shoulder pain	3	2	

Table 3.5 *continued*

Disorder	Female	Male	Unknown
Swollen knee	2	1	
Pain in hip	1	1	
Bad teeth	1		
Lip problem	1		
Eye problem	7	2	
Breast infection	5		
Whites	3		
Menstrual problems	10		
Eye cancer		1	
Breast cancer	6		
Cancer in yard (penis)		1	

Binns identified nearly 100 symptoms or disorders which patients brought to him for treatment [see Table 3.5]. For most of these (often quite specific, such as 'lip ulcer' or 'gored by a bull') he treated very few people: in most cases, fewer than five in the course of his thirty-year career. In more general categories, of course, the numbers are larger. Binns treated at least sixty-six cases of apostems. However, a numerical breakdown of his cases reveals that Binns had a minor speciality in the treatment of venereal diseases: 196 of his patients complained of gonorrhoea, whites or a combination of syphilis symptoms. In addition, he treated numerous cases of hernia and urinary retention in men. Although he did not cut for the stone, he acted as an early modern urologist, and patients apparently sought him out for this kind of treatment.

Most of the disorders Binns treated would have been considered specifically surgical problems in his own time. These included wounds, fractures, ulcers, fistulae, herniae, apostems (infected swellings), tumours, skin rashes and venereal diseases. However, sixty-one of Binns's casenotes refer to 'medical' problems such as ague, stomachache, headache, insomnia, diarrhoea, and epilepsy. Some of these patients, including two who were apparently given prophylactic purges, were Binns's relatives who may have chosen to consult him rather than a more expensive physician. In one case, Binns treated himself for ague. However, Binns gave internal medicines to non-relatives as well. These medical cases show that to some extent Binns was operating as a general practitioner, despite the monopoly granted to the

Royal College of Physicians over the prescribing of internal remedies.

Indeed, the distinction between internal and external preparations was one which the most scrupulous of surgeons would have had difficulty in making and applying to his own practice. Regardless of the multitude of medical theories available in the mid-seventeenth century, therapy depended upon the humoral principles of maintaining or restoring the body's internal balance through evacuation. Thus, even if the disorder treated were a wound or fracture of an extremity, happening to an initially healthy body, treatment invariably included purges and clysters (enemas) to keep the body 'soluble'. Surgeons also prescribed diets which were expected to prevent or reduce infection and help in the healing process.

Binns's therapeutic routine was based on humoral conventions. Regardless of the patient's disorder, a careful record was kept of the number, and sometimes the consistency, of his or her daily and nightly bowel movements. These were controlled by laxatives, enemas and suppositories. The prescription given depended upon the patient's age and his or her 'habit of body' (general health), as well as upon his or her ailment. The 80-year-old gardener, mentioned above, who had been stabbed, was given clysters and suppositories rather than laxatives because he was elderly and weak.[21] Binns tended to begin any sort of treatment by prescribing a laxative. This might be given on its own or as one ingredient in a general-purpose 'diet drink' or 'bolus'.

Like any medical practitioner, Binns had favourite preparations which he prescribed again and again, some of which he probably made himself. His 'pill fortis', one of the medicines most frequently mentioned in the casenotes, must indeed have been strong; in the case of a carpenter whom Binns treated for a knee injury, two pills each morning produced eight stools a day for at least six days.[22] Binns even treated 'looseness' (diarrhoea) with laxatives. A woman who complained of having had this condition for three or four years, giving her between four and ten stools a day, was prescribed three pills fortis six days after her diarrhoea had improved. The dose produced six stools, after which the woman was well.[23] Pill fortis was also used in a case which may be an early report of induced abortion. A maid who complained that she 'wanted her menses' was given, as part of her treatment, a dose of the laxative which produced twelve stools.[24]

Binns never bothered to write down the recipe for pill fortis; perhaps he wished to keep it secret. However, he did give details for other purges he used. Rhubarb and senna, commonly used laxatives, appeared frequently in his prescriptions. Binns also used mercury in both internal and external applications for many illnesses. In his employment of both herbal and metallic remedies he was typical of the surgeons, who were quicker to adopt the new Paracelsian remedies than were the physicians.[25]

In addition, and sometimes in preference to purges, Binns prescribed emetics or 'vomits'. Most frequently used ingredients were cream of tartar and antimony. These were used for prophylactic as well as curative purposes. Traditionally the English thought it good to take physic at least once a year, usually in the spring, whether they were ill or not. In one instance, Binns prescribed vomits, purges and 'stomach pills' to five members of his cousin Edward Griffing's family, including Griffing, his wife, his daughter, his maid and the maid's mother.[26] Vomits were also used as the preferred treatment for agues. In one case, Binns prescribed a vomit for a maid-servant with ague; the preparation produced fifteen or sixteen vomits! There is no record of whether or not the maid recovered.[27] Like laxatives, emetics were used to prepare patients for further treatment. Before operating on two cases of hernia aquosa (collections of fluid in the scrotum), Binns prescribed vomits.[28]

While laxatives and emetics were the common currency of all medical practitioners, other means of evacuation were performed chiefly by surgeons. Letting blood, cupping, scarifying, blistering and making issues or setons (artifically produced ulcers which were not allowed to heal), were specifically surgical methods used to help the body void unnecessary or evil humours.

Blood-letting, like vomiting and purging, could be either curative or prophylactic. It is interesting that Binns did not record a single case of prophylactic phlebotomy. Perhaps he left such matters to lower-status barbersurgeons or barbers. Indeed, despite the bloodthirsty reputation of pre-modern medical practitioners, Binns was remarkably sparing in his use of this procedure. He tended to use it under very specific circumstances. He routinely let blood in cases of head injuries and, indeed, criticised the St Bartholomew's Hospital staff for not letting blood in the case of one patient who died of a head wound.[29] He also let blood in cases where other sorts of wounds appeared to be becoming infected.[30] He drew blood for headaches.[31] And he let blood in cases where humoral tradition specifically required such treatment, such as the case of amenorrhoea mentioned above, where Binns drew blood from the saphena vein in the foot in order to draw the menses downward.[32]

Binns also used phlebotomy when the circumstances seemed to warrant it, even though he did not normally let blood for the condition being treated. He occasionally bled his syphilis patients.[33] In one desperate case of a gunshot wound which had bled much initially, Binns let the patient's blood after his wound was dressed, and again the next day. Unfortunately the patient died that evening.[34] In the case of an infected swelling of the arm which had been caused by unskilful phlebotomy, Binns opened a vein in the patient's foot as part of his treatment.[35]

Cupping or using boxing glasses was another means Binns infrequently used to bleed patients (through suction rather than incision). He employed this method for head and eye ailments, and appeared to prefer it when counter-irritation was called for. In one case of an ulceration in the eye he applied cupping glasses, blistered the patient's neck and made an issue in her arm, all on the first day of treatment. He repeated the blistering and applied boxing glasses every day for about six weeks thereafter.[36] Cupping was sometimes combined with scarification. This increased the flow of blood through a number of shallow incisions. Such treatment was usually applied to the shoulders or neck.[37] Binns also used scarification on its own. In the case of a syphilis patient whose foreskin was becoming gangrenous, Binns cut away the mortified flesh and scarified the remaining foreskin.[38]

Blistering and the making of issues were the methods of counter-irritation Binns used most frequently. These were expected to provide alternative means of evacuation for the surplus humours causing the patient's discomfort. They were also expected to draw such humours away from the primary location of the disorder, thus giving relief. Patients themselves requested issues. In one case, that of a serving-maid who had burned the left side of her face, the patient did not feel completely well until Binns had made an issue in her left arm.[39] In the case of another patient who was suffering from leg ulcers, Binns removed and cured an issue which was not helping the patient, and then made a new issue in her arm three months later. The patient recovered.[40]

Like his colleagues, Binns mainly named and treated symptoms. This is not surprising, since according to humoral theory it was quite possible for collections of symptoms to alter, becoming more or less serious depending upon the individual sufferer's 'complection'. Thus, when the diarist John Evelyn had smallpox in 1646, his physician believed that if he had not been let blood, the disorder 'would have prov'd the Plague or spotted fever' because Evelyn's blood was 'so burnt and vitious'.[41] Thus, although healers identified specific diseases as well as symptoms, the symptoms were the main targets for treatment.

While Binns occasionally identified diseases, such as lues venerea and 'fits of the mother', his casebook is a modern diagnostician's nightmare. For those interested in what Binns's patients 'really' had, his descriptions are not only confusing, but also misleading. For instance, for Binns gonorrhoea was a symptom rather than a disease; he used the term to refer to a discharge from the penis, combined with discomfort during urination. He either treated the symptom separately with preparations specific for its cure, or treated the patient with his usual remedies for syphilis if other symptoms were present. Conversely his treatment of apostems was essentially the same whether the infected swelling was the result of a wound or the manifestation of some disease. However, for the purposes of this study, modern diagnoses of Binns's patients are irrelevant. We are solely concerned with Binns's point of view and that of his patients.

Binns's cases may be divided into three major groups: conditions resulting from injuries, those brought about by disease states, and those requiring repair work, such as herniae. There are, of course, overlaps in this categorisation. For instance, apostems, ulcers and fistulae were produced by both injury and disease, and were, as indicated above, given the same treatment regardless of the cause. But, by necessity, most injuries were dealt with differently from most diseases and will be discussed separately. This study will examine first the injuries Binns treated, then his handling of cases requiring repair techniques, and third his treatment of a variety of diseases, concentrating upon his speciality, venereal disease.

I INJURIES

> In the sixteenth and seventeenth centuries tempers were short and weapons to hand. The behaviour of the propertied classes, like that of the poor, was characterised by the ferocity, childishness, and lack of self-control of the Homeric age. . . . Their nerves seem to have been perpetually on edge, possibly because they were nearly always ill. The poor were victims of chronic malnutrition, the rich of chronic dyspepsia from over-

> indulgence in an ill-balanced diet: neither condition is conducive to calm and good humour. Moreover, a gentleman carried a weapon at all times, and did not hesitate to use it.[42]

The sorts of injuries brought to a medical practitioner's consulting room or a hospital ward at any time can yield a good deal of information about the quality and risks of life for people living in that time and place. Binns's thirty years of practice spanned a particularly violent and dangerous period of English history, including as they did the years of the Civil War. Indeed, a number of Binns's cases – possibly as many as fifteen – dealt with patients wounded in battle. However, the casebook shows that London streets, shops and taverns were as dangerous as battlefields. While fourteen of Binns's patients were hurt in the course of their occupations and nineteen hurt by horses or coaches, some forty-one were wounded by violence.

Weapons varied. Binns treated nine gunshot wounds. Twelve people were injured with such instruments as rapiers, broadswords and a pack-needle.[43] One husband broke his wife's nose with his fist.[44] Several head and face injuries were dealt with pint pots.[45] And Binns treated three wounds caused by human bites. (He also treated three cases of dog-bite.)[46]

Often these violent injuries were crimes of passion, perpetrated when one or both of the participants were drunk. For example, on 25 February 1638 at 9 pm,

> One Mr. Robert Peyton of Donnington received a wound (by one Captain Nayle) with a pottle pot intercilium from the right eyebrow to the left, upon the very edge of the os frontis, the which fractured the cranium and depressed the lower part. . . . He was much in drink. With to do I dressed up the wound and stayed the bleeding & forced to hold on the medicines all night otherwise he would have plucked all off.[47]

In a similar case

> 7 June 1640 at night one Ellis Morgan a soldier received 4 several punctures (by his fellow soldier & kinsman in drink both) one in the middle of the sternum, one in the upper side of the left breast . . . , one near to the left shoulder . . . , one a little above the right arm pit going toward the end of the clavicle.[48]

Certainly passion, with or without the aid of alcohol, provoked the following assault:

> May 10 1643 at night Mr. Ashberry (a lutanist) was bitten by Gottier the French lutanist in Covent Garden had a piece of his cheek bitten out the breadth of an inch & longer on the left side from the corner of his mouth & neither lip down to the lower parts of his jaw, and as much tore up toward his cheek.[49]

Then as now, drunkenness and passion helped to explain, if they did not excuse, violent acts. But a number of the injuries Binns treated are harder to understand. It would be interesting to know why Mrs Chayre, the butcher's wife, was stabbed in the belly with a pack-needle by the porter.[50] And an almost modern impression of anonymous urban violence is given in the case of a servant of the trunk-maker who 'was shot in the shoulderblade through the bone with a pistol out of Pauls through 2 thick deals & he standing in the shop at work'.[51] The man died two days later, presumably without ever having seen or identified his murderer.

Social and economic tensions strained relationships between people. Husbands and wives, parents and children, masters and servants and apprentices abused each other.[52] A recent explanation for the increase in the number of witchcraft accusations in the Tudor–Stuart period cites as a reason for accusations and executions the annoyance and guilt produced by indigent old women who begged for alms or goods, and when refused, cursed the reluctant donor.[53] An echo of this situation appears in the case quoted above where Sergeant Major Jenkins stabbed 80-year-old Samuel Warde when the old gardener begged for alms and then 'replied some words' when refused.[54]

Even those whose duty it was to keep order were not immune from the violence they sought to control. On Boxing Day 1643 Mr Oram, 'a cook in Holborn' who was also serving as constable, 'was wounded over the head, cut over the first three fingers of the right hand to the joint next the hand, cut obliquely over the same elbow on the outside, incising the process of the' elbow joint.[55]

Wounds dealt in battle had a better reputation than others, imputing neither stupidity nor malice to either the giver or the receiver. Binns treated three soldiers wounded at the battle of Newbury fought on 20 September 1643. One, Captain Broomfield, was 'shot . . . with a brace of bullets', one passing through the left shoulder, the other entering the same armpit and lodging in the scapula.[56] Major Manwaring was more fortunate, merely having been 'shot through his gorget [a piece of armour protecting the throat] & so did but bruise his neck where the bullet lay'.[57] Binns's cousin, Edward Green, who served under the major, had both bones of his right arm broken just above the wrist by a splinter.[58]

Binns's tone in reporting all symptoms, whether caused by violence or disease, was that of detached objectivity. He displayed emotion very rarely, and this only in cases where patients refused to follow instructions or, in one case, where a patient neglected to pay a sizeable bill for his services.[59] Thus, it is impossible to obtain from Binns's casebook any attitude regarding the violence which surrounded him. Perhaps, then as now, it was so common as to be unworthy of comment.

Binns described eleven cases where patients were injured in the course of their occupations. The most dangerous trades he came into contact with were associated with construction. A carpenter, Mr Day, was injured on 23 October 1646, when in the course of 'breaking a board upon his right knee [he] struck a nail to the top of the rotula [kneecap]'.[60] Fifteen years later, Mr Day's man 'had [his] left arm hurt so with a crane that the minor fossil came through the flesh in the joint of the wrist the head of the fossil came all out we had much ado to reduce it'.[61] One Thomas Johnson, a joiner, fell off a ladder breaking both bones of his left leg below the knee, one of which 'broke through the flesh in the inside . . . w/wound of a finger's length'.[62] On 13 September 1653 the glazier, Launcelott Derrick, fell two storeys into a courtyard, breaking his left leg.[63] A bricklayer called Myllis was either unlucky or clumsy. On 27 November 1639 he

> had a severe fall near upon 3 storeys in the inside of a new building from the timber of one floor to another taken up speechless but within an hour spoke but not sensibly no hurt about him but his left clavicle broken close to the sternum & a little place contused in the occiput or pole behind his head.[64]

Binns reported laconically, 'Afterwards was killed in the same work, none knows how, found under a great window'.

Of course, other occupations had their hazards as well. Perhaps the most dramatic occupational injury Binns treated was the case of a young butcher on Saffron Hill who was gored in the left thigh by a bull. In a less dramatic case, a cutler in Holborn 'struck his first finger of his right hand against the hot tongue of an old knife which wounded him in the third joint which wounded the tendon in the inside'.[65] By the time Binns saw the wound, the tendon had 'rotted'. The man injured himself in May, but was not well until the end of July.

A number of Binns's patients were injured by horses or horse-drawn vehicles. One groom had his left leg broken 'by a blow of his horse heel'.[66] Others less occupationally qualified were hurt in similar ways. A woman 'had her left leg broke by a coach wheel'.[67] 'Mr. Payne broke his left collarbone . . . falling off a horse.'[68] A young man 'fell from a horseback & put his right arm out of joint in the elbow'.[69] Regardless of these cases, however, horses appear remarkably safe compared to the hazards of the age of the automobile.

The work of housewives and maid-servants was also dangerous. Mrs Carie, a goldsmith's wife, was treated for a badly infected hand and arm after pricking her finger with a needle.[70] Elizabeth Bemis, Mrs Brewer's maid, was 'burned with fire upon the left temple close to the eyelid and under the eye'.[71]

And the home itself was full of hazards. Children were particularly at risk. On 14 November 1648, 'Mrs. Swallow her daughter by the maid's carelessness warming the bed the girl being in bed, she burnt her left leg in the innerside in the small & the right leg her outer ankle'.[72] In another bed accident, 'A porter's child fell out of the bed and broke the left thigh bone'.[73] A 2-year-old, who tumbled even further, fell 'out at a window a storey high & bruised all the top of the head'.[74] Adults also hurt themselves at home. One Mr Balsom fell 'down the stone stairs in his garden upon a paving stone yard', bruising his left shoulder and suffering a compound fracture of his left forearm.[75] Indeed, it is remarkable that the casebook contains so few examples of accidents happening in the home, considering that in the seventeenth century open fires were the rule, building regulations were non-existent and tools conformed to no standard except the maker's own. To survive, one had to be careful.

Of course, even vigilance could not prevent some accidents. One poor woman, a servant at Gray's Inn, died after receiving a head injury 'being in a boat upon the Thames by a stick thrown from another boat'.[76] Another woman was wounded on the forehead by a tile, which presumably slipped off a roof.[77]

Binns did not describe the circumstances which produced many of the injuries he treated. Most of these were simple dislocations, fractures and cuts which he dealt with for very short periods of time. Typical of his commentary on such cases was the following: 'A girl in Shoe Lane put her right elbow out. Put it in. Well'.[78]

Joseph Binns was successful in treating most of the injuries he came across. What follows is a general description of his therapeutic approach to wounds, fractures, dislocations and bruises. Only brief mention will be made of the preparations Binns applied to the injured part. This study is only tangentially concerned with the seventeenth-century pharmacopoeia and whether or not it 'worked'. It will concentrate, rather, on Binns's routines which reveal both the results most important to the surgeon and the procedures patients willingly underwent.

In cases of stab wounds Binns first attempted to stop the bleeding with dressings which he called boulsters, pleagetts or rowlers. Sometimes he searched the wound with either a finger or a probe before dressing it, but he usually delayed this procedure for a day or two, presumably to avoid exacerbating the bleeding. He then usually prescribed a laxative or a clyster, to keep the body soluble, and a cordial to support the patient's strength and spirits. He also generally prescribed a light diet, often consisting exclusively of liquids such as broth and posset-ale. After the initial bleeding had stopped, Binns attempted to prevent infection by keeping the wound open. This he did by means of a tent (a roll of dressing or other material) inserted into the mouth of the wound to keep open a drainage tract.[79] If the wound were so small a puncture that it could not be easily searched, Binns might dilate it with an instrument he called a root before inserting the tent. Binns also occasionally injected medicines into puncture wounds.

Binns treated cuts or lacerations similarly to stab wounds, except that he usually stitched up the wound immediately after stopping the bleeding. In the case of a tailor in Postern Lane who cut his own throat, Binns sewed up the wound which did well for twelve days. At this point, it 'began to apostemate', so Binns reopened the wound and changed the ointment on the dressings. The patient recovered in spite of himself.[80]

Gunshot wounds presented special difficulties. Occasionally the bullet lodged in the body and had to be cut out. Sometimes there were powder burns to contend with. In one case part of the lining of the injured man's doublet was projected into the wound by the bullet and was removed three days after the man was shot.[81] Compared to most puncture wounds and lacerations, gunshot wounds were dirty, yielding 'a dirty black matter' for the first few days of treatment. They could also be foul smelling.[82] Some cases Binns treated similarly to his puncture wounds, keeping the wounds open with flamulae (fabric strips or strings) or tents moistened with medicines. Sometimes he used injections, as with puncture wounds; other gunshot wounds he simply dressed at the skin surface. Despite their difference from other sorts of wounds, Binns used no special medications for gunshot wounds. Once the bleeding had been stopped and foreign bodies removed from the wound, he adhered to his usual routine of frequent dressings, laxatives, clysters and occasional phlebotomy, watching for the signs of infection, and trying to prevent it if possible. It should be noted that Binns's definition of infection included swelling, the build-up of fluid, local heat or fever, and sometimes mortification. A moderate discharge from the wound was regarded as normal and healthy.

Binns used numerous preparations, both to bathe and annoint wounds and upon the different parts of his dressings. He expected wounds to heal in a certain fashion, and prescribed different preparations to aid in each stage of the healing process. If a wound were unusually painful, he applied a cataplasm (medicated poultice) to ease the patient's discomfort. He was then most concerned to bring the wound to 'digestion', that is to cause or facilitate the production of healthy discharge. If, in the process, 'proud' or 'spongy' flesh formed in the wound, Binns attacked it with spirit of wine or other preparations designed to remove it. Next Binns wished the wound to 'incarnate'. This involved a reduction of discharge from the wound and a generally healthy appearance of it. The final step was to cicatrise or close the wound. Binns was careful not to allow wounds to close until either the threat of apostemation had passed or, in the cases of compound fractures and incised bones, splinters of bone had emerged from the wound.

Of course, wounds very often did become infected. When they did, they were treated in the same way as other sorts of apostemations and fistulae. This treatment will be described below. Binns dealt with many infected wounds – cases so extreme that tendons and bones had become 'corrupt' or 'foul' and extremities threatened to become gangrenous. However, in only three cases did he resort to amputation.[83] One can only speculate about the reasons for Binns's reluctance to perform an operation which his colleagues certainly used more often than he did. The surgeon John Woodall, who had preceded Binns on the staff at St Bartholomew's and won a certain amount of lasting recognition for his publication of a handbook for naval surgeons, had written a detailed description of the procedure he used to amputate limbs, both gangrenous and otherwise.[84] Perhaps Binns did not consider himself to be sufficiently skilled in amputation to attempt the procedure even in desperate cases. Perhaps he considered the risks of amputation to be greater than those of the ills which might suggest it as a therapy. However, it is most likely that Binns's confidence in his ability to deal with infection made amputation seem unnecessary.

His success rate proves such confidence to have been justified. Out of seventy-nine injuries which involved open wounds, the casenotes report eight deaths, twenty-one unknown results and fifty cures. These injuries range from the most desperate, such as that of the servant of the trunk-maker, mentioned above, whose gunshot wound killed him within two days, to the most minor, such as that of the goldsmith's wife who pricked her finger with a needle.[85] These figures do not include all of Binns's patients who might have undergone amputation in the hands of another surgeon. Many of the apostemations of extremities Binns treated were very serious, possibly life-threatening, but were not the result of injuries. Indeed, the above figures do not include the case of one patient who did undergo amputation, because his disorder was caused, not by a wound, but by an aneurism in his arm which had developed after he had been let blood by an unskilful surgeon.[86] The figures also do not include the case of Binns's only patient who died of gangrene. This was Thomas Caswell, who on 25 June developed a little redness and pain in his toe. By 29 July his foot and lower leg were gangrenous. On 6 August he died. Binns apparently did not consider amputation.[87] None the less, the figures demonstrate that Binns was more than competent to handle the wounds which came his way.

Binns treated fifty-eight cases of fractures and dislocations, exclusive of head wounds.[88] In his treatment of these patients, his greatest concerns were to prevent or cure infection and fever, and to restore the use of the limb. He was not as interested in whether broken bones were properly set. Thus, in one case of a fractured leg where the bones refused to knit, 'the greater fossil being broken obliquely there start up a small corner of the bone towards the inner ankle so as it caused pain so I broke off the sharp point with my nail & applied mixt. ung. after which he had no pain'.[89] He did, of course, set bones, using splints, various sorts of plasters, rollers, laced stocking and pillows to immobilise the injured part. His approach varied from case to case. Concerning one leg fracture, where the initially applied splints caused much pain, Binns took the splints off and used linen and cotton ligatures with cotton 'stupes', tying the leg 'up close in a pillow'.[90]

64 *Explanation of the use*

The XXVI Table.

Of the extending of the Thigh broken into divers parts, and the setting of it; of the reducing of the knee that is disjointed; and of setting the whole foot in a mean posture.

Fig. I. represents the thigh broken extended by bands, when it cannot be extended with the hands, and *Hippocrates* his Form is not at hand: Let the Sick be laied on a common Form, with his face upwards; let the band be tied under his arm-pits, and put another band in the space that is between his privities and his fundament: Lastly, another band must be bound above his knee, and his ankle; these bands must be drawn by strong servants, the uppermost upward A, the undermost downward, till the Chyrurgian hath set the fracture. In the setting of the knee out of joint, when extension cannot be made with the hands, let the upper bands be bound alike, and the undermost above the ankles.

Fig. II and III. shews the mean figure of the members and muscles of the arm and the whole foot; which is necessary in the extension, setting, binding and placing of a part either broken or dislocated. But I therefore caused the figure of this configuration to be printed here, that young Chyrurgians, when it shall be often pointed at underneath, may at first sight learn it, and may imitate the same in their practice.

Of Chyrurgical Instruments. 65

TABULA XXVI.

Fig. I.

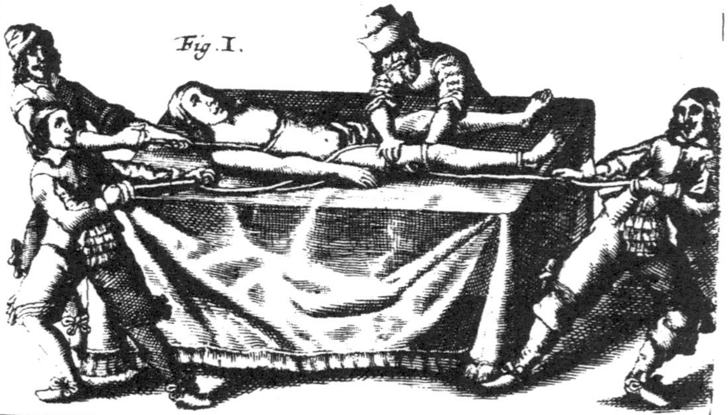

Surgeons were usually trained by apprenticeship. However, growing numbers of books on the craft were directed at young surgeons in the seventeenth century with the intention of improving their knowledge and skill. (J. Scultetus, *The Chyrurgeon's Store-house*, London, 1674.)

Binns regarded broken bones – particularly in the legs – as serious injuries, treating patients for months, applying plaster after plaster, and checking limbs for strength.[91] People who broke their legs spent a long time in bed. Mr Fisher, the innkeeper at the Star in Holborn, had his left tibia close to the ankle broken by a coach wheel in March 1640. It was a compound fracture and Binns feared gangrene, so he dressed it twice a day for the first two weeks. Mr Fisher was completely bedridden well into May, being laid on a pallet every two or three days while his bed was being made. Binns was still applying new plasters in August, when the casenote ended, incomplete.[92] Mrs Lynsie, whose leg was also broken by a coach wheel, was out of her bed only three times in the first twenty-one days after her injury.[93] Mrs Cromwell, who suffered a compound fracture of the tibia on 19 January 1645, was confined to bed for two months. She suffered so much pain in the first two days after her injury that Binns prescribed a sleeping draught – a very rare event in his practice.[94]

Less serious were broken arms, clavicles, ribs and noses. These Binns set, usually delaying application of the long-lasting 'restringent' plaster for a few days until the swelling had gone down.[95] He applied warm dressings to ease pain and reduce swelling. As in other injuries, he occasionally let blood, prescribed clysters or laxatives, and recommended a light diet.

Dislocations were usually regarded as less serious than fractures, except when they were accompanied by a wound.[96] Binns reduced the dislocation, then immobilised the limb. His treatment of the following patient is quite typical.

> Jonathan's son the carman fell from a horseback & put his right arm out of joint in the elbow so I put it in, myself with little extension by pulling the cubitus & withall bending it inward & thrusting up the eminence of the advitorium all at once & so it slipped in. It slipped out again by putting his arm out at length: it went in again as it did before.[97]

After some twenty days of treatment, during which two plasters were applied, the patient found his joint a little stiff so he could not straighten it, but 'by carrying it out & motion it came again, all praised be God'.

Head wounds – particularly those involving fractures – were among the most serious disorders Binns treated. Of the thirteen cases for which we have some details, four patients died, five got well and four casenotes were incomplete, so the outcome is unknown. The four patients who died experienced a similar pattern of symptoms. Each seemed reasonably well after the initial dressing of the wound and remained well for at least a week. After between nine and fourteen days each patient developed symptoms – vomiting, fever and/or paralysis – which became increasingly severe until the patient's death between thirteen and twenty-five days after injury.[98] In three cases Binns and the other surgeons consulted laid the cranium bare in order to determine whether the skull had been fractured.[99] In two cases the trepan was applied.[100] This procedure was obviously reserved for the most desperate cases, when the patient was expected to die in any event. Both of Binns's patients who underwent trepanning died within twenty-four hours after the operation.

Not all patients suffering skull fractures died. In August 1649,

> Frank the drawer at the Castle Tavern in Paternoster Row . . . received a blow with a pint pot upon the frons near the edge of the left temporal muscle, which made a little depression with a fracture round the depression and a piece of the depressed bone carried away to the side of the wound.[101]

Binns gave Frank the treatment he routinely used for head injuries. He opened a vein and gave Frank a suppository. He dressed the wound, using warm medications and bandages. He then prescribed a suppository every other day, changed the medicines used on the dressings as healing progressed, rolled the bandages loosely and watched Frank's daily progress. Frank recovered quickly.

Binns regarded this treatment regimen as necessary. In the case of Will Evims, a patient who died thirteen days after receiving a knife wound on the left side of his forehead, Binns, who merely consulted, criticised the attending surgeon for 'neither [having] given him clyster nor opened vein nor applied anything to his wound more than pleagetts coplaster'.[102] Binns was, however, flexible enough to learn from what he perceived as his own mistakes. In the case of a boy who died twenty-five days after having been kicked in the head by a horse, Binns apparently felt he was partly to blame for the patient's death, for he wrote, 'Let it be your care not to roll the head too hard'.[103]

In addition to the serious injuries described above, Binns treated a number of patients for sprains, bruises and relatively minor burns. One sprained ankle yielded quickly to several days of hot ointments and soaking, combined with a stiff

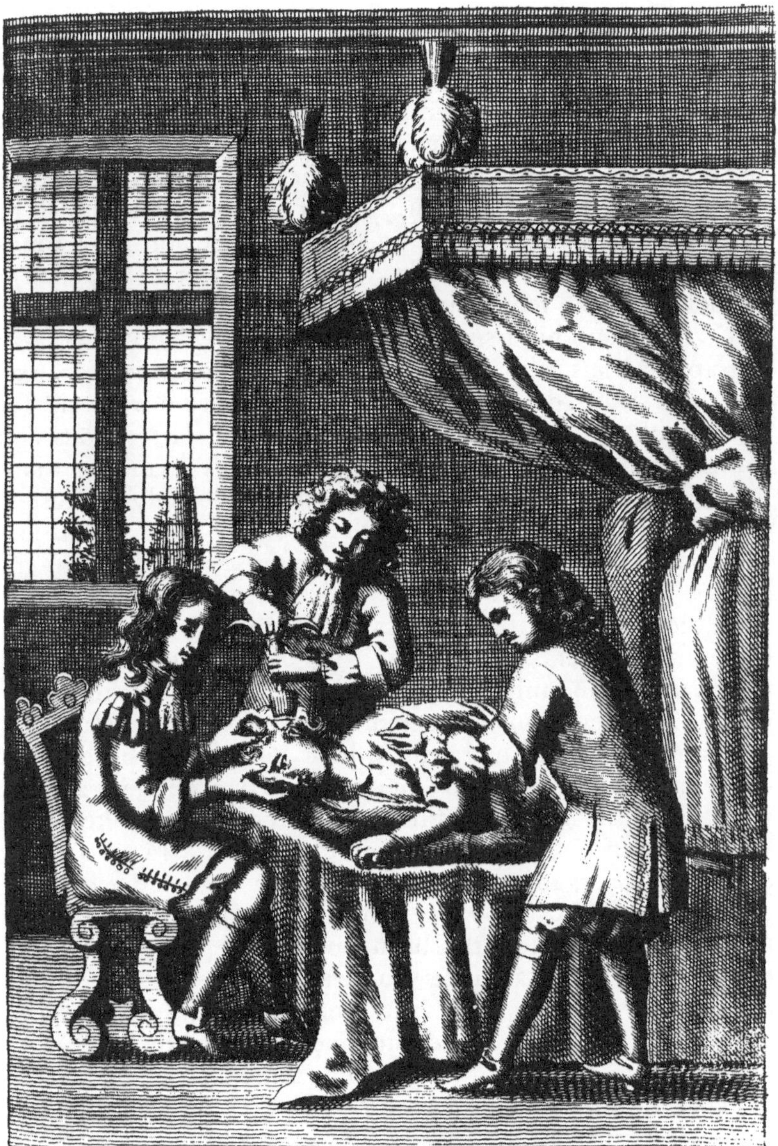

Engraving of a surgeon trephining a patient's cranium, 1678. (Anon., Wellcome Library)

plaster.[104] A more stubborn case of a repeatedly sprained ankle resisted a long and varied course of treatment which included fomentations, purges, plasters, a laced stocking and a trip to Bath. The patient remained uncured.[105]

Bruises usually responded after several applications of oils and plasters.[106] However, some bruises became infected. These Binns treated similarly to apostems, which will be discussed below. The most remarkable case of bruising Binns treated, however, was that of Mr Lower, 'an ancient gentleman [who] fell & bruised his arm & shoulder' in January 1647. Binns and his assistant treated Mr Lower with a series of hot applications and soaking, plasters, fomentations, an ox's belly and a diet drink, until April. They were never paid for their trouble.[107] Lower owed them 30*s*. for plasters, oils and fomentations, and £5 'for my pains and my man's constant pains for 3 months'. This case is remarkable only because it was one of the few appearing in the casebook where Binns lost the cool objective style which characterises the bulk of his entries. His outrage at being denied his fee is apparent.

In the course of his long career, Binns recorded treating only five patients for burns. In each case the patient recovered.[108] In only one instance was Binns called immediately after the injury occurred. In this case, that of a maidservant who scalded her arms in June 1651, Binns produced a cure within three weeks by the use of warm unguent applied with a feather and lawn (fine linen or cotton) rags kept wet with another ointment laid over the burn.[109] In two other cases Binns began treating burn victims only when other efforts had failed. When he 'began cure of Elizabeth Bemis Mrs. Brewer's maid', the burn on her left temple near her eyelid had caused an ulcer so deep it was 'almost to the cranium'. During his first visit Binns opened a vein, applied cupping glasses, ordered a clyster and fomented the ulcer with whey. After several of these fomentations, he applied an unguent until the burn had healed. However, after healing had taken place, 'her eyelid began to draw up within a month . . . so that the inside was turned out, it became very painful and swelled like a bladder'. This the patient treated by stroking her eyelid 'with a dead hand', thereupon finding relief. (Binns did not comment upon this therapy.) However, 'she had not perfect ease till she had an issue in her arm on the same side'.[110]

In the less serious case quoted above, Binns was called in a week after Mrs Swallow's daughter had received leg burns as a result of the maid attempting to warm a bed while the girl was lying in it. Mrs Swallow had been treating the child herself, and called in the surgeon only after a yellow salve she had applied had made the 'leg rise all in little blisters red and itching'. She treated the blisters with a red balsam she had obtained 'formerly' from a Dr Wright to treat a similar condition caused by a 'plaster of burgundy pitch'. Binns decided to continue using the balsam, adding two other ointments and a barley water application to the treatment. Within two weeks, the patient was cured.[111]

In the case of a young man who had burnt his face and hands with gunpowder, Binns appears to have been called in by 'young Mr. Plummer', the patient's surgeon, because the case might have proven to be serious.[112] Treatment, including blood-letting, a clyster, unguents and milk fomentations, was uneventful, however, the burns being nearly healed within ten days.[113]

The above discussion has shown that Binns's treatment of injuries followed predictable patterns and was quite successful. The following sections will turn to what might be referred to as repair jobs (such as his treatment of hydrocephaly, herniae, tumours, apostems and fistulae), and his approach to illnesses.

II SURGICAL REPAIRS

A significant part of Joseph Binns's practice was concerned with the surgical repair of such conditions as ulcers, herniae, apostems, fistulae and tumours, in addition to an assortment of less commonly encountered ills, such as hydrocephaly. Again, difficulties exist with regard to terminology. For instance, an apostemation, or infected swelling, might also be described as a tumour, since Binns used the word 'tumour' to refer to any swelling. Also, apostems frequently developed into fistulae. Equally, after opening, they might become ulcers. Thus, any figures mentioned in connection with these terms must be approximate. However, a rough breakdown of Binns's own references to these conditions indicates that he treated thirty-one patients for ulcers (excluding those caused by syphilis), sixty-six for apostems, twenty-five for fistulae, eighteen for herniae, thirty-five for tumours and nineteen for other disorders requiring repair.

These patients came to Binns hoping to obtain relief from pain and disability. Many also hoped to have their appearances improved. Consider the case of Mrs Storye, a coachman's wife, who had a 'tumour varicosus in the right cheek & coming out at her mouth, in her neck to her shoulder, no bigger than a cherry when she was born but increased as she did grow'.[114] The tumour was only occasionally painful: from time to time it apostemated and required surgical intervention. However, Mrs Storye must also have been concerned about the disfigurement it caused. When Binns saw her, the tumour 'was apostemated from behind her ear to the temple very big'. He was able to cure the apostem and leave 'the tumour less than it used to be, praised be God'. Another woman, 'one Goodwife Lewis', had 'a wen on the inside of the right arm in the armpit & so along the arm for almost a hand's length fastened up to the muscles of that side the scapula where it was rooted & hanging down as big as a child's head'.[115] Binns was able to remove the growth. Still another patient, 'One William White . . . had been troubled with hernia carnosa in his left stone . . . the whole body of the testicle dilated & grown the bigness of a mushmelon'.[116] This casenote was incomplete, so we never learn whether this poor man found relief.

These three sufferers must surely have worried about the unsightliness, as well as the pain, of their disorders. Despite the ubiquitous hazards of smallpox, syphilis, rickets and other diseases which disfigured those they did not kill, seventeenth-century Englishmen and women valued a good appearance. They bought or coveted luxurious fabrics and extravagant styles of dress. They used elaborate wigs and coiffures. Both men and women applied make-up. Thus, it should be remembered that surgeons, then as now, were required to repair the appearance as well as the function of the body.[117]

In any case, surgical repairs were more often required by people who were in pain and who, often justifiably, feared the possibly fatal consequences of allowing a condition to continue. Many such patients sought a return to their previously stable state, rather than a complete cure. For instance, Mr Arthur Rudle had worn a steel truss to control his rupture for many years. When, after having taken cold, he found he could not replace the rupture in the truss, he first called for the truss-maker, Mr Bostocke, and later for Joseph Binns to help him. Binns, through a series of clysters and warm applications to the rupture, was finally able to replace the rupture in the truss twenty-six days after he was first consulted. Mr Rudle was satisfied.[118] He was also fortunate. Mr Sadler was not so lucky. He bruised his old rupture, and all the efforts to replace the rupture in his truss made by Binns and the patient's friends were useless. Sadler died five days after he was injured.[119]

Some patients and their families were in the unenviable

position of deciding to alter a reasonably stable condition in the hope of getting permanently rid of a disorder. Consider the sense of guilt and responsibility which must have burdened Mrs Wilson. When her baby was born,

> it had a little knot or tumour soft in the nape of the neck upon the skull. This grew bigger every month so that in September 1648 it was as big as one's fist, I was satisfied that it was water, the child's head was larger much than children of that age usually are (it was then some 8 months old) I perceived there was a perforation in the skull. I was fearful to open it because of the accidents which might follow [,] but being earnestly desired of the mother of the child, she being well resolved concerning the child, the 15th of September, 1648, I opened this tumour by incision.[120]

There followed a month during which Binns repeatedly opened the baby's head. The child was feverish and sick most of the time. On 16 October it died.[121]

Not all surgical repairs of congenital disorders were so dangerous. Binns reported that 'Mr. Webster of Chesterfield his son was cut of a wry neck the 19 June 1640. It was skinned in 5 days. (Mr. Harris his way of cutting)'.[122] Binns made no suggestion that such an operation was either dangerous or unusual. However, Mr Webster was concerned enough to travel a long way in search of expert surgical help. He was not alone. London was used as a medical centre for the whole of England, and Binns's patients had often travelled long distances to consult him.[123]

Another sort of condition Binns was occasionally called upon to repair was the disorders caused by unskilful or unlucky surgery (not necessarily performed by a trained surgeon). Binns treated at least eight patients for iatrogenic illnesses ranging from an aneurism caused by blood-letting, which eventually led to the amputation of the affected arm, to an apostem in the anus caused by the passing of a clyster pipe 'through the skin close to the verge of the anus, and so through the gut into the rectum'.[124] These problems illustrate the hazards of prophylactic medicine. Seventeenth-century preventative health care required, in addition to a moderate diet and good sleep and exercise habits, regular use of purges, clysters and phlebotomy. Binns did not indicate how many of the eight patients mentioned above had been well before they had undergone the procedures which made them consult him. However, they had certainly been willing participants in operations which they expected to do nothing but good.[125]

Since Binns treated their problems in the same way as he treated other apostems, fistulae and skin irritations, we will not discuss them further here.

The repair job Binns most frequently undertook was the treatment of apostems and fistulae. As indicated above, these ailments resulted from various causes. Sometimes wounds apostemated.[126] Sometimes patients developed apostems and fistulae as complications of conditions such as haemorrhoids, tooth-decay, childbirth, breast-feeding and ague.[127] Anal fistulae were very common.[128] Sometimes these were complications of haemorrhoids. Sometimes they resulted from apostems in the pelvic region. Another frequent location of apostems and fistulae was the mouth. Rotten teeth usually caused these.[129]

Whatever the cause or location, Binns's approach was either to open and drain the infected swelling, making certain that all infected matter had issued before he allowed the orifice(s) to close, or to open the fistula (a hollowness left by earlier infection), cleanse the area, and make sure the flesh as it grew again was sound. His usual method of opening both apostems and fistulae was to apply 'the caustic stone' for several hours, which either opened the affected place on its own or made it easier for Binns to open it by incision. A typical case was that of

> One Mr. Francis Tilney of Grays Inn [who] had a large apostem under his chin, of 10 days collection, the 7 Feb [1642] I laid on the caustic stone & opened it an hour after, there came out much matter, there remained a hollowness some days after being cut . . . & not likely to join. I laid the caustic stone upon it for one hour so it cast all & became an open sore, which healed in 10 days, but the siccatrix girte down his chin.[130]

Binns also used 'suppurative cataplasms' which occasionally opened apostems on their own.[131] Very rarely he opened apostems by incision alone.[132] And sometimes apostems obligingly opened spontaneously.[133]

Once an apostem was open, Binns assisted drainage of matter by inserting a tent into the opening. If the orifice was not large enough, he dilated it with a root. He then assisted drainage by the use of various medicines, either applying them to dressings, bathing the affected area or injecting them into the orifice.

In cases of fistulae where Binns could find two orifices, he sometimes drew a 'frenum' or string through both openings and tied the string progressively tighter. After several days he was usually able to open the fistula by incision quite easily.[134] After opening a fistula, he used similar preparations to those he used for apostems to cleanse the hollowness of matter, scar tissue and spongy flesh, before assisting healing.

The cure of apostems and fistulae was often a long, frustrating business. Just when it seemed that healing was about to occur, a new swelling would develop, or a new hollowness be found, and the whole process of treatment would begin all over again. In May 1645, after suffering from an ague, John the carman's son developed an apostem in his right calf. Binns opened and treated it in his usual manner, but John developed a fistula which became reinfected (that is 'full of matter') at least four times before it finally healed in April 1646.[135] He was unusually fortunate. Mrs Hodge's youngest son, who developed an apostem in his hip and buttock in December 1650, two years after having been kicked by a horse, was treated for his gradually deteriorating condition until he died in October of the following year, 'a very skeleton'.[136] Such patients required frequent visits for dressing changes, assessment of the healing process (often requiring alterations in prescriptions), and monitoring of the general physical state, including pain, sleep, appetite and bowel movements. Many of the working hours of Binns and his assistants or apprentices must have been occupied by visits to apostem and fistula sufferers.[137]

This section would be incomplete without mention of the most remarkable case of fistula Binns treated. A servant, Elizabeth Woodward, was admitted to St Bartholomew's Hospital in July 1650, suffering from a fistula which opened three fingers below her sternum and voided material from her stomach. She recovered enough to leave hospital in April 1651, but was admitted again in November of that year. She died in March 1652.[138]

From apostems and fistulae we will now turn our attention to ulcers. Binns treated many sorts of ulcers. Some, as indicated above, came about in the course of treating apostems and fistulae. Many (which will be discussed elsewhere) resulted from syphilis. Some were cancerous. Some were symptoms of scurvy. Some were complications of other disorders, such as tumours and corns. And still others appeared spontaneously on their own.

Binns kept a number of medications which he used mainly for the treatment of ulcers. He had his own 'ulcer water' and 'unguent mixt'. He also touched ulcers with strong preparations composed of such substances as mercury, antimony and vitriol. His aim was first to cleanse the ulcer of 'escars', discharge and unhealthy spongy flesh, then to promote healing.

His success in healing ulcers varied. Although he tried a number of different preparations on Mrs Lightfool's facial ulcers between May and July 1633, each new ointment caused much pain, but did no good.[139] Some ulcers, such as the apthas Mr Hutchinson's girl Sarah had on her gums and tongue, would almost certainly have disappeared on their own. (Sarah was well in ten days.)[140] Others of Binns's cures seem almost miraculous. On 4 April 1655 a 14-day-old infant developed an ulcer on the navel after the umbilical cord had fallen off. Despite the efforts of Binns and the physician Dr Bathurst, the ulcer grew until 'it spread as broad as a xx piece'. At this point Binns used his unguent with an antimony preparation, and reported 'good digestion'. The ulcer healed by 20 April, 'Laus soli deo'.[141]

Although Binns treated a number of ulcers he described as cancerous, he never approached them with much hope of success. Indeed, he reported a cure in only one case of cancer. This was that of Goodwife White of St Giles in the Fields. Binns removed her cancerous breast in St Bartholomew's Hospital on 3 February 1648. She was alive and well in 1653.[142] Binns attempted another breast removal seven months later. This patient was also in St Bartholomew's Hospital. Binns

> used a double ligature upon the woman's breast the 9 August at morn 1648. Tied it harder the 11th at morn & the 12, & the 14th it had gained much – the 16th & the 18 – the 22nd the lower string was through the bigness of a finger, the upper one near to an inch . . . so with string cut it off in the ligature. It bled pretty freely. Died a week after.[143]

Thereafter, Binns treated breast cancers more cautiously, dealing with the tumours and ulcers as he did non-cancerous ones. In addition to breast cancers, he treated cancerous mouth and tongue ulcers. Regardless of the therapy applied, patients with cancer usually died.[144]

Binns also treated several leg ulcers which had been caused by scurvy. These began with swelling and spots in the affected leg. The spots turned to pustules or blisters, and these eventually became ulcers. Binns treated such patients with juice of scurvy grass, purges and a variety of ointments (depending on what had the best result).[145]

Despite his lack of optical equipment, Binns was able to diagnose and successfully treat three cases of ulcers in the eye. In one case he described the affected eye in detail:

> I found her eye much inflamed [,] upon the pupilla a little whitish dint in the outward coat of cornea like the pressure of a pin's head with little towes from it as if it had been a little piece of flock of wool, which seemed to be an ulcer. Her pain was great pricking & burning.

Binns characteristically treated the woman's whole system, blistering her neck, purging her with pills, applying plasters to her temples and dropping medicines into her eye. The ulcers got worse at first, so Binns changed the eye medications (including woman's milk in the second preparation) and cupped and scarified the patient's shoulders. After this the eye improved. The woman was relieved of her pain and left with 'some weak sight' in her eye.[146]

Perhaps more clearly than with other types of disorder, Binns's approach to ulcers illustrated both the seventeenth-century surgeon's empiricism and his willingness to try his hand at any sort of problem which was brought to him, however frustrating. If one medicine failed to produce the desired effect, Binns tried another. If cancerous ulcers appeared hopeless of cure, he attacked them anyway. Despite both surgeons' and physicians' understandable unwillingness to accept 'incurable' cases, Binns and his colleagues did take them on, applying their skills as best they could. This perseverance reflects not only the surgeons' patience and dedication, but also the patients' demands. It is not surprising that the barbersurgeons were the most numerous among full-time medical personnel in seventeenth-century London.[147]

Binns's practice included the treatment of many tumours. As indicated above, he used the word 'tumour' to describe any swelling, rather as the modern practitioner might use the word 'oedema'. However, he also used the term more specifically, referring to growths which were not apostemated swellings. He also used other terms, such as 'wen', 'polyp', 'ficus' and 'ascites' to refer to such growths.

Some tumours were easier to treat than others. Polyps in the nose, for instance, were not difficult to remove, but tended to recur. Binns wrote in 1650,

> I extracted a pollipus out of Mrs. Cooper's daughter's nostril & made her an issue in her left arm. I had extracted it out of both nostrils 2 years afore this . . . (I expected it again in 1654). They

> are in both nostrils like a bunch of grapes, injected after a restringent medicine.[148]

Likewise, Binns had no difficulty treating a 'ficus' in the anus of one Mr Lucas. On 2 February he 'made ligature' upon the tumour. He reported that 'it looked deadish the next day and flaccid, it came off going to stool the 6 February at morn'.[149]

However, other sorts of tumours were harder to deal with, and Binns approached them with caution. Indeed, Binns's casebook reveals nothing more clearly than this surgeon's reluctance to use the knife. Even when opening the flesh was necessary, Binns preferred gradual (and hopefully bloodless) means, such as the caustic stone and ligature. One can only speculate about the reasons for this reluctance. Perhaps Binns feared infection. Perhaps he feared making a bad condition worse.

The following case illustrates his caution. On 16 March 1661 he and the surgeon Mr Arris were called to see a Mr Chilsonne who had

> a great tumour on the inside of his right thigh very large in length from the middle of the thigh to the knee in thickness from the forepart of the thigh so to the underside of the thigh to the outside.

They judged that 'it was a schirrus cancerosus' and ordered a cataplasm to be applied. Their prescriptions were used for some two weeks. At this point, a Dr Williams was called in. He was in favour of opening the tumour by means of a 'sympathetic specific medicine' of his own composition. This was first applied on 8 April. On 10 April incision was tried, but 'there came blood trickling out pretty fast, so clapt on a dosell [dressing] . . . and bound it up till the 11 April, cut a little deeper till blood came', dressed it again, and continued this pattern of treatment until the physician could insert a probe two inches into the incision. At this point the patient died (16 April). The next day the tumour was opened. Binns reported 'there was nothing in it but coagulated blood & a substance like rotten liver, & but little thin blood, & a hollowness from it up to the groin full of black grumous blood'.[150] Binns obviously felt the patient would have been better off without the physician's radical help.

Binns attempted to remove only certain sorts of tumours. These were not always small. In a case mentioned above, Binns removed a wen from a woman's shoulder-blade which was 'hanging down as big as a child's head'.[151] In a less successful case he 'incised' a cancerous tumour on a man's thigh on 12 February 1652. He then treated the resulting ulcer and a new tumour which developed on the patient's ribs until 29 August, when the man died. Despite this sad outcome, Binns reported 'his thigh is even cicatrised'.[152] He obviously felt that his course of treatment was appropriate.

Other sorts of tumours Binns dealt with by using surface applications and internal medicines. In a case of scrofulous tumours of the neck, for instance, Binns prescribed a course of vomits, purges, salves and plasters. This patient was under his care on and off for four years. Her condition did not heal permanently, so she left Binns and looked elsewhere for a cure. Binns noted laconically, 'She was after touched by the King'.[153]

Most of the tumours Binns treated were easily visible, occurring on the extremities or the neck and head. Tumours of the abdomen and chest were more difficult, both to identify and to treat. Many patients with such internal growths must have taken them to physicians, since surgical excision of them would not have been possible and, in any case, the formal division between surgery and medicine would have placed such ills within the physician's sphere. Binns did undertake treatment of an 'ascites' tumour of the belly. He opened this swelling on 24 June 1655, releasing a gallon of fluid the first day and a similar amount on the two following days. The fourth day he released three quarts and the patient felt better, but was very restless. He died that evening.[154] As in the case of hydrocephaly discussed above, and one of another infant who was born with an 'aqueous tumour on the small of the back', Binns was able to drain the swelling, but could not stop production of the fluid.[155]

The last major type of repair job Binns undertook was the treatment of hernia. He treated eighteen male patients for hernia. Eight of these suffered from 'hernia aquosa', a condition during which one testicle filled with a watery fluid. Ten patients had other sorts of herniae.

Binns's treatment of hernia aquosa followed a routine which was usually successful. The day before surgery, the patient was prescribed a vomit. The next day the swelling was opened by incision. The following case was typical.

> 1652. Dr. Bennet hath had a hernia aquosa 12 months in his testicle [.]. I opened it the 8th of April in the afternoon the stone lay to the seam in the middle of the scrotum, & I made incision on

> the outside towards the thigh an inch from the stone, and toward the bottom of the tumour. There came out of clear water three parts of a pint, I used a restringent & warm fomentation for 5 or six days, morn & night, with a hot stupe.

The patient recovered.[156]

The problem with hernia aquosa was that it tended to recur. Poor Mr Samuel Davison had had a hernia aquosa opened by the surgeon, Mr Will Moollins, in the spring of 1653. After the operation, Moollins had given him a diet drink and pills which made his mouth and throat sore. Mr Davison developed a fever. His hernia grew again. This time he consulted Binns, who opened the hernia 24 October 1653; half a pint of fluid issued. Binns prescribed a purge and a new diet drink. However, the hernia grew again.[157]

Binns treated other sorts of hernia with surface applications and trusses. Mrs Benfield's son, who had had an inguinal hernia as a baby, developed an intestinal hernia as a young man. Binns treated it with purges and the application of hot ointments and dressings. The patient was cured in two weeks.[158] Mr Robinson's old intestinal hernia fell down so that it filled the scrotum. Binns and two surgical colleagues, Mr King and Mr Heath, tried to reduce it without success. They treated the patient with clysters, fomentations and cataplasms, but the patient died seven days after he became ill.[159]

In his treatment of hernia, as in his other repairs, Binns's very mechanical approach to disorder can be clearly observed. He treated symptoms. Although he prescribed purges, clysters, issues and phlebotomy, these procedures were designed to keep or produce a humoral balance in the body, rather than to attack primary causes of disease, about which Binns seems not to have speculated. He aimed merely to get rid of an unwelcome manifestation of disease or to return the patient to a bearable stable condition. He frequently succeeded. Of the approximately 194 repair jobs he undertook, 92 left the patient well, 22 resulted in improvement of the condition, and only seven left the sufferer no better than before. In forty-four cases the outcome is unknown, and thirty-one patients died.

In reporting the outcome of an attempt at surgical repair, Binns's casenotes frequently ended with the statement, 'Well laus deo'. Yet his personal definition of the word 'well' seems limited at best. Patients were well when they could function more or less independently. Thus, people who could walk on their broken legs when the legs were still in plaster were well. Hernia aquosa sufferers were well as long as their recurring ailments did not inconvenience them. Binns's surgical repairs were, therefore, conservative measures. His was no miracle surgery which could restore lost beauty or promise permanent cures. Rather he attacked the immediate problem, hoping to produce stability in the patient's condition.

III DISEASE STATES

Joseph Binns treated many ailments which were produced by disease states. Some conditions, like the spots, ulcers and swellings which appeared on the legs of scurvy sufferers, fell properly within the surgeon's sphere of operation. Others, such as diarrhoea, sore throat, agues and coughs, might more appropriately have been taken to a physician.[160] Binns treated internal problems with purges and vomits, sometimes adding a typically surgical remedy, such as an issue, to the course of treatment. His general approach to illness has been more fully discussed above, and need not concern us here. What we will investigate at length is his handling of venereal disease, which called upon all of his medical and surgical abilities at once.

Binns was consulted in 133 cases of gonorrhoea or syphilis.[161] In addition, twenty women brought to him problems which might be called 'female disorders', including whites (copious and unpleasant vaginal discharge), suppression of the menses, inordinate menstruation, and 'fits of the mother' (seizures produced by a wandering womb). Some of these patients may have had syphilis.[162] Several men called upon him to treat urinary retention which may or may not have been caused by venereal disease.[163]

Syphilis marked its victims both physically and morally. The disease was a chameleon, changing its manifestations during its course, and becoming dormant for years at a time, reappearing when its unsuspecting host had thought him- or herself long since cured. Dr Thomas Sydenham described the progress of syphilis as follows:

> The patient is affected with an unusual pain in the genitals . . . a spot, about the size and colour of a measle, appears on some part of the glans. . . . A discharge appears from the urethra . . . the aforesaid pustule becomes an ulcer. . . . Great pain during erections pathognomic of the disease. . . . Ardor urinae. . . . Bubos in the groin. . . . Pain in the head, arms and ankles. . . . Crusts and scabs appear on the skin. . . . The bones of the skull, the shin-bones, and the arm-bones, are raised into hard tubers. . . . The bone becomes carious and putrescent. . . .

> Phagadaenic ulcers destroy the cartilege of the nose. This they eat away; so that the bridge sinks in and the nose flattens. . . . At length, limb by limb perishing away, the lacerated body, a burden to earth, finds ease only in the grave.[164]

Symptoms of advanced syphilis were well known, and even lampooned by the dramatists of the time. In the sad tale of a man who fell first into the arms of a harlot and then into the hands of a radical surgeon, the sufferer complains,

> I am a knight, Sir Pock-hole is my name,
> And by birth I am a Londoner,
> Free by my copy, but my ancestors
> Were Frenchmen all, and riding hard this way,
> Upon a trotting horse my bones did ache
> And I faint knight to ease my weary limbs,
> Light at this cave, when straight this furious fiend,
> With sharpest instrument of purest steel,
> Did cut the gristle of my nose away,
> And in the place this velvet plaster stands,
> Relieve me gentle knight out of his hands.[165]

However, the 'saddle-noses' and pain-racked limbs were no joke to the victims of the pox, whose only hope was in a course of treatment nearly as savage as the disease itself.

Binns adapted the remedies he prescribed to the severity and types of symptoms presented, the sufferer's previous experience of 'cures' and the patient's reactions to the means tried. The first manifestation of the disease which Binns saw most frequently was gonorrhoea, which involved discharge from the penis, 'smarting' during urination, and uncontrollable erection or 'standing'. Binns routinely began treatment with a dose of 'pill Barbarosa', which purged the patient, and an injection into the urethra of his 'green water'.[166] To this he often added a diet drink which contained the purging herb senna. If the condition continued, he moved on to one or both of the two courses of treatment favoured at the time – a month's prescription of either guaiacum or mercury. The guaiacum cure was considerably more pleasant for the patient. Sometimes it apparently succeeded.[167] However, Binns used mercury far more often.

The mercury treatment of syphilis involved taking mercury internally, applying it in ointments to rashes, scabs and ulcers, and in 'waters' injecting it into apostems, noses and genitalia. Side effects of treatment were a sore mouth and throat, sometimes involving ulceration, spitting great quantities,

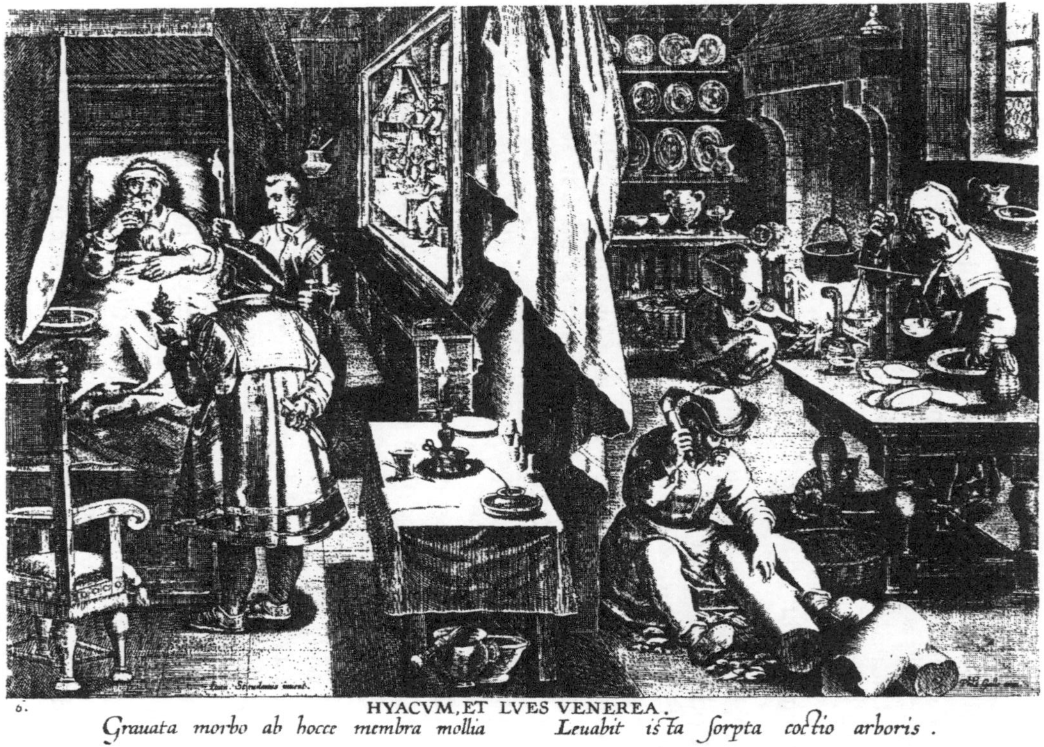

The preparation and use of guaiacum in cases of syphilis. Guaiacum and mercury were the preferred medicines for venereal disease in seventeenth-century England. (Philip Galle *c.* 1600, after J. van der Straet, Wellcome Library)

occasional nausea and frequent bowel movements. In the hands of an unskilled or unscrupulous practitioner, the cure could be worse than the disease. On 8 May 1639 Binns first saw Joan Carter,

> who hath the lower mandible corrupt (& the teeth fallen forth) all the chin from the one cheek to the other, her cheeks & chin much swollen & hard, she was fluxed by Kixton the Quack 3 years ago, & she continued spitting at times ever since, & at that time where her cheeks were ulcerated for want of looking to they grew so hard cicatrised that she could not well open her jaws so he cut them & after that she had a contraction of some branches of sinews down her neck, that she could neither open well her mouth nor lift up her head much.[168]

By October he could report that 'she [was] very well praised be God, & no great blemish, only her chin a little shrunk in'.

Binns himself was very careful about mercury doses and patients' reactions to them. If the patient had too extreme a reaction, he either reduced the dose or withdrew the mercury for a time. By the same token, if doses did not seem to be working, he increased them.[169]

Binns apparently experimented with different mercury doses and preparations. His 'guinea pigs' were patients in St Bartholomew's Hospital. During one February he gave three men the same number of 'precipitate pills' on three successive days and compared their reactions. On the first day, five grains gave one man four stools and the others two stools apiece, with no vomits. Eight grains on the second day produced two, five and four stools respectively. On the third day, sixteen grains gave the patients two stools, four stools and two vomits, and six stools respectively. One man had begun to spit at this point.[170] The mercury preparation Binns used most frequently was called manna mineralis. However, he also experimented with a recipe which included mithridate and one called Sampson's Turbith.[171]

In addition to careful monitoring of mercury doses, Binns treated the symptoms which the mercury produced. Mr Thomas Mazeine had first consulted Binns in May 1635, at which time 'the diet' removed all his pains. In March 1637 he had nodes in both shins. Binns prescribed a mercury course which relieved the pain in his legs, but caused ulceration of his tongue and cheeks 'with white sloughs'. Binns treated this problem with 'lotion of barley, althea roots, licorice and violet leaves which cleansed the ulcers in the 7th or 8th day'.[172]

Characteristically Binns combined a mercury flux with

other prescriptions designed to improve the patient's general health. He almost always prescribed a diet drink, and recommended healthy eating habits. He blamed a repeat patient, Mr John Malett or Merett, for the fact that his ulcerated forehead was slow to heal, writing 'but sometimes it would be all cicatrised, & he keeping no good diet, but disordered, so it would ulcerate by places & some little pieces of bones cast out'. Several months later the patient 'took pills, & became temperate so, he grew fat & in very good health & all his forehead healed save a little moisture came out above his nose, very well in April 1655'.[173] Binns also prescribed sweating for syphilis patients, as did other practitioners.

The nature of the disease required the healers who treated syphilis to apply their skills to particular immediate problems as well as to the disease as a whole. Most distressing to both sufferer and practitioner were the ulcers on the foreskin which rapidly became gangrenous and caused patients to lose all or part of the penis.[174] In one case Binns applied 'a strong cataplasm to revocate the spirits and hinder putrification', and twice scarified the foreskin. When these measures did not work, Binns cut away the mortified flesh.[175]

Another manifestation of syphilis which was particularly difficult to treat was its invasion of bones which caused tumours and the eventual rotting away of the bone itself. In 1645 Mr Fotiley was cured 'of a pain in his left leg nocturnal a little tumour upon the bone' by a Mr Sase. 'In 1651 he had pain again. The bone foul which Quince [another surgeon] took off with a mallett and chisel & the diet. Took away his pains'. Binns first saw the patient in April 1659, when the bone was 'like a rotten post'. Binns applied dressings to the bone itself and gave mercury internally. In August Mr Fotiley went down stairs 'and coming up again he turned a little awry & broke the rotten part of the maior tibia in sunder so keeps his bed wholly'. By October he was feeling a bit better, but still had to return home to Berkshire in a horse litter.[176]

Other symptoms of syphilis which Binns treated separately were ulcerated throats, palates, noses and lips, bubos in the groin, obstructions in the urethra, nodes in the shins and the skull and various pains in the joints and the head. His treatment was remarkably successful. Of the 133 patients he treated for gonorrhoea or syphilis, 60 recovered and 15 got better. He left only ten uncured. Two patients died. In forty-six cases the outcome is unknown.

These figures indicate that Binns knew what he was doing, but they do not tell the whole story. Some patients, disheartened by long and inconclusive courses of treatment decided to consult other practitioners.[177] Some who had apparently been cured became ill again years later. Binns's casebook contains references to quite a few repeat patients who consulted him along with other practitioners in their interminable efforts to rid themselves of the pox. The most faithful of these sufferers was one Mr Brooks who underwent some seven courses of treatment in four years.[178] Thus the number of 'cures' indicated above is probably an overestimate of the patients who were permanently healed, and the small number of deaths recorded is probably an underestimate.

Binns and his patients were clearly convinced that syphilis was sexually transmitted. Mr Baker, a bookseller's man, developed pustules upon the glans 'by dealing with a pocky woman'.[179] Mr Henry Richards 'the 20 July in the night suffered much pain bet. glans & praepution having lain with a wench some 5 or 6 days afore'.[180] Indeed, Binns was puzzled about the possible origins of Mr Millbank's 'Fistula in Scroto', writing

> these two years past we can understand no venereal cause, but, nocturnal pollutions & sometimes a forcing of his seed to flow & so caused some disorder & caused the flux at first & so from an ill habit in the parts & so communicated to the whole habit.[181]

This suggestion that masturbation could cause syphilis is surely novel.

Because of its associations with unclean sexuality, syphilis affected people's attitudes and behaviour concerning marriage. Mr Baker was aghast when his syphilis re-emerged shortly after his marriage in the summer of 1655. He had thought he had been cured five years earlier.[182] Mr Egas apparently felt he had been unfairly treated by the pox when the disease returned after four years' dormancy. He protested 'that he had not dealt with any but his wife who was then very well & had been for long time'.[183]

None the less, people with syphilis married and had children. William Bemis and his wife were not the only husband and wife that Binns treated as a couple for syphilis.[184] And Mrs Rud, who was 'troubled with the whites . . . , ulcer in pudenda & tumours in labias pudenda' and had 'much smart in making her water' was treated with pill Barbarosa, the green injection and other local applications until she had stopped breast-feeding her baby girl. Thereafter her symptoms were cured with mercury prescriptions. She had no trouble until she developed nodes in her shins three years later, having recently married again.[185] One wonders what her first husband died of.

As the above discussion has amply indicated, syphilis was a loathsome disease. It disfigured its victims and lasted a dreadfully long time. A severe case of the pox could impoverish the sufferer. In one year of treatment, Mr John Merett or Malett ran up a £35 bill at the apothecary's. And, due to its associations with sexual vice, it was also an unrespectable disease. While a person suffering from smallpox or scrofula (also disfiguring ailments) was an object of pity, a pox-ridden sufferer was more likely to be ridiculed – and avoided.[186]

Therefore it is not surprising that many of the people Binns treated for syphilis complained of more innocent-sounding individual symptoms, such as chronic headache or sore throat. 'My cousin Spooner's sister' consulted Binns for 'extreme pain in her head . . . it being all her head over & as much by day as night but somewhat worse in the night'.[187] Several days later she developed nodes on her forehead and pains in her shoulders. Binns prescribed a mercury flux. Considering such attempts at concealment, it is possible that more of Binns's patients were syphilitic than the numbers quoted above indicate.

Certainly the women who consulted Binns for amenorrhoea, too small an amount of menstruation and the whites may have had the pox. Mrs Elin Barker, who complained of amenorrhoea, 'sloughs & stench', falls within this category.[188] The unfortunate 5-year-old girl who had the whites in very great quantity was another possible victim. Binns wrote 'it was feared [that] one that had the gonorrhoea spent his sperm betwixt the child's legs upon her pudenda, but this was not certainly proved'.[189]

There was, of course, another possible explanation for amenorrhoea. On 20 July Binns treated 'Mary at Mr. Barham's' who 'wants her menses' with laxatives and emetics. He also let blood from the saphena vein in the foot – a treatment for this complaint which was used in classical times. Nine days later her menses 'came down very well'.[190] This sounds very like induced abortion.

Binns also treated other 'female problems', such as inordinate menses, fits of the mother and swelling in the hand and arm which occurred after childbirth. For all of these conditions he prescribed laxatives and/or emetics which usually produced the desired result.[191] One interesting case of 'fits like fits of the mother' may shed some light on this now-archaic disease. Binns treated 'My sister Gray's sister' for such fits with the usual emetics until, nearly a month after beginning treatment, she voided a worm. He then prescribed one dose of the mercury preparation manna mineralis, after which the patient was well.[192]

Binns's treatment of syphilis and other genito-urinary disorders was mechanical and conventional. His choice of this area as a speciality, if choice it was, was also conventional. Surgeons had been undertaking the cure of venereal diseases since the early sixteenth century at least. Binns left related areas of surgery alone. He did not cut for the stone. Neither did he act as a man-midwife. He apparently found his own area of expertise sufficiently demanding and rewarding. Indeed, his regular syphilis patients alone must have provided him with a good living. For services and medications for the year 1658, Mr Edward Carothorne paid him £29 9*s*.[193] St Bartholomew's Hospital paid him only £30 a year for acting as a staff surgeon. Binns's therapeutic methods did not change over the entire thirty years covered by the casebook. Venereal disease provided him with an arena where his own special talents – patience, caution, conscientiousness and persistence – paid off.

IV CONCLUSIONS

There is much Joseph Binns's casebook does not tell us, both about his own practice and about the ordinary practice of surgery in seventeenth-century England. Only tantalising hints are given about Binns's 'man' – the servant, apprentice or assistant who is occasionally mentioned in a casenote. Since surgical training was invariably by apprenticeship, and since Binns was an active member of London's surgical community, it is more than likely that he kept a series of apprentices in the course of his career. It is equally likely that, as a well-to-do man, he employed one or more servants. However, the casebook deals almost exclusively with Binns's own contacts with patients; the identity, function and status of his 'man' must remain a mystery.

In addition, the casebook provides little information about the prices Binns charged for his services. Money due or received is mentioned only under unusual circumstances. Thus we know nothing about the surgeon's ordinary rates, or whether he charged on a sliding scale, according to the patient's ability to pay.

It is more than likely that Binns did not record details of every case he dealt with during his thirty-year career. Even considering this factor, the number of patients Binns treated was small, compared to the thousands who consulted the astrological physician, Richard Napier, during forty years of practice.[194] How accurate a picture of seventeenth-century surgical practice does Binns's casebook provide, considering the size of the sample?

It seems probable that Binns was far more typical of surgeons than Napier was of physicians. Because Napier provided a very specialised service, sufferers travelled for many miles to consult him in his own home. His national reputation inflated his clientele. Furthermore, Napier dealt with his patients' problems in the course of fairly brief conversations; thus he was able to treat as many as fifteen patients a day.[195]

Binns, on the other hand, visited his patients in hospital or in their own chambers. His duties often involved time-consuming procedures, and usually required repeated visits – sometimes more than one a day. Thus, the demands on his time prevented him from treating large numbers of patients at any one time. Furthermore, although he was respectable, Binns did not command a national reputation. His reputation was closely tied to that of the Company of Barbersurgeons and London surgeons generally.

Although Binns's casebook was intended simply as a record of treatment given and reactions achieved, a great deal can be inferred from it about what being a seventeenth-century surgical patient was like. It was anything but pleasant. In reading Binns's matter-of-fact observations, it is easy to lose sight of the fact that all of his operations were performed without anaesthetic, that the ulcers produced by his mercury cures were painful, and that the desired reactions to purges and emetics were unpleasant. People did not expect to feel good while undergoing medical and surgical treatment.

Why did they seek out such torture? Part of the answer lies in popular ideas about illness. The more suffering illness caused, the stronger were the measures needed to combat it. Thus, the sufferer in the midst of a mercury cure could take comfort in the very discomfort he or she felt. At least something was being done. Surgeons were so frequently consulted because the service they provided was highly specialised. While lay-people often made and prescribed medicines and advised therapeutic regimens, they less frequently used surgical instruments.

In addition, if Binns's casebook is an accurate indicator, surgeons frequently succeeded in relieving their patients. In those cases for which information is available, 265 patients emerged well from Binns's treatment and 62 got better. Twenty-two patients failed to improve and fifty-three died. This was an impressive achievement. Most of his patients did not consult Binns until they had spent some time treating themselves or receiving treatment from friends and/or relatives. Thus, by the time he undertook their cases, their conditions had already become acute.

It must be reiterated that Joseph Binns was in no way unique. He did not obtain unusual wealth or fame in the course of his career. Neither was he ever censured by his own Company or the Royal College of Physicians for irregular practice. He published nothing. His casenotes indicate that he was cautious and very conventional. His career very probably paralleled the careers of many of his colleagues. Thus, his casebook testifies to the great service provided by seventeenth-century surgeons. Modern medical historians have underrated them because of what they could not do, ignoring the value of what they did.

4

THE PHYSICIAN'S TALE

Seventeenth-century medicine has received more attention from historians than has seventeenth-century surgery. Biographies of great physicians form the backbone of traditional medical history. Studies focusing on the day-to-day practices of physicians are rare, but they do exist. Michael MacDonald's recent *Mystical Bedlam: Madness, Anxiety and Healing in Seventeenth-Century England* is based on the voluminous casebook of the astrological physician Richard Napier.[1] MacDonald's work provides an excellent example of the kinds of information such sources can yield. Napier's life, thought, techniques and clientele are investigated in great detail and related to the more general question of mental illness in the period.

However, useful as it is, MacDonald's study tells us little about the practice and experience of physic in seventeenth-century England. His focus upon madness leaves the vast territory of 'physical' illness, even within Napier's practice, unexplored. And Napier was himself obviously untypical. MacDonald calls him 'one of the last Renaissance magi' who attracted patients, one suspects, partly because the service he provided was relatively hard to find elsewhere.[2] Napier, as an astrological physician, was a specialist. Although astrology was used as a diagnostic and therapeutic tool by many seventeenth-century healers, it was secondary to other methods.

At present, no studies comparable to MacDonald's exist of 'conventional' seventeenth-century physicians. Having examined Joseph Binns's surgical practice, therefore, we will take a briefer look at some physicians' casebooks in order to provide a basis for comparison of the experience of physicians and their patients with those of Binns and his clientele. As indicated above, a number of physicians' casebooks are available.[3] For example, the great mid-century physician, Sir Theodore Turquet de Mayerne, who served the Court and

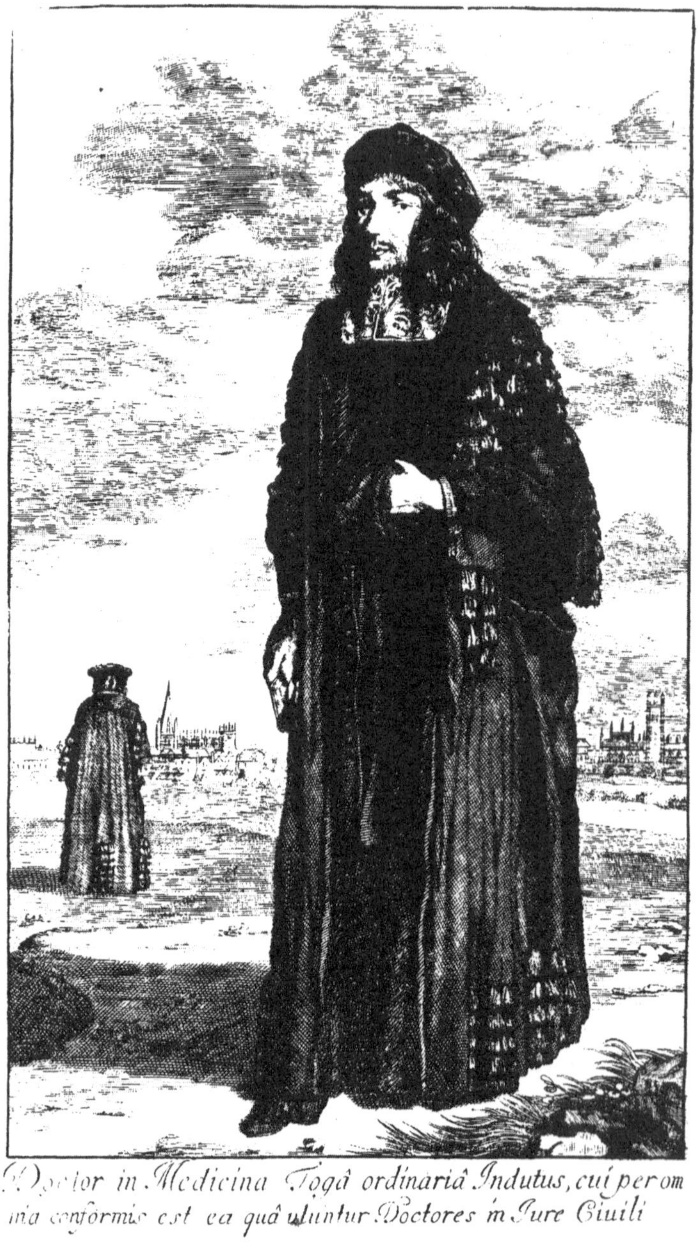

The seventeenth-century physician's gown was the same as that worn by the practitioner of Civil Law. (Wellcome Library)

numerous upper-status families, left extensive records, beautifully written and bound.[4] However, analysis of Mayerne's casebooks, interesting as it might be, would leave many questions unanswered and might, indeed, prejudice our viewpoint by supporting old stereotypes. For instance, it is generally assumed that physicians' services were more expensive than those of other healers and that physicians were therefore patronised only by the well-to-do. Neither Mayerne's casebook nor that of the late-seventeenth-century London physician, Sir Edmund King, could yield fair evidence regarding this issue.

The casebooks of less-well-known physicians, then, provide more suitable source material for this study. As indicated above, extensive 'physical' casebooks, such as Napier's, do exist. However, for purposes of comparison, three shorter casebooks kept during different periods have been selected for study. We will examine the casebook of Dr Barker of Shrewsbury for the years 1595 to 1605, that of a physician probably practising in Cambridge between 1619 and 1622, and the notes and correspondence of John Symcotts for the years between 1633 and 1660. Through comparison of these records kept by provincial healers, both among themselves and with those kept by the urban healer Binns, some conclusions may be drawn about occupational healing in seventeenth-century England.

I JOHN SYMCOTTS

The records kept by the physician John Symcotts are particularly appropriate for our purposes.[5] Symcotts was an almost exact contemporary of Joseph Binns. Born *c.* 1592 and dying in 1662, his practice spanned the same period as Binns's. Because Symcotts was a rural practitioner, his casebook will allow us to compare rural with urban circumstances. It will also allow us to identify similarities and differences in the practice of medicine and surgery in the same period.

Inevitably Symcotts's casebook differs from that of Binns. It is by no means as rich a source, giving information about only 83 patients in contrast to the 671 whom Binns mentioned. Further, unlike Binns, Symcotts noted only sporadically the outcome of the treatment he prescribed. However, the Symcotts papers include a collection of correspondence which reveals much about his relationships with his patients – an element notably lacking in our knowledge about Binns. In addition, due to the efforts of F. N. L. Poynter and W. J.

Bishop, who edited the Symcotts papers, we know far more about Symcotts's biography than will ever be known about Binns's.

John Symcotts was one of seven children born to John and Elizabeth Symcotts, who settled in Sutton, Bedfordshire. Not much is known about the Symcotts' economic and social status. However, the physician's brothers George and Thomas became London merchants, his twin, Robert, a minister, and John himself undertook a long course of study at Cambridge at about the age of 16, information which suggests that the family was reasonably well-to-do. John Symcotts was admitted as a pensioner at Queens' College, Cambridge, in 1608, matriculated in 1610, received his BA in 1615 and his MD in 1636, after he had already been practising medicine for many years.[6]

After leaving university, Symcotts settled in Huntingdon where he lived until his death in 1662. His medical practice extended over Huntingdonshire, Bedfordshire and Cambridgeshire. He worked closely with Gervase Fullwood the elder, who was most likely his assistant. Fullwood himself kept a 'man', Edward Johnson, who collected fees and carried on some correspondence for the practice.

During the Civil War Symcotts's sympathies lay with the parliamentarians. Indeed, Oliver Cromwell was the most famous of his patients.[7] Although he apparently never joined the army, Commonwealth and Protectorate governments frequently called upon Symcotts to serve on commissions for the regulation of financial, military and other civic affairs in Huntingdonshire.[8]

Poynter and Bishop write of Symcotts's appearance and medical history:

> His brother Thomas refers to his lean and spare body. In early life the doctor suffered from headaches, which he eventually cured with a diet drink. On his own statement he had three attacks of smallpox, and he was, during the last ten years of his life, a martyr to gout.[9]

He never married. Since his brothers predeceased him, the bulk of his property was bequeathed to his nephew, Dr William Symcotts, only son of his brother Robert.

Notwithstanding Poynter and Bishop's judgment that 'His fortune was not large, considering his "painful indeavours" during forty or more years of practice', John Symcotts became prosperous, if not wealthy, as a result of his exertions.[10] His will indicates that he left nearly £200 in cash to friends and relations. He also left property in Huntingdonshire, Cambridgeshire and London, which included arable land, meadow, an inn, six houses, a dovecot yard and an adjoining hog-yard.[11] Symcotts, like Binns, did well in the medical marketplace, although he certainly never charged fees on the scale of those commanded by well-known London physicians.[12]

His casenotes, few as they are, indicate that Symcotts was truly a general practitioner. Although he treated more cases of consumption than any other disorder, sixteen cases out of a total of eighty-two do not demonstrate a speciality. Indeed, one suspects that Symcotts kept his casebook, not as a record of all the cases he dealt with, but as a way of noting the sorts of treatment he applied to various kinds of ailments, perhaps for future reference.

Symcotts's records demonstrate that the conventional division between surgery and medicine applied as little to provincial medical practice as it did to London surgical practice. He treated many ailments which might more appropriately have been dealt with by a surgeon, including apostems, sore eyes, haemorrhoids, itching, skin rashes, tumours, urinary retention and disorders resulting from issues.[13] He also treated menstrual problems and disorders related to childbirth which might equally well have been treated by a surgeon or midwife.[14]

However, his approach to such ailments was sometimes different from that of a surgeon. For instance, in November 1641 he was summoned by the midwife Mistress Willis to the bedside of Mistress Lewis of London who was in labour. The child had died, and the midwife sought medication which would hasten its delivery. Symcotts prescribed and then went home. After twenty-four hours, when the patient was nearly at the end of her strength, Symcotts prescribed again and the woman was delivered, 'Deo soli laus sit'.[15] A surgeon would very likely have tried to deliver the child by the use of instruments, which almost certainly would have mutilated it.[16] Perhaps the midwife consulted Symcotts for this very reason.

Sometimes Symcotts approved typically surgical treatment, although he did not perform most surgical procedures himself. For instance,

> 1652. Mr. Cater of Kempson, having an issue in his left arm, and purged too little, had a hard glandulous tumour in his left armhole very painful, attended with a feverish distemper. Then was

> applied poultices ex apio and other emplasters as friends advised. It grew worse and worse, would not be dissolved, but tended to maturation, to which at length it came. I forced out at a little orifice much purulency, and it was laid open by a London surgeon and healed by him.[17]

He was also interested in surgical problems which he may not have treated himself. For instance, he reported successful treatment of two cases of gaping navels. In the first,

> Mr. Corbet's child of Huntingdon (a girl), by the unskilful cutting of her navel string, her navel gaped and would not come together, seemed an omphacele, and so continued for three years at least. The mother found a receipt in an old English physic book which she adventured with success.[18]

Symcotts then repeated the 'receipt'. In the second case,

> 1651. Mery Herby his son of Thurleigh had a gaping navel for a year and more. Mistress Child (the musician's wife) applied to it parsley (and (she) (Mistress Herby) thinks some knotgrass and plantain withal) stamped and made into a plaster with butter and so applied it. The child voided great store of urine and thereupon the navel closed perfectly.[19]

None the less, the majority of Symcotts's patients suffered from problems which were, by definition, medical. The list of their ailments includes gout, cachexy (defined by the *Oxford English Dictionary* as 'a depraved condition of the body in which nutrition is everywhere defective'), asthma, worms, ague, fits (including fits of the Mother), jaundice, palsy, apoplexy, mania, constipation, looseness (or diarrhoea) and a variety of aches and pains. Symcotts also saw a single case of bubonic plague.[20] One wonders if he would have attended this patient had he and the other healers consulted known beforehand what they were dealing with.

Often, neither the patient nor Symcotts appear to have put a single name to the disorder from which the patient suffered. Rather, Symcotts listed symptoms in his casenotes as his patients described them. The following report is typical.

> Mistress Christian Tenum of Cambridge, fifty years of age, could sleep so little that for fifteen years she had scarcely two and only rarely three hours sleep each night. For twenty years she had a pulsing of the arteries and when she first lay down to rest many images of things passed before her eyes. Ringing in the ears. She

> felt as if a heavy burden or weight was continually pressing down upon the top of her head. She had a feeling of intense heat at the back of the head. She was usually delirius once a day. Pain in the left abdomen. In colic a concentration of wind. Weakness of the back. During her menses (which had stopped five years earlier) her face had swollen, and it was followed by several stools. Three years ago she was stricken with paralysis and from this she still has a numbness of the head.

This patient consulted several other healers before seeing Symcotts. He prescribed a regimen of diet drinks, a vomit, purges and diuretics. About a year after he began treating her, Mistress Tenum 'made much bloody water and voided many stones which she dreamt not of before, and so was cured'.[21] In this case, although Symcotts prescribed diuretics, he obviously did so as a matter of routine. It is notable that both Symcotts and his patient appear to have been surprised when she passed stones with her urine.

In other cases both Symcotts and his patient determined that a collection of symptoms belonged to a single condition. For example, under the heading 'De Asthmate 1637' he wrote:

> Goodwife Usher of Dunton was extreme short winded, oft times wheezed, was much fallen away and in a consumptive state of body, insomuch that her mother and others feared she could not hold out one month at most, being in likelihood to be choked of a sudden for want of breath.[22]

Of course, like all healers, Symcotts found that he was occasionally wrong about a diagnosis. In one case a young girl exhibited the following symptoms:

> There seemed a great compression of a sudden of the midriff and spirital parts which made her cry lamentably and struggle with hands and feet for breath and pain. At last, fetching a large breath, she came to herself again; then she fell into another, and so into a third and fourth or more; then, upon a little rest, she would be as well as ever, eat heartily and walk strongly.

Although he noted that 'It of all diseases most resembled the Mother' (that is fits or suffocation of the Mother or womb), he 'conceived it to be from worms'. He treated the girl with remedies specific for worms, but she grew no better. Then, 'upon application of black soap (taught by Sir Rowland St. John's lady as the best remedy for fits of the mother) to the soles of her feet, the fits went off'.[23]

Like Binns, Symcotts's therapeutic techniques were based upon humoral theory. To restore the body's humoral balance, he purged, sweat and vomited his patients. He also frequently ordered bleeding, clysters and issues – procedures often requiring consultation with a surgeon. Sometimes the courses of treatment he ordered were quite radical, as we shall see. However, they were never irresponsible. Symcotts believed firmly in the 'means' he used. In one case of sore eyes he wrote, 'Nothing prevailed till an issue was made in both arms, by which means she stands perfectly cured'.[24] In another case a patient died because he unwisely had an issue healed.

> Sir Thomas Nevill of Holt, having had an issue in his leg which ran much, he would need have it healed by a surgeon about Michaelmass 1635. About Christmas following he found his stomach ill and all parts out of order. He had a vomit and purgatives but nothing availed. After, he fell into asthmatical fits, and was hectical, grew weaker, his urine utterly confused, and so continued for 11 or 12 days. . . . At last after a great draught of ale (upon which he was at first refreshed) he fell into a great quivering and within seven hours after died. The only cure had been the opening his issue in time.[25]

Symcotts routinely ordered his patients to be bled. However, he did not resort to this treatment 'in almost every case of disease or injury', despite Poynter and Bishop's observation.[26] Like Binns, he used blood-letting sparingly, ordering it in only twenty-two out of eighty-three cases. Sometimes he apparently considered phlebotomy a last resort. In the case of Larance Gunnill, who suffered from a painful skin eruption, he prescribed several inward and outward preparations from which the patient 'presently' found ease. Symcotts noted, 'If not I had opened a vein'.[27]

Regardless of his caution, however, Symcotts let blood plentifully when he felt it was necessary. When Mr Egerton, youngest son of Lord Bridgwater, lay unconscious 'in an apoplexy' in 1648, Symcotts first 'cupped his shoulders and head without scarification'. Later the patient was 'cupped again and scarified on the shoulders and crown, where, by deep scarification, a vein bled as it had been from the arm'. At the same time, 'leeches were set to the fundament'. All in vain, for the patient died shortly afterwards. Even in this case, the physician was cautious. He commented, 'I omitted opening of a vein in his arm, lest it might have been blamed as the cause of his death, and so also the bleeding of the jugulars, for want of skill in the surgeon'.[28]

Symcotts's papers, like Binns's casebook, make clear that the conventional treatments of the time were powerful. Even good treatments must be properly applied. Symcotts warned against 'too much confidence in issues alone without due purgatives'.[29] He noted that

> Colonel Herby of Thurleigh, trusting to his issue in his arm (made at London) neglected the taking such usual course of physic (as his rheumatic and nephritic case required) this last fall of the leaf, and thereby a tumour arose under his armhole, induced much pain, but brake within 9 or 10 days after poulticing.[30]

In another case, Symcotts had prescribed a seton as part of his treatment for severe pain in the lower back.

> At last, wearied with her complaints, I caused a large seton to be made in the ham of the same leg, with a skein of silk (drawn through by the eye of the great long needle that was red hot at the little end), wetted in oil of elder to fetch out the fire. This in a fortnight's space gave her admirable ease; her sleep and appetite returned. By unskilfulness she lost the seton, and thereof made a fontanella by putting in a piece which was not of that efficacy that the former was, and so about a quarter of a year after died.[31]

Even properly applied treatments sometimes proved too powerful. Two of Symcotts's patients died after taking the vomits he had prescribed.[32] In such cases, where the patient was very weak, the physician took a calculated risk in prescribing the remedies he felt were necessary.

Symcotts preferred herbal remedies above all others. In only one recorded case did he use mercury.[33] He used herbal preparations internally, usually as purgatives, diuretics and emetics. He also applied them outwardly on poultices, plasters and in baths.

He obtained recipes from many sources. Thanks to Poynter and Bishop's careful reading of the Symcotts papers housed in the Wellcome Library (not included in their edition of Symcotts's records), some information is available about the physician's reading. As one might expect, he made no reference to popular medical and surgical works, but he did consult

> recognised medical authorities of the time. Among them are Riviere, Joel, Croll, Guillemeau, Garencieres, and Forest. The first three were prominent spagyric or chemical physicians, followers of Paracelsus (1493–1541).

Thus, Symcotts's reading was in advance of his practices.[34]

Symcotts also obtained medical recipes and advice from English physicians, although these were imparted, not from published writings, but by correspondence and word of mouth. Several letters from other physicians to Symcotts are printed in Poynter and Bishop's edition. In one, apparently written by a William Vylan, Symcotts received information about bubonic plague. Symcotts had asked four questions: first, whether a patient with plague should be purged regardless of his or her general physical condition; second, 'whether a pestilent botch [bubo] can wholly go back without any mark or hardness left in for guide'; third, 'that a man dying of the plague having no botch or rising appear, is he not apt to have spots appear, being rubbed, laid by the fire, etc.'; and fourth, 'that if a man die of the plague and lie two days and two nights, whether that body will retain the natural stiffness as others of common diseases'.[35] This letter is particularly interesting, for it reveals Symcotts's belief or suspicion that plague was a disease different from all others – a feeling he shared with his contemporaries, both healers and lay-people.

Again like his contemporaries, Symcotts collected medical recipes from non-medical sources. While most of his informants were relatives and friends, he was receptive to almost any account of a cure. For instance, he noted the following treatment:

> My Lady Cotton, being about 13 or 14 years old, had so great a bleeding at nose that nothing would stay it. She being brought into a desperate condition, Sir John and her mother having gone from her that they might not see her die, the cook-maid boldly took a cloth wet in cold water (vinegar it may be had been better) and made her sit upon it, and so her bleeding was stayed.[36]

A similar report concerned

> Goodwife Viccar of Sutton, being stricken with a palsy all one side, after the taking of a purge or two and some other small remedies, a woman gave her counsel to lie close covered with two large sheep-skins new taken off for 24 hours together. She endured 17 hours of her task, sweating exceedingly all that time, and so was recovered.[37]

Symcotts cited such examples, not as curiosities, but in a respectful uncritical manner.

He frequently noted recipes given to him by gentlewomen.

Thus, he recorded directions for the making of a 'spleen plaster' given him by Lady Pickering and 'Mrs. Rolt of Pertenhall's Medicine for the Ague'.[38] Indeed, he apparently respected such amateur female healers as colleagues, noting in one case that an ointment had 'been proved singular good by the Lady Frances Somerset for fourteen several infirmities'.[39] Sometimes he shared his patients with such ladies. For instance, when Goodwife Finsam of Eyworth three weeks after childbirth developed 'great swellings in her hands, feet and other parts about her', complicated by a feeling of numbness in those parts, 'Mistress Anderson gave her first diascordium, then bezoar'. Only when a swelling in one of her breasts 'brought her to extremity of pain night and day' was Symcotts called. He was not in the least critical of Mrs Anderson's treatment. Indeed, the first poultice he himself recommended did no good. However, the second poultice he prescribed caused the apostemation to break, 'and all her pains ceased'.[40] The physician apparently felt quite comfortable with this informal system of referral, as is demonstrated in the case cited above where a midwife summoned him when she was unable to hasten the delivery of a dead baby.

In some cases medically knowledgeable gentlewomen were also Symcotts's patients. His correspondence with Mrs Anna Carr provides a good example of the mutual respect such a relationship could generate. Mrs Carr wrote to the physician, thanking him for his 'choice receipts which I highly esteem of'. She went on to send Symcotts her recipe for a poultice for a bruise, writing about it,

> If it were for my life I would not use anything else, for with this only I have cured those that carts have gone over, whose water was been gore blood; one that a loaded cart pressed in that sort that blood issued out at all passable places; an old man that was by a bull tossed up, and by the fall lighting on his head and back, and both made and spat blood.

She also sent Symcotts a calcined toad which he had requested, asking him 'what powder of toads calcined is good for. I only use it to staunch blood, but then I do not calcine them'. In addition, she sent word to Mr Fullwood that she had received three dozen vial glasses and two dozen pots which she had requested. Symcotts apparently wrote to her, saying that calcined toad stopped bleeding 'by holding it in the party's hand, so smelling to it; or else hanging it against the pit of the stomach'.[41] More will be said below about Symcotts's relationships with both patients and other healers.

As the above examples make clear, Symcotts used some medicinal substances which fell outside the categories of herbal or chemical remedies. One can only guess at the mechanism by which calcined toad stopped bleeding. The same can be said about the bullet he directed to be swallowed as part of his treatment for fits of vomiting.[42] More familiar, but equally mysterious, was his application of 'pigeons sprinkled with salt' to the feet of a man who was dying of apoplexy.[43] Obviously, although Symcotts had no respect for unlearned healers, he approved of some techniques borrowed from traditional medicine. Indeed, this physician demonstrates why rigid demarcations between academic, popular and magical healing techniques are anachronistic in a discussion of seventeenth-century English medicine.

Symcotts also used diagnostic techniques which were becoming old fashioned even in his own day. The Royal College of Physicians disapproved of uroscopy and many of its members frowned upon astrological medicine.[44] Symcotts used both, although he was sceptical about astrology. For instance, he wrote to his patient Mr Powers, who dabbled in that science,

> I am sorry for your bearing an unnecessary pain by forbearing the use of the plaster, which might have been safely laid on today, notwithstanding your skill in the passage of the sign, which (for anything I know) is nowhere else to be found, but only in the Almanack. The ancient co[nceit] of it is but a fancy, and the ominous events thereof either lies or false positions.[45]

Although he sounds sceptical, warranting Poynter and Bishop's observation that the physician 'scorns such beliefs', he either belied his scepticism or humoured the patient when, in later correspondence, he wrote that 'this season is not propitious to eradicate physic'.[46] Symcotts also examined urine. A patient, John Williams, sent the physician a urine sample, together with a description of his symptoms. Symcotts himself wrote that he was concerned about a patient who subsequently died because the patient's 'water was thick and yellow which intimated the great oppression of the stomach and heat of the liver which had made so much choler'.[47]

None the less, neither of these techniques are mentioned frequently in Symcotts's notes. More important were the patient's appearance and description of his or her sensations.

Also significant was Symcotts's own knowledge of the patient's medical history. For instance, he prescribed for a lady who was not his patient, excusing his breach of occupational ethics in the following way:

> without any derogation from that knowing man, your present physician . . . , but for my long experience I have had of your constitution from your childhood.[48]

Symcotts's methods were rewarded. Of the cases for which the outcome is known, thirty-five patients recovered, seven improved and only thirteen died.

Symcotts's relations with other physicians were, on balance, harmonious. Certainly he was much respected by his assistant or partner, Gervase Fullwood the elder. As Poynter and Bishop say, nothing is known about Fullwood's qualifications. 'That he was named with Symcotts on commissions between 1647 and 1660 indicates that he was of good family and position.'[49] Fullwood deferred to Symcotts's judgment in the correspondence the two healers carried on with Mr Powers, which will be discussed below. His letters to that difficult patient frequently state that the prescriptions sent were directed by 'the doctor'.[50] The impression given by this correspondence is that Symcotts was the senior member in the practice.

Symcotts was sometimes critical of other physicians. Edward Adye, who received a Cambridge MA in 1628 and was an extralicentiate of the Royal College of Physicians, was Symcotts's contemporary and competitor. The two physicians shared at least two patients.[51] Symcotts disapproved of Adye's therapeutic and diagnostic techniques. Concerning Adye's views on smallpox, he wrote 'Therefore in these cases [of the disease in strong adults] in which Mr. Adye by urine gives a warrant of security, he may be deceived'.[52] Symcotts was more outspoken in a letter to Mr Powers dated 19 February 1641.

> For Adye's conceit of bleeding at the beginning, you have it commonly in any case, sex or age whatever [unless] these do contraindicate. That noddy little thinks what an adventure it is to take blood from an old withered man, whose fountains of blood-making may be justly suspected of weakness and some unsoundness.[53]

More frequently Symcotts mentioned the successes of other

healers and adopted their methods. Thus, when Mr Taylor of Clapham was cured of haemorrhoids by a surgeon who advised him to take tobacco, Symcotts 'upon this example' prescribed the same treatment for Mr Boner of Hail Weston.[54] He also approved a course of treatment prescribed by Mayerne.[55]

As indicated above, Symcotts consulted with his colleagues by mail. This correspondence reveals that he gave advice in addition to soliciting it. In a letter addressed to a Mr Templer from Lawrence Wright (1590–1657), physician in ordinary to Oliver Cromwell during the 1650s, it is clear that Wright's interpretation of a particular case is partially based upon information given him by Symcotts and Dr George Bowles, another provincial physician.[56]

Symcotts was a self-consciously respectable physician who recognised the importance of having a good reputation. In one case he actively defended his own by mail. He wrote to a Dr Francis of London in order to give his version of the death of one of his patients, Mr Elms.[57] It is, perhaps, significant that this case was also known to Mr Powers.[58] Mr Elms died after having taken a vomit prescribed by Symcotts. The physician's defence of his methods says much about his feelings about his medical colleagues, his concern about his reputation in the lay community and his contempt for unlearned healers. Thus, his letter to Francis will be quoted at some length.

> D. Francis. Your verdict of Mr. Elms his death, I believe much wrested from your own meaning, is still kept up by two empirics (they who lived on each hand of Lilford) to render me odious to that side of the country and raise their own credits by blasting mine. For them, as the testimony of my conscience bears me above their malice, so do I contemn to give accounts unto them (for their sakes) or make an apology for myself. My desire is to satisfy you or be satisfied by you.
>
> They report you to say Mr. Elms had not a pleurisy, that the cupping glasses were improper for drawing humours to the place affected, that bleeding did more hurt than good.
>
> In my description of the cause, symptoms, and remedies applied, which was sent up to London, I set down . . . with all fidelity what was applied and in what order. The second day after he was clearly sick, I gave a vomit which, though it wrought fully, yet the night following he slept soundly and awakened comfortably, and sent me word he was very well, but thirsty and desired beer, whereof (drinking plentifully) taking a great draught and cold, contrary to my directions, within two hours after he felt a sharp pain at his left breast which, increasing quickly to an

> insufferable height, I first laboured to mitigate with useful fomentation.

Symcotts then applied cupping glasses to the patient's chest – a treatment he continued to feel was warranted. Later, to ease the pain, he applied hot bread with mithridate. Notwithstanding these measures, the patient died.

Symcotts felt that Mr Elms was partly to blame for his own death. Unbeknownst to the physician, Elms had been 'tampering' with mercury sublimate six weeks before his final illness, which had caused inflammation of his mouth. When he became ill, he spent an entire day 'setting his house in order, disquieting himself all the day long . . . and infinitely weakening his spirits thereby'. Another contributing factor was Elms's general condition. Symcotts wrote that

> a strong disease fell upon weak principles. He had a dry cough for three months before; his flesh was wasted almost to skin and bones . . . his eyes sunk, his face more than ordinary swarthy, and the vivid colour of his lips decayed.

Finally Symcotts maintained that another practitioner had interrupted his own course of treatment, to Elms's disadvantage:

> I might justly allege Mr. Resburrow with his apothecaries constant interrupting for near three days together (in my absence) the course I had prescribed, though upon those remedies they saw his pains abated.

Such an interruption was clearly in violation of Symcotts's understanding of proper medical ethics.

Although the physician's feelings about his licensed colleagues varied depending upon the circumstances, his disapproval of unlearned healers never altered. He wrote of one such practitioner who had been treating Powers, 'For your doctor his advice, I like it not; such roweling, drawing and slabbering smells too much of his barber's shop from whence he went out Dr.'.[59] In a later letter he wrote

> I hear your Dr. there is much offended with me for inveighing against him. I pray stop the rumour. I assure you I have been ever silent in the censure of wandering practitioners, and so of him, but for a few words I inserted into a letter to you. I suffer such to weary out themselves. I think him worthy of contempt, not of

> opposition, which would make the world think there were something good in him that might disadvantage me. Let him therefore not think of me, as I do not of him, being neither sorry for his stay nor glad for his removal.[60]

Symcotts's contempt for his unlearned competitors echoes that expressed by the anti-quack writers.[61] He also singled out unlearned barbers, empirics and wandering practitioners as particularly harmful. However, his ire, like that of the anti-quack writers, rarely extended to amateurs who dabbled in medicine. For instance, one of the physician's patients, Mistress Cosens of Croxton, 'being seven months with child, had a severe haemorrhage for two days together'. Symcotts 'ordered that her legs should be rubbed and bound . . . that a cupping glass should be placed on the region of the liver and a plaster of vinegar and true bole on her forehead'. He also prescribed a 'julep . . . of plantain water, oil of vitriol and syrup of violets'. These measures helped, but did not totally check the patient's blood loss. Then, 'a beggar woman told the patient that she would recover if she took shepherd's purse in her broth'. Symcotts ordered a broth with this herb in it, and the patient was cured.[62] Indeed, the remedy worked so well that he prescribed it for a girl with excessive menstrual flow shortly afterwards.[63] Perhaps Symcotts, like the anti-quack writers, only felt threatened by other healers if they charged for their services.

The basis of any healer's success or failure is his or her clientele – how large it is, the prices it can afford, and its opinion of the healer's services. Because we become acquainted with relatively few of Symcotts's patients (surely only a fraction of those he actually treated) we know rather less about his clientele as a whole than we know about that of Binns. The physician treated forty-seven female and thirty-three male patients. The sex of three patients is unknown. There is no obvious explanation for the slight predominance of females in his practice as there is for the predominance of males in that of Binns. Like Binns, Symcotts treated people in every social class except royalty. Of the eighty-three patients whose cases were recorded, twenty-seven were upper status, forty-one of middling status and thirteen of lower status origins. Again, as in our analysis of Binns's clientele, these figures can be only approximate. Categories for each patient were determined either on the basis of information provided by Poynter and Bishop or according to Symcotts's own mode of address. As a general rule, a title such as 'Lord' or 'Sir' suggested upper status, 'Mistress' or 'Mister', middling status, and 'Goodwife', 'Goodman' or a name without any prefix, lower status.

Comparison with Binns's clientele reveals that, while the great majority of his patients were middling status or below, the majority of Symcotts's patients were middling status or above.[64] Such an observation provokes a number of questions. Is it possible that relatively few lower status people consulted Symcotts because his services were too expensive? This seems unlikely. For instance, Symcotts's patient Mr Powers paid only £1.2*s*.8*d*. for two months of treatment in 1641. Even considering the effects of inflation, the £29.9*s*. one of Binns's patients paid for a year's treatment in 1658 suggests that urban surgeons could command fees as high as, or higher than, those charged by provincial physicians.[65] While one could, with little probable profit, debate the relative spending power of poor people in rural and urban settings, perhaps another line of inquiry would be more appropriate.

In Chapter 2 the different statuses of physicians and surgeons were discussed. These differences were perceived by both healers and their patients. Despite the fact that the status of physicians was not as high as they could have wished, they were well educated and certainly at home with 'high culture'.[66] The skill physicians sold in the medical marketplace was authority based upon familiarity with the theories encapsulated in medical writings, both published and unpublished. Surgeons, on the other hand, were more akin to expert craftsmen. No one else could provide their service as well as they did, but they used their hands rather than their mouths.

Physicians' patients could receive not only a prescription, but also a humoral explanation of their ailments. Physicians gave these explanations with the same seriousness and conviction ministers of the time gave to sermons on sin. Perhaps this very seriousness and the verbal aspect of their occupation made physicians easy to mock.[67] In any case, one suspects that patients must have had to be of a certain social and educational level fully to avail themselves of the physician's services. For instance, Symcotts wrote to Mr Powers:

> Your high coloured urine is an apparent sign of inflammation of blood and multitude of choleric humours, which (nature not rightly disburthened of by the common ways) are carried upwards, fixed in the bordering parts of the brain, cause that pain, noise and impostumous matter which you complain of.[68]

Mr Powers suffered from headache and sore eyes.

Those who most appreciated the physician's academic attainments were people of backgrounds similar to, and more elevated than, the physician's own. While the anti-quack writers accused unlearned healers of talking pretentious gobbledegook in order to impress ignorant patients, better educated people would have known the difference. In consulting physicians, they hoped for a cure, but expected knowledge. Thus, Symcotts's patients reflected elevated social statuses disproportionate to their presence in the population at large.[69]

As indicated above, Symcotts's patients were drawn from a wide area. The map of patients' residences shown below, drawn from the casenotes, demonstrates that virtually all of Symcotts's clients lived within a twenty-mile radius of Huntingdon, with the exception of the patients who came from London. Although the physician and his assistants did travel to visit clients, much of the practice's business was

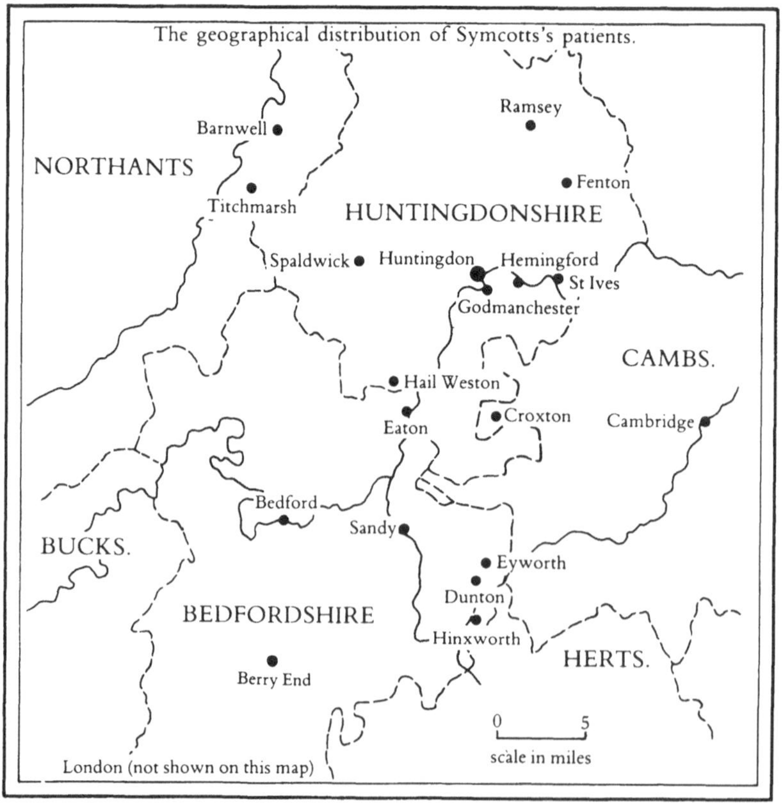

The geographical distribution of Symcotts's patients.

conducted by correspondence, regardless of how far from Huntingdon the patient lived.

The correspondence printed in Poynter and Bishop's edition of Symcotts's papers provides an excellent opportunity for us to explore the physician's relationships with his patients. The Powers correspondence is particularly useful, spanning as it does nearly ten years of treatment. There can be no doubt that Symcotts got on well with his patients. Their trust in him is reflected in the fact that although Mr Elms died during the summer of 1641, his wife consulted the physician when her young daughter was suffering from fits in September 1642. Obviously Mrs Elms did not believe that the vomit Symcotts had prescribed had killed her husband.[70]

None the less, the correspondence makes clear that Symcotts's patients were demanding and by no means uncritical of the treatment they were given. They also had sufficient confidence in their own medical judgment to suggest possible treatments to the physician. Thus, John Cotton wrote,

> Mr. Doctor,
>
> It being now three weeks since my wife was delivered I think it now convenient for her to use some abstersive physic, for though she finds herself very well, yet I think after such a time it will not be amiss to use evacuation. Pray consider what you think may be most proper for her, and, if you think it convenient, we shall be very glad to see you here.[71]

Cotton's tone is similar to that taken by John Evelyn in his relations with physicians.[72] Both gentlemen consulted with physicians on more or less equal terms. Less arrogant, but perhaps even better informed is the letter quoted above from Anna Carr. Indeed, she made no mention at all of any illness for which Symcotts was treating her. Her letter reads less like that of a patient consulting an expert physician, and more like a note from one colleague to another.[73]

The physician's letters to his patients reveal both his respect for their knowledge about medicine and their own bodies and his concern that they accept his judgment. Thus, he explained the reasons for the therapy he advised in addition to sending prescriptions and directions for their application. To Mistress Halford he wrote a long epistle which, although it does not tell the modern reader what specific symptoms the patient suffered from, it does illuminate Symcotts's diagnostic methods and his determination that Mistress Halford understand the rationale behind her treatment. He proposed to heal her:

> first, by a gentle purgative way to abate such serous and waterish humours which must necessarily abound in the first region by your sedentary life and are the antecedent matter of those which (abounding in the (liver) veins and other inward parts and likewise in the whole habit of the body) have now by long custom found an irregular vent for themselves. . . .
>
> In the second place, I should prescribe bleeding (necessary indeed to the cure, if the opinion of impropriety of the season did not reclaim) in regard of the hotter temper of your liver, the fountain of redounding choler which, insinuating into the veins, sharpens the blood and humours thereof and causeth by turns that inflammatory humour of your eyelids, moradicty of urine, and those small eruptions on your nails and suchlike . . . symptoms, all which are dulled if not quite removed by this remedy. . . .
>
> After this, I shall proceed to things rather of a drying than astringent nature, as the disease requires. . . .
>
> Last of all, for the absolution of the cure, much and great exercise by degrees is requisite. . . .[74]

The casenotes indicate that Symcotts at one point treated this patient for 'fits of vomiting, great pains in her stomach and the whole abdomen, which sometimes together, sometimes successively, followed the pains of her back; which being all most incessant, soon wasted both her flesh and spirits'.[75] It is not clear whether the above letter concerned this illness.

As his letter to Mistress Halford indicates, Symcotts, in true humoral fashion, treated whole patients, not merely diseases. He took into account the sufferer's age, mental state, body type and general physical condition, in addition to the specific complaints the patient made. Nowhere are these concerns more obvious than in the Powers correspondence.

Mr Richard Powers kept a shop in Ramsey, which was about ten miles from Huntingdon. He is referred to as 'an old and withered body', who was about 60 years old in 1633, when the surviving correspondence began. He suffered from a multitude of disagreeable symptoms, chief among them gout. Symcotts and Fullwood were not the only healers he consulted. As indicated above, he was treated by Dr Adye and a wandering practitioner to whom Symcotts took exception. In addition, he talked to friends about his ailments. In an early letter the physician defended his own prescriptions against 'whatever your neighbours talk against physic'.[76] In another letter he wrote, 'Your friends that tell you this will not cure you full little know what your case had been by this time if you had not taken this course you have done'.[77] Regardless of Symcotts's impatience with the ignorant medical advice Powers received, however, he did not wholly dismiss it. In one letter he wrote, 'The counsel of your two friends I approve of, to be careful of that pain in your neck'.[78]

Repeatedly the physician reassured Powers that the course of treatment he advised was the best possible. In answer to Powers's worries that the therapy he received was too violent, considering his age and weakness, Symcotts wrote,

> Considering the symptoms laid down before my eyes I found some proper to the scurvy, others peculiar to the old gouty humour which whirls about and if you look not to it may fall upon some inward part as the stomach, guts, sides, etc., or unto your foot, as very lately upon my old father (before that as healthful a man as lived) and that so suddenly that in three days it corrupted so his foot to the bone that daily flesh deaded and putrified parts of bones were taken out. I spared not his age, 77, but advised bleeding and purging above 40 times in less than seven weeks space, or he had been in his grave.[79]

On a later occasion, Powers had been told by an acquaintance that his illness would kill him. Symcotts wrote,

> The Londoner spake like a pothecary, or himself, to determine such an event. I have seen it oft cured in as old as you, especially in two but last year; the one was old goodman Church of our town, the other Mr. Chessam of Brampton, who was all over like a dried leather skin, his legs as black as the stock and as sore and lame as a cripple. It was within the compass of my skill and God his blessing to help these.[80]

Despite the physician's long-suffering patience with Powers's complaints and doubts, he occasionally showed annoyance. When in 1633 Powers had been reading a popular medical work by Sir William Vaughan, *Natural and Artificial Directions for Health* (1600), he wrote to Symcotts, citing Vaughan in his criticism of the treatment he was receiving. Symcotts replied,

> The crick of your neck, the pain of your toe, the swelling of your knees and the trembling of your joints which you call the palsy are all from one and the same cause.

He went on to explain the humoral origins of these symptoms for which, 'I have . . . prescribed you a regular course which, if you follow, I make no question but your author Vaughan his prognostic vain and frivolous'.[81]

Regardless of Powers's incessant queries and criticisms of Symcotts, he grew very dependent upon his physician. Indeed, he consulted Symcotts about each detail of his personal life, becoming unable to make the smallest decisions without worrying about their possible medical consequences. In the autumn of 1642 Symcotts advised him

> to keep your chamber . . . and there to maintain a constant warm air day and night. . . . For the [question?] of keeping your chamber whether all or part of the winter I cannot determine. That will be longer or shorter as you get strength and the disease weakens.

Powers must have asked if it was safe for him to go to church, for the physician wrote, 'You need not take care for going to church. God in this case will have mercy and not sacrifice'.[82]

Powers obviously preferred Symcotts to Fullwood. In one instance he complained bitterly about a remedy Fullwood had prescribed: 'This physic put me to intolerable pain and gripings in my breast, back, stomach and sides'. He suffered with this medicine for three days.

> Then the doctor [Symcotts] must amend Fullwood's stuff and he sent me three pills which I took in hope the pills would take away the [evil?] of Fullwood's physic, and so I hope it did for it wrought very well and gently; but for Fullwood I had neither ease nor sleep . . . in three days and three nights, but lay in miserable torments.[83]

A likely reason for Powers's dislike of Fullwood was Fullwood's obvious impatience with Powers. Fullwood apparently handled the financial business of the practice. Characteristically Powers quibbled over paying in full several of the bills he was sent. In June 1639 Fullwood wrote indignantly,

> Mr. Powers,
> I thank you I have received the 13*s*.3*d*. by Mr. Peacock and have given him acquittance in full. But I much wonder you should yet so much question the dueness of the 4*s*.8*d*.. I thought I had satisfied you about it when you was to Huntingdon and we spoke about it last; but for the most part of it you deceive yourself in this present letter, for that drink which you say Mistress Willis brought you was certainly made with the plantain water and juice

> of barberries and mirabilons etc., by your description of it to me. That you took it was not my fault, nor is it good reason why I should bear the loss. Directions for the use of them was also sent with them, howsoever it miscarried. For the glass, you say right: it's most like we had charged it, for we could not send the water without a glass. For the lenitive electuary and ointment, I know not what became of them afterwards, but I am sure your messenger had them all from me; and all were sent, not by my freeness or forwardness, but by direction from Dr. Symcotts for you, as he himself can yet remember, and will tell you if you will believe him.[84]

Neither Fullwood nor Edward Johnson, Fullwood's 'man', had much sympathy for the cantankerous old man. Compare with Symcotts's tone of patient reassurance Johnson's remark, 'You need not wonder that your cure is no further on foot, you may rather wonder that you was not in your grave long before this'.[85] Indeed, it is quite possible that Fullwood and Johnson actually had more contact with Powers than did the physician. Many of the 'physic directions' for Powers's use came from Fullwood, and he and Johnson had the unpleasant duty of collecting Powers's fees. It might follow that Powers actually blamed Fullwood and Johnson for the medical bills he paid. Certainly Powers resented these bills. On a wrapper he used to enclose his papers was written, 'Dr. Symcotts' letters, physic [directions] and apothecaries' bills; from which God deliver us'.[86]

The financial dealings between Powers and Symcotts's practice leave no doubt that the administration of physic was charged for in a way similar to that of surgery. The major difference between the bills of Binns and Symcotts was that Binns named a specific fee for his own labour and that of his man. It may be that this was one way physicians sought to demonstrate their claims to professional status. By charging only for medications, physicians could demonstrate their disdain for the 'trade' connotations of charging for services rendered. One can only speculate about whether prices for remedies were padded in order to include an unspecified fee for expert advice. In their introduction Poynter and Bishop mention that 'there is a record of a purge being rewarded with £65' – a princely sum in the seventeenth century.[87] While Symcotts never charged such enormous prices, he managed to prosper on the basis of the fees he received, which suggests that there was a healthy profit margin attached to the remedies he prescribed. It is also likely that patients offered him payments after consultations which were not noted in the practice's records.

How typical was Symcotts of seventeenth-century provincial physicians? For purposes of comparison, we will take a brief look at two other 'physical' casebooks from the period.

II TWO PROVINCIAL HEALERS

Little is known about Dr Barker of Shrewsbury. The local record office has no specific record of him, but suggests that he might have come from London. As indicated above, his casenotes are drawn from the period 1595 to 1605. Thus, his is the earliest healer's practice examined for the purposes of this study.[88] There can be little doubt that Barker was, indeed, a physician, although his qualifications are unknown. Many of his case-descriptions and most of his prescriptions were written in Latin. Like Symcotts and Binns, his orientation towards diagnosis and therapy was humoral.

Barker's casebook refers to some 145 patients, of whom 70 were men and 75 women. Less can be inferred about the social status of his patients than is the case with the practices of Binns and Symcotts. This is true for several reasons. Barker's is a difficult hand to read. Thus, the deciphering of names and titles is more difficult for his casebook than for the others considered. We are also without the sort of background information provided by Poynter and Bishop for the Symcotts papers. As far as can be determined, Barker's clientele came largely from middling and lower status backgrounds. Only five of his patients were titled; eighty-three were designated Mr or Mrs; fifty were called Goodwife or Goodman, or simply named with no prefix.

Like Symcotts, Barker was a general practitioner, treating a large variety of ailments. Some disorders were named, as was the case with vertigo, arthritis, ague, dropsy, green sickness, epilepsy, apoplexy, melancholy, lues venerea, asthma and gout. However, as with Symcotts, Barker usually began his notes by giving a list of the patient's symptoms. Thus, Mr Bownes had a cold brain, pain in the left side of his head and neck, a disturbance in the bottom of his stomach and a feeling as if cold water were in the region of his left 'stone'. He spat much phlegm, and had weak joints and 'windiness' of the stomach.[89]

Like Symcotts, Barker dealt with a number of problems which might have been treated by a surgeon or midwife. He was consulted for the stone, bruising, purulent bloody flux from the uterus, menstrual problems, pimples, itching, syphilis, ulcers, fistulae and complications of childbirth. Indeed, 29 out of 145 cases might properly be considered 'non-medical'. Barker treated such ailments by using internal remedies to purge the patient. He also applied medication to the skin in the form of ointments. However, he did not use surgical instruments. Thus, he treated a fistula by ordering the patient to be bled, and treated an apostem by purging, then rubbing, washing and anointing the affected place.[90] One suspects that Binns would have had little time for such methods.

Unlike Symcotts, Barker treated several patients for emotional illnesses. In the seventeenth century no rigid demarcation was made between physical and mental ailments. Thus, patients with emotional problems were usually treated for physical symptoms as well. For instance, Mr Aron the younger was given a purge for wind in the genital region, 'nocturnal pollutions' and impotence.[91] Mr Clyve was also purged. He was

> Very melancholic delighting in solitariness. He thinketh that he speaketh foolishly and vain. And imagineth that he is weak and that his legs and body is worn away. When he is worst he is gotten to be most heaving and lumbering. . . . He eateth and sleepeth well. His skin is rough and is dry, stiff and cleaveth to his flesh.[92]

Barker treated nine patients for melancholy. He also dealt with one phantom pregnancy and one case of 'disturbance of reason often speaking vain things and idle' associated with 'convulsive pains within her body, left arm and that side of her head and neck'.[93] In the latter case the physician obviously suspected true lunacy, for he noted the moon signs throughout the long description of this patient's case.

Indeed, it should be noted that Barker was more serious about astrology than any of the other healers whose casebooks have been consulted for the purposes of this study. His notes are dotted with astrological signs which aided him in both diagnosis and treatment.[94] Barker also routinely examined his patient's urine.[95] This is not surprising, considering that the Royal College of Physicians did not officially disapprove of this practice until 1601 and, as we have seen, many respectable physicians employed uroscopy well after it became controversial.[96]

Unlike the other healers whose casebooks are consulted,

Barker was interested in the prophylaxis of plague. He visited one Mathew Warrow in Turk's Hill on 20 August 1603. There he prescribed preventative treatment for Mathew which consisted of purging, sweating and weekly 'pestilent pills'. He also prescribed the pills for Mathew's wife. In addition, on the same day he prescribed pestilent pills for Owen Meredith's wife, his servant and three maids.[97] Barker also treated several who had survived plague but suffered from secondary effects. One patient was left with a sore knee.[98] P. Yonge's wife, 'being recovered of the pest and the apostem being not well cleansed and . . . healed, after three months a humour fell into her hips and knees . . . with stiffness . . . and weakness of stomach'.[99] There is no record of the physician treating an active case of plague.

Because Barker treated a number of women who suffered from menstrual disorders and other 'female' problems, this area of his practice is worth some consideration. In keeping with the humoral orientation which considered the body's general condition before determining treatment, an adult female's menstrual history was frequently mentioned by seventeenth-century healers, regardless of the symptoms the patient presented to the healer. For instance, Dr Symcotts treated Lady Howard for symptoms including a dry cough, which had lasted for ten or twelve years, griping in her body, weakness and thinness. In his description of her condition he noted that her menses had been suppressed for many years.[100] Barker made similar notes. For instance, he treated one woman for headache, fever, backache, pain in the side, melancholy and 'trembling of the heart'. He also mentioned that she had inordinate menses.[101]

However, Barker treated a number of patients whose chief complaint was gynaecological. He dealt with a 'purulent flux from the uterus', retention or suppression of the menses, green sickness, irregular menstruation, inordinate menstruation and 'whites'.[102] In these cases, he invariably prescribed an herbal purge, frequently containing betony.[103] He occasionally ordered other remedies. For instance, for green sickness he anointed the patient's side, purged her, ordered that she sit in a bath for three days, then purged her again.[104] Although several of his gynaecological patients may have been suffering from syphilis, actually named in only two cases, there is no record of Barker prescribing mercury. In only one case did he order guaiacum. For Mrs Berk he prescribed a purge, then a diet drink of guaiacum, sweating every fifth day and a vapour bath. He also ordered cloths moistened in honey and guaiacum water to be applied to Mrs Berk's body.[105]

Little can be inferred from Barker's casenotes about his relationships with his patients. That the Pilstor family, for instance, consulted him on several occasions suggests that he had a loyal clientele.[106] As was the case with other healers, Barker's patients sometimes helped to determine their own treatment. Mrs Coderington received treatment for a mysterious quartan ague which kept returning about the time of her menstrual period. She told the physician that all hot medicines offended her.[107]

Equally little is known about Barker's relations with other healers. One example suggests that he consulted amicably with his colleagues:

> Dr. Turner sayeth that before Mr. Cole fell into . . . [that disorder] he had a troublesome cough through a distillation and I know he had divers . . . fits through tartarous matter and once after a clyster by P. Pena his counsel he avoided many stones.[108]

However, in a case of phantom pregnancy, he implied criticism of the physician Dr Davis, who prescribed 'a strong vomit . . . which made her weak and a fortnight after she fell into a grievous and continual vomiting'.[109]

Considering his casebook as a whole, Dr Barker appears to have been a conventional physician of his time. He used astrology, examined urine and prescribed quantities of herbal remedies. While it is possible that his clientele came from a relatively lower social status than did that of other physicians, it is equally possible that his patients were higher status than this reading of his casenotes suggests.

The third 'physical' casebook which will be examined in this chapter was kept by a healer who probably practised in Cambridge during the years between 1619 and 1622.[110] It is assumed that he was a physician, because of the kinds of cases he undertook and the therapeutic methods he used. However, it is possible that he was an empiric. Some of his prescriptions were unorthodox, as we shall see. His hand, although easy to read, seems relatively uneducated. None the less, his prescriptions were routinely written in Latin, which suggests that this healer had at least a basic medical education. He noted treatment of eighty-two patients: forty-eight male, twenty-seven female and seven whose sex is unknown. Thirteen of his patients were titled, forty-one of middling status and twenty-four of lower status. The social status of four of his patients could not be identified. A large number of his patients resided in Cambridge colleges. This may account for the relatively large number of males in his clientele.

His casebook, like those of the other physicians, is not as detailed as that of Binns. Often, he merely noted the name of the patient and the symptoms complained of. Never did he indicate the outcome of the treatment he applied. Like Symcotts and Barker, he treated numerous 'surgical' cases including bruising, the stone, itching and haemorrhoids.[111] He treated these with internal remedies combined with phlebotomy and clysters. He also dealt with five cases of gonorrhoea in men, for which he sometimes prescribed 'pillulae chimica' (a mercury preparation?) and guaiacum in addition to other remedies.[112] Considering that the total number of his casenotes is relatively small, it is possible that this healer treated gonorrhoea as a minor speciality.

Like Symcotts and Barker, this healer most often described symptoms rather than naming a single disease. Even when a disease was named, the healer was himself cautious about diagnosis, implying that the patient had suggested it. The following casenote is typical:

> The young lady Maynard
> Her liver obstructed. Her stomach clogged with phlegm. Her body waterish. Subject to toothache. Her eyes swollen or puffed up. She hath had fluxum menstruam abundant but now little. But often and waterish. She fears most a consumption, or dropsy.[113]

Occasionally his diagnosis was more definite. Specific diseases named are gonorrhoea, the stone, jaundice, worms, frensy, palsy, dropsy, haemorrhoids, 'The Mother' (that is fits or suffocation of the mother or uterus) and epilepsy.

This healer mentions using neither astrology nor uroscopy. He was fonder than was Barker of phlebotomy and leeches. He rarely prescribed a clyster. He is unique among the healers we have examined for having ordered a course of treatment at a spa. His directions for Mr Samuel Cutler of Ipswich include nine prescriptions of internal remedies, a special diet, liniment to be applied by a barber to the neck, arm and hand, and instructions for the use of 'the Cross Bath'.[114] Presumably Mr Cutler was going to Bath to find relief. The detailed directions he was given included the following warning:

> The weather growing cold use the King's Bath but beware of that

> I told you. As you find good, use it. In any case, never go into the bath but after a stool either naturally or by a suppository.

We are not told Mr Cutler's symptoms.

The area in which this physician most differed from the other healers examined was his marked attraction to remedies and ingredients which were neither herbal nor chemical, but which were either animal or exotic in nature. To Mr Standish, who suffered from the stone, he gave numerous directions including the following:

> To make a powder for yourself, take a young male hare quick. Kill it and save all the blood in a dish. Pull all the hair off the skin. Mix it with the blood. And dry it in an oven. Beat it to fine powder and sear it. Take of this the weight of [illegible] in like order as the former powder.[115]

Goodman Kettle, who suffered from nosebleeds, was told to take 'his own blood, dried between two tiles, beat to fine powder and often blowed into his nose'. He was also directed to 'make a tent of cobweb and fresh hog's dung to put into your nose' – presumably in order to drive the blood away from the evil smell. In addition, to draw the blood inward and downward, Kettle was advised to eat calves' feet, neates' feet and sheep's feet.[116] This healer suggested that

> for preserving your sight, take of woman's milk that bore and nurseth a man child iii spoonfuls: of the urine of the same child iiii spoonfuls, beaten with a new-laid egg with some camphor added. Set to steep all night in a closed glass in a warm oven. Soak little linen cloths in the mixture and apply them to the eyes all night. This to be done three nights running four times a year. Also the eyes are to be washed in the morning with white wine.[117]

In three cases he prescribed the eagle stone for women in labour. This object, a round or egg-shaped stone, hollow in the middle, which rattled when shaken, was attached to the mother's thigh in order to hasten delivery. So powerful was it that midwives were warned not to leave it in place once the child was born for fear that it might cause prolapse of the uterus.[118]

It is obvious that occasionally this healer dabbled in sympathetic magic. Apparently he did not use other magical methods, such as incantations, spells or amulets. However, his techniques would certainly have been frowned upon by the more conventional healers Binns, Symcotts and Barker. These healers also avoided the use of such exotic substances as mummy and unicorn's horn, prescribed by the Cambridge practitioner.[119]

This healer used some methods which reflected classical medical traditions. No case provides a better example of this than his treatment of 'the Mother'. Rather than prescribing the standard purges and vomits, he returned to the classical notion of the wandering womb which must be lured back to its proper place. Thus, he had the 'Gentlewoman, Mr. More's friend' use sweet applications on her genitals and introduce foul smells to the nose: 'Let her smell to partridge feathers burnt: smell to asafoetida'. He also ordered her to sneeze in order to drive the rising womb downwards.[120]

We know little about this practitioner's relationships with other healers. In one case he apparently consulted with two other 'doctors', Goslin and Forthow.[121] However, these are the only colleagues mentioned in his casebook. Equally little is known about his relationships with patients. The Maynard family consulted him on at least three occasions.[122] That his university patients resided in six colleges suggests that his reputation among the scholars there was reasonably good. Neither he nor Barker made any reference to the charging and payment of fees.

III COMPARISON AND CONCLUSIONS

Comparison of the physicians' casebooks examined here reveals a number of similarities. All three practised outside London. Although each healer was based in a relatively populous town, the patients of each were drawn from a large rural area surrounding the town. The physicians were all general practitioners. They all subscribed to humoral theory. They prescribed herbal remedies, in the main, although the Cambridge physician also used animal and exotic ingredients. Their prescriptions were usually written in Latin, though case descriptions were usually in English. Although they used some surface applications in the form of ointments and baths, they largely depended upon internal medicines. Some of these remedies were sent to patients already prepared; occasionally patients were expected to follow the physician's instructions in preparing the remedies themselves. While the physicians prescribed such measures as blood-letting, issues, blisters and clysters, they did not perform these procedures themselves.

Each of the physicians used some relatively old-fashioned techniques. As indicated above, it is not surprising that

Barker, the earliest physician studied, routinely employed uroscopy and astrology. Appropriately Symcotts had less frequent recourse to these methods. Indeed, the correspondence he received suggests that he occasionally examined urine and paid attention to astrological indications at the patient's request.[123] The Cambridge physician used neither uroscopy nor astrology, but dabbled in natural magic. His was the only casebook encountered which reveals strong links with traditional medicine.

These findings confirm the suspicion that the anti-quack writers attempted to create the impression that there was a more definite line of demarcation between reputable physicians and 'quacks' than really existed. A combination of personal interest and patients' demands could make a 'piss prophet' of the respectable Symcotts. Physicians were by no means inflexible in their adherence to academic authorities and the guidelines laid down by the Royal College of Physicians. Again, Symcotts's papers indicate that even a conventional physician was willing to try unconventional methods if such methods seemed likely to produce a cure.

How did the physicians studied differ? The records kept by our nameless Cambridge healer are of the utmost help here, for they permit us to see the tremendous similarity between Barker and Symcotts. Barker and Symcotts were the earlier and later sides of the same conventional coin. Their responses to the symptoms presented were predictable. They took the patient's medical history, then prescribed several herbal preparations designed to produce evacuation. Rarely did they record either the outcome of the treatment prescribed or the necessity of a return visit by the patient.

Barker's use of uroscopy and astrology was relatively insignificant. He was neither a 'piss prophet', depending totally upon signs in urine for prescription and prognosis, nor an astrological physician, relating all diagnosis and treatment to signs found in the sky. The differences between his practices and those of Symcotts reflect the changes in conventional medical treatment in the first half of the seventeenth century.

The Cambridge healer's notes do not conform to the pattern followed by Barker and Symcotts. He was lavish in his prescriptions, apparently ordering remedies in proportion to the patient's wealth. For instance, Sir William Maynard was directed to take some twenty medicines for gonorrhoea. Sir Oly of Clare College received only four prescriptions for the same disorder.[124] Often the remedies he prescribed were unconventional. And the traditional notions which underlie these remedies offered him an alternative to the manipulation of humours produced by conventional techniques. His use of the eagle stone, for instance, provides a direct contrast with Symcotts's use of internal remedies to provoke delivery. It also served as an alternative to consultation of a surgeon with his instruments.

It is tempting to see this healer as a minor medical renegade, operating dangerously near to the territory of unlearned healers. Yet his use of Latin, his upper status and university patients and his apparently amicable relations with at least two local 'doctors' suggest that he was also reasonably respectable. Although his qualifications are unknown, it is quite possible that he himself had pursued a course of university study. Thus, while he does not quite fit the pattern of the conventional physician of his time, his practices demonstrate the spectrum of medical care available within the fold of respectable medical practitioners.

Comparison of the physicians' casebooks with that kept by the surgeon Binns adds to our knowledge of this spectrum. Binns's therapeutic routines were similar to those followed by Barker and Symcotts. Like them, he depended upon purges, emetics and diuretics to promote evacuation, thus keeping the patient's body in a 'soluble' state. Like them, he used surgical procedures such as blood-letting and issues responsibly and sparingly.

With hindsight, it is possible to see Binns as the most modern of these three very conventional healers. He did not use uroscopy and astrology at all. His prescriptions reveal a wide knowledge of the relatively new chemical remedies popularised by the disciples of Paracelsus. Unlike Barker and Symcotts, he applied all of the treatments he prescribed himself, not depending upon additional lesser healers to act according to his orders.[125] And, unlike Symcotts, he charged both for remedies provided and services rendered, thus directly recognising his place in the medical marketplace.

In addition, because of the sorts of problems Binns treated, he dealt more with specific disorders than did the physicians. While the surgeon used evacuative medicine to treat the whole patient, he focused his attention on localised symptoms in a way the physicians rarely did.

What did physicians and surgeons think of each other? Judging by the casebooks analysed here, there was much tolerance and little prejudice on both sides of the occupational divide. Binns apparently respected physicians generally, although he recorded one case in which he disagreed with a physician's judgment.[126] Correspondingly Symcotts respected surgeons, although he felt a surgeon was unskilful in one instance.[127] None the less, there can be no doubt that physicians regarded surgeons as subordinate to themselves, and surgical procedures as essentially menial. On the other hand, no impression is given in Binns's casebook that the surgeon felt inferior to any other practitioner. He took independent charge of his patients, worked with physicians as colleagues, and saw himself as rendering an expert service.

It is not possible to compare Binns's success rate with that of the physicians. While the surgeon conscientiously noted the outcome of his treatment, the physicians did so only erratically. Symcotts reported the outcome in only fifty-five cases. According to this meagre sample, he did well; thirty-five patients recovered, seven improved and only thirteen died. Barker and the Cambridge practitioner reported the outcome of a case so rarely that consideration of their success rate is impossible. Thus, one cannot make an informed statement about the relative efficacy of 'physic' and surgery in seventeenth-century England. In this area, as in many others, the perceptions and preconceptions of sufferers and patients were more important than any demonstrable expertise. As we shall see below, at least one patient, Samuel Pepys, had greater regard for surgeons than he had for physicians.[128] One can only speculate about how general this feeling was.

Concerning relations between healers and patients, certain generalisations are possible. Symcotts's correspondence and the diaries of lay-people confirm that seventeenth-century sufferers knew a good deal about their own ailments and took a large amount of responsibility in their courses of treatment.[129] Very often, people attempted to cure themselves and sought medical advice from relatives and friends before consulting healers. Symcotts and Binns each had many patients who had come to them as a last resort. The remedies prepared by lay-people – particularly women – were valued by people beyond their own social circle. As indicated above, Symcotts knew a number of gentlewomen who acted as amateur healers with his entire approval and respect. Further, their medical recipes were collected by lay-people and healers alike. Robert Hooke's collection will be discussed below.[130] Symcotts's has already been mentioned.

Whether or not they acted as healers, lay-people were often required by healers to make or apply their own remedies. Ingredients frequently came from their own larders, cellars and gardens. For instance, Symcotts's 'restorative water for any that is in weakness' contained the following:

> Take 3 pints of new milk, 1 pint of red wine, 24 yolks of new laid eggs. Beat all these together, then put to it as much fine white manchett [bread roll] as will soak up the aforesaid milk and wine. Distill it with a soft fire.
>
> Take a spoonful in any spoon meat you eat and in each draught of drink. This hath recovered one wasted to skin and bone in a month's time.[131]

Patients and their servants also performed minor surgical tasks such as applying leeches, giving clysters and making up medicinal baths and fumes. Sometimes physicians' prescriptions were made up by people other than either the patient, the physician or an apothecary. For instance, Mistress Willis, a midwife, brewed a diet drink for Symcotts's patient, Mr Powers.[132] Thus, patients and many lay-people surrounding them were intimately involved with illness and medicine.

Patients and their families sometimes asked healers for particular services and remedies. This was usual in the case of prophylactic physic, often taken once a year, when an individual would purchase a purge or ask a surgeon to let blood. Equally usual was the preventative medicine aimed against a specific disease. We have seen that Barker on one occasion provided 'pestilent pills' for two families and their servants. However, medical and surgical services were often specified for other disorders. Mr Cotton asked Symcotts for a purge for his wife after she had given birth.[133]

Further, patients felt free to consult more than one healer. As we have seen, Mr Powers, loyal old nuisance though he was, sought treatment from at least two other practitioners during the course of his relationship with Symcotts. In this, he was quite typical. Each of the casebooks examined makes references to patients who had consulted other healers before coming to the one writing the notes.

Thus healers, competing in the open market, had to justify treatments prescribed, hoping to be vindicated by success. Symcotts's correspondence is full of letters from him to patients, explaining the advice he has given in terms of the patient's own needs. For instance, to Mr Powers he wrote, 'I am in haste yet I will not grudge to give you a short account of my intention in the late prescribed course'.[134] This was followed by a full page concerning his prescription of a purge. Such letters show great respect for the patient's understanding.

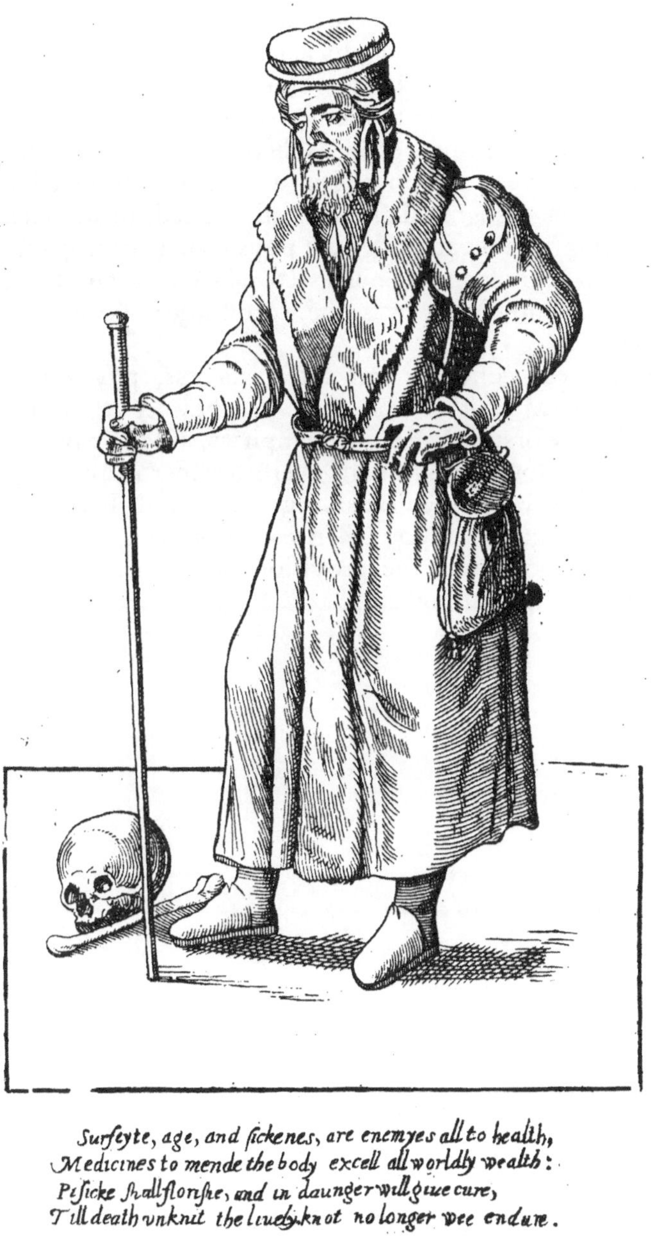

This sixteenth-century woodcut both praises physic and reminds the reader that no physic can prevent death. (W. Bullein, *Bulleins bulwarke of defence against all sickness* . . ., London, 1562.)

They also show the healer's concern that his methods appear to be correct, regardless of the outcome.

Herein lies the core of the physician's problem. Unlike other learned authorities, such as ministers and lawyers, the physician was expected to demonstrate his knowledge in a concrete way by curing people. Whether the patient recovered or died, however, the physician wished his knowledge and expertise to be recognised and trusted. Indeed, to some extent, actual curing was regarded by the physician as irrelevant, since the medical knowledge he possessed was felt to be of intrinsic value. This knowledge was the commodity he offered the community.

In terms of economic and social success, physicians as a group achieved neither the rewards they coveted nor the failure their worst enemies, the empirics, might have wished them. Physicians like Symcotts were prosperous members of the community, living satisfying lives and helping their patients through a variety of crises. However, they did not have a monopoly over the provision of internal medicine in seventeenth-century England.

5

SUFFERERS AND PATIENTS: THE DISEASES OF THE PEOPLE

In 1651 Thomas Hobbes wrote that 'the life of man is solitary, poor, nasty, brutish and short'.[1] While this statement was inaccurate for many living in his own time, it does reflect a comparative truth which historians and demographers have been eager to enlarge upon. Dietary, sanitary and housing conditions have been held accountable for a great deal of misery, including disease.[2] High infant and child mortality, and a relatively short expectation of life at birth have been meticulously determined and duly regretted.[3] However, it must be remembered that, while the seventeenth-century English criticised the conditions they lived with, they had not the standard of comparison which blesses (or curses) late-twentieth-century scholars. This study is concerned with seventeenth-century perceptions and expectations. Thus, it will try to avoid implicit (and self-congratulatory) comparisons between then and now.

No attempt will be made below to make causal associations between living conditions and illness. Such associations necessarily refer to the hypotheses and discoveries of modern science, and are thus irrelevant for the understanding of seventeenth-century experience. The same objection applies to efforts made to diagnose the diseases seventeenth-century sufferers 'really' had. They *knew* what they had. Our presumptuous diagnosis of the green sickness as chlorosis, for instance, has nothing to do with their understanding and treatment of the disorder – nor with our understanding of their behaviour. Neither will any assessment be made of whether or not the treatments people underwent 'worked'. In this area, as in others, the sufferer will speak for him- or herself.

People suffered from a multitude of discomforts and disorders in seventeenth-century England. Some scholars maintain that most people felt unwell most of the time.[4] None the less, historians, demographers and epidemiologists have concentrated their attention on epidemic diseases, particularly plague.[5] While this concentration is understandable in view of the tremendous mortality and social dislocation caused by epidemics, it distorts our perception of the diseases people suffered and died from in the period.

In the sixteenth and seventeenth centuries London underwent six major outbreaks of plague. These occurred in the years 1563, 1593, 1603, 1625, 1636 and 1665. These outbreaks were sometimes, but not always, reflected in provincial epidemics. For instance, Bristol suffered severely from plague in 1563 and 1603, but not in 1625 and 1636.[6] And, it must be remembered, most people lived in villages or hamlets in the countryside: areas much less susceptible to plague infestation. Gregory King, the pioneer demographer, calculated that nearly 80 per cent of the population was rural.[7] Thus, although dread of the plague was certainly a part of general seventeenth-century English mental furniture, it was quite possible for an individual – particularly someone living outside London – to live out a long lifetime without ever personally experiencing a plague epidemic. Thus, other diseases, although not carrying the dramatic impact possessed by the very word 'plague', were as or more significant in the lives and deaths of members of the general public.

One way of estimating the incidence of serious diseases in a population is to obtain a numerical breakdown of the causes of death. This method has its faults, which will be discussed below. However, it is such a good indicator of both the disorders people died from and contemporary popular diagnoses of symptoms that it cannot be ignored.

Perhaps unfortunately, the following discussion is based largely on London records. It is widely repeated that the London experience was untypical. London was many times larger than any other seventeenth-century English city and contemporaries and historians agree that it was an unusually unhealthy place to live.[8] However, the medical casebooks and lay diaries which are cited elsewhere in our discussion support the conviction that both diagnostic categories and individual experience of endemic diseases were similar throughout the country. The Josselin family, living in deepest Essex, and the Hobys, living in remote Yorkshire, suffered from conditions which were all too familiar to Londoners.

The two best seventeenth-century sources giving causes of death are the London Bills of Mortality and those parish burial records which record the disease the newly deceased was suffering from.[9] A superb work which serves both as a provider of new information and as a guide to the London Bills of Mortality is John Graunt's *Natural and Political Observations Made upon the Bills of Mortality* (1662). On the basis of these sources, a profile of killing diseases can be drawn over a long period of time.

As suggested above, the widest fluctuation is seen in the incidence of epidemic diseases. For instance, in 1625 the plague killed 35,417 people in London. In 1648 it killed 611. In 1629, 1633 and 1635 no plague deaths were reported at all.[10] A similar, though less dramatic, fluctuation appears in the incidence of death from other diseases recognised as infectious. For instance, smallpox killed some people every year in seventeenth-century London. However, it was worse some years than others. In 1659 smallpox killed 1,523 people, while in 1660 it killed 354.[11] Even non-infectious killers exhibit fluctuations which are more difficult to account for. For example, in 1648 only 106 London women died in childbirth; in 1652 the number had jumped to 213.[12] Even allowing for population growth, that increase is extreme, particularly considering that only 194 women died in childbirth in 1660.

Despite the fluctuations observable in the incidence of all the disorders recorded, however, it is possible to identify the diseases which had the most significant impact on the population. From this information one can make inferences about some of the disorders which disrupted the lives of the survivors, as well as those of the deceased. Among the most consistent killers were unspecified 'fevers', consumption and the simple experience of being born, usually labelled as 'chrisoms' or 'infants'. In a comparison of the Bills of Mortality for 1632, a non-plague year, and the plague year, 1665, over 1,000 people died in each of these categories. Other major killers were smallpox, abortion and stillbirth, 'teeth' and old age, which claimed between 450 and 1,000 deaths in each year.

Certain changes can be observed over a period of years in the incidence of a number of non-infectious disorders. These changes can be viewed either as alterations in diagnoses of conditions which had always been present, or as indications of the advent of new diseases. John Graunt wrote about both of these alternatives. For instance, he felt that deaths in infancy had been reported differently early in the century than they were later, writing,

> Of convulsions there appeared very few, *viz.* but 52 in the year 1629, which in 1636 grew to 709, keeping about that stay, till

> 1659, though sometimes rising to about 1000.
>
> It is to be noted, that from 1629 to 1636, when the convulsions were but few, the number of chrysoms and Infants was greater: for in 1629, there was of Chrysoms, and Infants 2596, and of the Convulsion 52, *viz.* of both 2648. And in 1636 there was of Infants 1895, and of the Convulsions 709, in both 2604, by which it appears, that this difference is likely to be only a confusion in the accounts.[13]

He goes on to say that deaths put down to teeth and worms are also interchanged with the categories Infants, Chrysoms and Convulsions, which further confuses matters. The indication of convulsions as the cause of death became increasingly common in the course of the century, judging by the burial records of St Vedast parish, London. For the years 1674–83, convulsions was the single most frequent cause of death, followed closely by consumption, fever and gripes. Although the ages of those dying of convulsions is not usually given, the burial register often indicates that the deceased were children by identifying them as 'son' or 'daughter' of certain parents.[14]

One disease which is generally regarded by both historians and contemporaries as new in the seventeenth century is rickets. Graunt pointed out that rickets is not mentioned in the Bills of Mortality until 1634. However, he was undecided whether rickets was a new disease, or whether it was simply a new way of reporting deaths from the conditions 'livergrown' and 'spleen'. None the less, he leaned toward the judgment that rickets was a new disease, since the numbers dying from it steadily increased, while the numbers of those dying livergrown remained constant.[15] He made the same decision about another apparently new disease, the stopping of the stomach, which was first mentioned in the Bills in 1636.[16] While he did not view scurvy as a new disease, he observed that it was rapidly increasing in incidence, having killed but twelve in 1629 and twenty-five in 1660.[17]

Determination of the cause of death was made by the searchers. Graunt described the procedure as follows:

> When any one dies, then, either by tolling, or ringing of a Bell, or by bespeaking of a Grave of the Sexton, the same is known to the Searchers, corresponding with the said Sexton.
>
> The Searchers hereupon (who are ancient Matrons, sworn to their Office) repair to the place, where the dead Corps lies, and by view of the same, and by other enquiries, they examine by what Disease or Casualty the Corps died. Hereupon they make their report to the Parish-Clerk.[18]

Graunt, who was, after all, himself a haberdasher by trade, was not unduly concerned about the medical ignorance of the searchers, maintaining that most determinations of the cause of death were simply matters of 'sense', and that underlying causes for conditions such as old age (affecting persons who died at ages above 60) baffled even learned physicians.[19] For example, he wrote,

> As for Consumptions, if the Searchers do but truly Report (as they may) whether the dead Corps were very lean, and worn away, it matters not to many of our purposes [that is those of the Statisticians], whether the Disease were exactly the same, as Physicians define it in their Books. Moreover, in case a man of seventy five years old died of a Cough (of which had he been free he might have possibly lived to ninety) I esteem it little error (as to many of our purposes) if this person be, in the Table of Casualties, reckoned among the Aged, and not placed under the Title of Coughs.[20]

However, he mentioned one disease, the diagnosis of which the searchers often deliberately falsified. This was syphilis. About the pox he wrote,

> Forasmuch as by the ordinary discourse of the world it seems a great part of men have, at one time or other, had some species of this disease, I wondering why so few died of it, especially because I could not take that to be so harmless, whereof so many complained very fiercely; upon inquiry I found that those who died of it out of the Hospitals . . . were returned of Ulcers and Sores. And in brief I found, that all mentioned to die of the French Pox were returned by the Clerks of Saint Giles's, and Saint Martin's in the Fields only; in which place I understood that most of the vilest, and most miserable houses of uncleanness were: from whence I concluded, that only *hated* persons, and such, whose very Noses were eaten off, were reported by the Searchers to have died of this too frequent malady.[21]

Graunt observed that most who died of syphilis died 'emaciated and lean'. Thus, the searchers, 'after the mist of a cup of ale and the bribe of a two-groat fee', were nearly justified in reporting as the cause of death consumption, hectic-fever, atrophy or infection of the 'Spermatick parts'.[22]

It is, perhaps, more significant for the purposes of this study than it was for Graunt that the searchers were lay-women. Although they were occasionally told the cause of death by the attending physician, more often they made the determination themselves, aided by the family and friends of the deceased. The diseases or 'casualties' noted in the Bills of Mortality and parish records thus reflect popular categories for diseases.

A consistent killer with strong associations with humoral medical theory was surfeit, which killed between 63 and 371 people in each year between 1629 and 1660. Still another consistent killer was dropsy or timpany, which killed between 185 and 931 people a year in the same period. Apoplexy and 'sudden death' was far less deadly, in some years killing no one at all and at most, in 1658, claiming but 138 deaths.

Disorders which might be viewed as mental rather than physical in origin also killed. A condition identified simply as grief accounted for the deaths of between seven and twenty-two people a year in the period 1629–60. Suicide, under the heading 'Hanged, and made away themselves', was the cause of the deaths of between three and thirty-six people in each year of this period except one, 1633. Lunacy killed between two and eighteen people a year.

It is interesting that, in a time period renowned for both aggressive behaviour and dangerous living conditions, more people did not die as the result of violence or accidents. Between 1629 and 1660 there were three years in which no murders were reported – 1629, 1630 and 1633. And in only two years were there more than ten murders in all of the parishes contributing information to the Bills of Mortality. One wonders what was going on in 1660, when twenty were murdered, and in 1659 when seventy died by violence. These numbers do not include criminals who were executed; between seven and twenty-nine people died in this way from 1629 to 1660. More people died from accidental injuries than were killed by other people. These accidental deaths are reported under two headings – 'killed by several accidents' and 'sores, ulcers, broken and bruised limbs'. In only two years, 1650 and 1659, were more than a hundred people killed accidentally.

While the Bills of Mortality are an unrivalled source of information about the diseases people died of, this study is more concerned about the disorders people lived with. In this area as well, John Graunt is of some help. His comments about syphilis, quoted above, indicate that the pox either was or was thought to be a more common disease than the Bills of Mortality would lead one to believe. He also explained that gout, from which many people suffered, did not show up very frequently in the Bills because 'those that have the Gout are said to be Long-livers, and therefore, when such die, they are returned as Aged'.[23] Indeed, both Graunt's book and the Bills of Mortality can be seen as of unique value because the information they give cuts across class lines. Unlike medical casebooks and other sorts of private papers, parish records report the diseases of rich and poor alike.

This is not to say that the rich died of the same diseases as the poor did. Those reported as having been 'found dead in the streets' are unlikely to have been members of the upper classes. The same holds true for the few who were diagnosed as 'starved' in each year 1648–60. By the same token, a poor man or woman might have been considered fortunate to die of surfeit. Regardless of these observations, the Bills of Mortality provide a helpful insight into seventeenth-century interpretations of the always-democratic activities of the Grim Reaper.

More useful information about the ailments middle- and upper-class people suffered on a day-to-day basis can be obtained from the many diaries which have survived the last 300 years. These diaries are a veritable gold mine of evidence, not only about illnesses, but also about what the writers thought and did about them.

Inevitably diarists provide a one-sided view of the disorders people suffered from. Samuel Pepys, because of his personal experience, was very interested in bladder and kidney ailments, reporting not only his own sensations, but also those of acquaintances and relatives, as well as lectures and conversations with medical experts on the subject.[24] The Essex vicar, Ralph Josselin, greatly feared smallpox, and reported any local outbreaks of the disease, even though no one in his immediate family suffered very acutely from it.[25] The ever-ailing Robert Hooke's life revolved around how well or ill he slept.[26] None the less, the diaries and collections of correspondence available for the period can be examined and compared for indications of both commonly experienced ailments and disorders which could seriously affect an individual's life, whether or not a sizeable percentage of the population died of it.

Then as now, the most ubiquitous ailment was the common cold. All of the writers consulted had colds. However, while today this disorder is usually confined to the head and the chest, for seventeenth-century sufferers the term 'cold' retained more of its original humoral connotation and the ailment could attack any part of the body. Thus, Pepys often described his recurring pain during urination as being due to cold. Hooke complained of catching cold in his 'pole'.[27]

Colds were usually dismissed as minor ailments, treated, if at all, with casual remedies.[28] For instance, on one occasion Pepys asked Lady Batten for a spoonful of honey for his cold while dining at her home.[29] The sufferer, although inconvenienced, usually did not take up a sick role. However, sometimes colds were taken more seriously. In April 1649 Ralph Josselin took both mithridate and a stybium vomit for a cold.[30] John Evelyn was cupped and scarified for a cold he picked up in Italy.[31] And it was recognised that any illness, however minor, could suddenly become fatal. Mr Clerke, a solicitor of Pepys's acquaintance, died of a cold, having been ill for only two days.[32] In addition, colds in children were far more worrying than in adults.[33]

Nearly as common as colds were eye problems. Many diarists, including Pepys, Josselin, Evelyn and Hooke, suffered from either eyestrain or rheum in the eye or both. Indeed, Pepys gave up writing his diary for fear of exacerbating the eyestrain he worried might eventually blind him.[34] Eye problems, like colds, tended to be treated as minor annoyances – inconvenient, but not life-threatening.

Only in Pepys's case did the problem become serious enough for the sufferer to seek out a specialist. Pepys eventually consulted Dr Daubigny Turberville, who was 'the most successful practising oculist of his day', according to the editors of Pepys's diaries.[35] He also used a preparation advised by a fellow-sufferer, one Mr Cooling, and had his eyes dressed by his belt-maker's wife, 'an oldish woman in a hat'.[36] John Evelyn, who apparently favoured phlebotomy, was bled four times for his sore eyes in May 1647.[37] The other diarists simply waited out their eye ailments, which eventually passed.[38]

More serious than either colds or eye problems were the agues or intermittent fevers which afflicted many of the diarists and their relatives and friends. The Josselins' experiences with ague will be discussed below.[39] They, like others, found ague worrying and debilitating, but not fatal. The exception to this general observation is Dorothy Osborne's father who never really recovered from a severe attack of ague. Even after the fits ceased, he remained in his chamber. His attentive daughter wrote, 'I cannot say that he is at all sick but has so general a weakness upon him that I . . . do extremely apprehend how the winter may work upon him'.[40] Her fears were justified, for her father died soon after. Dorothy's brother, who came home to recover from an ague during her father's illness, was more fortunate. He eventually recovered, as did Dorothy herself, who had a relatively mild attack in April 1653 while her brother was recuperating. She wrote of her own illness, 'I have gotten an ague that with two fits has made me so very weak that I doubted extremely yesterday whether I should be able to sit up today to write to you'.[41] The following month she, her brother and her father had finally 'lost' their fits, 'but we all look like people risen from the dead'.[42]

Ague afflicted children as well as adults; like other diseases, it was more worrying in children. Lady Anne Clifford's daughter, Lady Margaret (at that time referred to only as 'The Child') had an ague during the February and March of 1617, when she was a toddler.[43] Lady Anne, who seems to have spent little time with her baby before the illness, reported spending 'most of her time . . . in going up and down to see the Child'.[44] Lady Margaret recovered. John Evelyn's first-born son, Richard, was not so lucky. He died of ague at age 5 years and 3 days.[45]

The cold and hot fits of ague were very unpleasant. And the intermittent character of these fits made agues particularly frustrating, since the sufferer felt fairly well between fits and could convince him- or herself that the illness had passed off. For instance, when Samuel Pepys's patron, Lord Sandwich, had an ague in January 1663, Pepys described a visit during which he found Sandwich 'not sick, but expecting his fit tonight of an ague'.[46] Later in the same illness, Lord Sandwich 'missed his fit' and hoped he was well.[47] His hopes were groundless, for the ague returned nearly a month later.[48]

In addition to agues, the diarists and their family members suffered from toothache. Elizabeth Pepys and Jane Josselin were particularly plagued with that painful disorder. In November 1661 Elizabeth Pepys had her teeth 'scaled' by Peter de la Roche, the operator for the teeth to the Royal household, in an attempt to improve her appearance and prevent further attacks.[49] However, as a preventative measure the operation did not succeed, for Elizabeth had yet another tooth drawn in May of that year.[50] Jane Josselin treated herself for toothache with tobacco.[51] She also suffered from pain in her gums.[52] However, like colds and eye problems, toothache, even when it ended in extraction, was regarded as being of minor significance.

Another widespread type of disorder were the various digestive ailments which attacked almost everyone at one time or another. Responses to these usually brief illnesses were mixed. Generally speaking, constipation was regarded as being more serious than either vomiting or diarrhoea (usually described as looseness or scouring). In the autumn of 1663 Pepys suffered from a disorder he described variously as wind, colic and being costive. It seemed very ominous to him that he could neither break wind nor produce bowel movements as 'naturally' and frequently as he would have liked.[53] While he complained of 'great pain' and took an enormous amount of purging medication for this problem, his main concern stemmed from the conviction that a constipated state was unnatural and fundamentally unhealthy.

Pepys's attitude was quite consistent with the humoral view of disease which regarded evacuation and a 'soluble' state of the body as beneficial. It was reflected in Hooke's relief upon vomiting after eating pullet and cheesecakes and Josselin's belief that the diarrhoea he suffered from in December 1648 had done him much good.[54] Such responses are certainly understandable, considering that most of the medicines people took were expected to cause evacuation of one kind or another. Natural vomiting, diarrhoea, sweating, expulsions of phlegm and even bleeding (from the nose, or in menstruation) may often have seemed merely the body's attempts to cure itself.[55] Thus, despite the evidence given by the London Bills of Mortality that, although no one died of constipation *per se* (although some died of surfeit), and many died each year of flux and scouring, the prevailing preference was for vomiting and diarrhoea as opposed to constipation.

Colds and disorders of the eyes, teeth and digestive tracts appeared in all of the diaries examined. Other conditions, although less ubiquitous, made frequent appearances. Not all the women who wrote or figured in the diaries consulted underwent pregnancy and childbirth. Lady Margaret Hoby and Elizabeth Pepys were childless. Dorothy Osborne was unmarried at the time she wrote her famous letters to William Temple, whom she later wed. However, Lady Anne Clifford had two pregnancies during the period in which she wrote her diary, and Mary Evelyn, Jane Josselin, and Alice Thornton were exceptionally productive, Mary having eight live births, Jane, ten and Alice, nine. Mary miscarried three times and Jane approximately five.

Of the fertile women mentioned above, only Lady Anne Clifford and Alice Thornton described their own experiences. Thornton's childbearing will be discussed below. Lady Anne did not describe her first pregnancy and the birth of Lady Margaret Sackville (born 1615). She did mention her second pregnancy, during and after which she was ill. She reported feeling herself quick with child in August 1619. In mid-October she wrote that she 'began to be ill'. From about this time she stayed in her chamber until the end of March 1620. The only specific symptom she reported was on 8 November 1619, feeling 'so ill that I fell into a swoon which was the first time I ever swooned'.[56] The child, Thomas, died soon after birth.

The experiences of Jane Josselin and Mary Evelyn were reported by their husbands. Jane's childbearing will be discussed below at some length.[57] Suffice it to say that her pregnancies were uncomfortable and her deliveries straightforward. Although she dreaded her labours for months before they occurred, she apparently accepted her frequent pregnancies as her natural lot and took an interest in them which is revealed in the predictions that she made early in at least five of her pregnancies about the sex of the unborn child.[58]

Mary Evelyn's pregnancies and deliveries were reported in far less detail than Jane Josselin's. The overwhelming impression given by her husband was that her fertility was desirable (indeed, expected) because of dynastic considerations. For this reason, too long a gap between babies was deplored.[59] Partly for this reason, her miscarriages were regretted.[60] John Evelyn did not indicate whether his wife's pregnancies were comfortable or uncomfortable. Nor did he describe her deliveries.

Mary's childbearing life was long. Married at 12, she miscarried at age 16, having been given a dose of physic which she took, unaware that she was pregnant.[61] Thereafter, she was more careful. She had five sons, born in 1652, 1653, 1655, 1657 and 1664, and three daughters, born in 1665, 1667 and 1669. She miscarried in October 1660, after falling from a stool.[62] Her last miscarrage occurred in April 1666, only six months after her daughter Mary was born.[63]

Unlike Jane Josselin, Mary Evelyn breast-fed none of her own children. This was undoubtedly due to the class difference. The Josselins were middle class by any definition of that inexact term; the Evelyns belonged to the landed gentry. While breast-feeding was increasingly acceptable and practised among the middle classes in seventeenth-century England, upper-class mothers did not usually feed their own babies.[64] John Evelyn had himself been put out to nurse immediately after birth and did not return home, weaned, until he was 15 months old.[65] His own children were also fed by wet-nurse. Jane Josselin almost certainly fed all of her babies herself. Comparison of the experiences of the Josselins and Evelyns make unavoidable the conclusion that the Evelyns suffered the consequences of wet-nursing. Of their five sons, three died within the first three months of life – one possibly having been overlain by the nurse.[66] The Josselins lost only one baby immediately after birth. That child died, aged 10 days, of a condition which could not possibly have been related to the care taken of him.[67]

Both Jane and Mary were comparatively fortunate in their childbearing. Although Jane complained of many more ailments during her childbearing years than she did in the twenty years after those years ended, she sustained no permanent handicap or illness through carrying and bearing children.[68] She lived to be at least 66 years old. Mary Evelyn died aged 74. Although her husband's account of her medical history must be regarded as sketchy at best, she apparently lived a remarkably healthy life, suffering hardly any illness at all until she was over age 50.

Both the Bills of Mortality and the diaries indicate that their contemporaries were not always as lucky as Jane and Mary. Many women did die in childbirth. In 1646 two neighbour women of the Josselins died giving birth.[69] John Evelyn's sister died at age 20 as the result of giving birth to a baby six months before.[70] Miscarrying caused problems as well. Pepys's Aunt Wight became very ill after a miscarriage in March 1662; his Cousin Scott died as the result of a miscarriage in February 1664.

Gynaecological disorders appear less frequently in the diaries than do conditions relating to pregnancy and childbirth. It is probable that this paucity of evidence reflects female modesty and male ignorance and disgust more than it does as actual absence of such disorders. Fortunately Samuel Pepys was interested in and sympathetic with his wife's 'female problems', and described them in some detail. Elizabeth Pepys had three distinct gynaecological disorders. She suffered from painful menstruation; according to her husband, she was infertile; and, most serious of all, she had recurring abcesses and eventually a fistula in her external genitalia.

The very first page of Pepys's diary referred to the couple's disappointed hopes of having a child. He wrote in January 1660,

> My wife, after the absence of her terms for seven weeks, gave me hopes of her being with child, but on the last day of the year she hath them again.[71]

By 1664 he was obviously more than resigned to their childless state, writing that Elizabeth thought she was pregnant, 'but I neither believe nor desire it'.[72] The fact that she had not borne a baby did not bar Elizabeth from helping out at the confinements of women of her acquaintance. Samuel reported that she was summoned to their labours; in one case he wrote that 'the midwife and she alone have delivered poor Betty of a pretty girl'.[73]

It is an open question whether the Pepys' married life would have been happier had they had children. Possibly Elizabeth would not have felt as isolated and bored as she increasingly did. And Samuel might have demanded less of her artistic and musical talents had she been busy with a young family. However, their childlessness gave them opportunities for companionship and communication denied to partners in more fruitful marriages. Pepys took a great interest in his wife's appearance and her artistic endeavours. And although they argued frequently, they also depended on each other for support. For example, in March 1668 Samuel's mind was troubled because of office business. Unable to sleep, he asked Elizabeth to talk to him 'to comfort him'. This she did; it eased him somewhat.[74] Thus, despite their spats and Samuel's infidelity, the Pepys marriage might be viewed as having been more 'companionate' than some modern scholars have maintained.[75]

Elizabeth's dependence on Samuel is certainly reflected in his description of her recurring bouts of pain in her external genitalia. Pepys first mentioned this problem on 2 August 1660. He wrote,

> When I came home, I find my wife not very well of her old pain in the lip of her *chose*, which she had when we were first married.[76]

This bout lasted only until 8 August, when Elizabeth was well enough for the couple to have sexual intercourse. However, the pain returned. By 21 October Elizabeth was complaining of boils in the 'old place'. She improved after using remedies sent by Dr Williams, the physician who had treated her before for this ailment.[77] This time she remained fairly well until May 1661, when the swelling returned. On 12 May it broke spontaneously and Samuel 'put in a tent (which Dr Williams sent me yesterday) into the hole, to keep it open till all the matter be come out – and so I question not but she will soon be well again'.[78]

After this episode, Elizabeth's 'old pain' mercifully stayed away for nearly three years. However, she was apparently not cured, for on 16 November 1663, Pepys wrote,

> and in the evening Mr. Holliard [a surgeon and friend] came, and he and I about our great work to look upon my wife's malady in her secrets; which he did, and it seems her great conflux of humours heretofore, that used to swell there, did in breaking leave a hollow, which hath since gone in further and further, till it is near three inches deep.[79]

Holliard decided to open the fistula by incision the following night. He arrived, prepared to operate, but found Elizabeth

> so fearful, and the thing will be somewhat painful in the tending, which I [Pepys] shall not be able to look after but must require a nurse and people about her; so that upon second thoughts, he believes that a fomentation will do as well.[80]

This decision relieved both Samuel and Elizabeth. Elizabeth had begged Samuel to stay with her and see the operation done, partly for moral support, partly because she refused to allow anyone else to 'see it done; no, not her own maids; and therefore I must do it, poor wretch, for her'.[81] Samuel was pleased that surgery was unnecessary, 'for I confess I should have been troubled to have had my wife cut before my face – I could not have borne to have seen it'.[82] The painless fomentation Holliard prescribed could be administered by Elizabeth's maid without the maid 'knowing directly what it is for, but only that it may be for the piles – for though it be nothing but what is very honest, yet my wife is loath to give occasion of discourse concerning it'.[83] Thus, Elizabeth's worries about both impending pain and the shame of having her malady generally discussed were dispelled. The fomentation was apparently a success, because Elizabeth never again complained of her 'old pain'.

She did complain of menstrual cramps which sometimes sent her to bed for a few days. These were frequently very bad indeed. On the occasion of the death of Samuel's brother, Tom, Elizabeth stayed at Tom's house to see the deceased laid out; her menstrual period arrived, causing her such discomfort that she had to be taken home and put to bed.[84] Despite the pain, however, Elizabeth seems to have had a fairly regular menstrual cycle. It should also be remarked that her period was not always painful. In no year from 1660 to 1669 did menstruation send her to bed more than four times.

Pepys's diary provides unique documentation of one woman's menstrual history over a long period of time. Samuel did not note Elizabeth's menstruation each time it occurred. He seems to have reported it only when it caused her discomfort. For instance, 1666 must have been a reasonably good year for her, since Samuel made no mention of her menstrual periods at all. None the less, Pepys's diary was the only one located which regularly referred to menstruation at all. It even provides somewhat conflicting information about sexual behaviour during menstruation. On 25 May 1668 Samuel and Elizabeth 'lay long making love', despite the fact that she was ill enough with her menstrual period to have stayed in bed the previous day.[85] However, Pepys was unable to talk Mrs Daniel into a little sexual play at the office the following summer because she was menstruating.[86] Pepys's diary is also informative about some of the terms used to refer to menstruation in mid-seventeenth-century London. He called it Elizabeth's '*mois*' or 'months', '*ceux la*' or simply 'those'.

The exclusively female experiences of pregnancy, childbirth and menstruation were the only subjects relating to health and illness about which the seventeenth-century diarists and correspondents were at all reticent. Certainly these writers were not as inhibited about male genito-urinary troubles. Ralph Josselin suffered for a week in 1647 with swellings in both sides of his groin.[87] As indicated above, Robert Hooke complained of having caught cold in his 'pole'.[88] And, more seriously, Samuel Pepys's father had an old rupture (of at least twenty years' standing) which occasionally escaped the truss which supported it, and caused him intolerable pain. Samuel described one horrifying occasion when he and his father had spent the day together away from home. When he returned after a brief absence from the room, he found his

> father unexpectedly in great pain and desiring for God sake to get him a bed to lie upon; which I did, and . . . I stayed by him, in so great pain as I never saw, poor wretch, and with that patience, crying only: 'Terrible: terrible pain: God help me, God help me' – with that mournful voice, that made my heart ache.

After a time, Samuel got him into a coach and drove home, stopping only once, in 'Paul's Churchyard . . . the jogging and pain making my father vomit – which it never had done before'.[89] Fortunately, after a half hour's rest in bed at home, the sufferer's 'bowels went up again into his belly, being got forth into his cod, as it seems is usual with very many men – after which he was at good case and so continued'.

Perhaps more common than ruptures, and certainly more deadly, were the kidney and bladder stones which plagued both women and men. Women both suffered and died from this disorder. Pepys's mother had a fit of the stone late in 1660.[90] And his Aunt James died of the stone in 1666.[91] However, if the (largely male) diarists are to be credited, most of those who had this disorder were male.

John Evelyn's brother Richard died of 'the stone in the bladder' after having suffered increasing agony for well over a year, refusing surgical intervention.[92] John described his pain as 'such exceeding torture . . . that he now began to fall into convulsion fits'.[93] John Evelyn himself suffered from kidney stones toward the end of his life. He first reported pain in his kidneys in March 1682.[94] By March 1692 he 'feared gravel in my kidneys'.[95] In July 1705, seven months before his death, he reported 'I had this night a very severe fit of [cold] trembling & heat after, with very great pai[ne in my] sides & back & all over my body, all symptoms of the stone'.[96] And by late December, in addition to his pain he was making 'bloody water'.[97] It should be remembered that he was 85 years old at this time.

Robert Hooke visited Sir Christopher Wren when he lay ill of the stone.[98] Pepys mentioned the death from the stone of the Lord Treasurer in May 1667.[99] He also marvelled at the size of the stone cut from the body of Sir Thomas Adam during the autopsy performed on his body. The stone was

> very large indeed, bigger I think than my fist, and weighs above 25 ounces – and which is very miraculous, never in all his life had any fit of it, but lived to a great age without pain, and died at last of something else, without any sense of this in all his life.[100]

By contrast, Robert Hooke described the death of the Bishop of Chester. Everyone had assumed the bishop had the stone, which had caused the urinary retention which finally killed him. However, the account of the autopsy given by Dr Needham indicated that the bishop had had

> no stoppage in his ureters nor defect in his kidneys. There was only found 2 small stones in one kidney and some little gravel in one ureter but neither big enough to stop the water. Twas believed his opiates and some other medicines killed him, there being no visible cause of his death.[101]

Without a doubt, the most famous sufferer from the stone of all time was Samuel Pepys himself. He was successfully cut for the stone by the surgeon Thomas Holliard on 26 March 1658. Thereafter, he held an annual celebration to commemorate the event. He maintained a special interest in genito-urinary problems, conversing with medical specialists on the subject and at one point attending a lecture about it at the Surgeon's Hall.[102]

He also made of himself a minor celebrity among his wide acquaintance on the basis of his recovery from the 'disease of the stone'. He visited people who were suffering from that disorder, urging them to undergo surgery, and displaying the stone which had been removed from his own body as an inducement. John Evelyn took Pepys to visit his brother Richard nine months before Richard's death. He wrote that Pepys 'carried the stone (which was as big as a tennis-ball) to shew him [Richard], and encourage his resolution to go through the operation'.[103]

It should be said that Pepys's enthusiasm for the operation had a sound basis, not only in his personal experience, but also in the evidence given by the London Bills of Mortality. In most years many more people died of the disease than died of the operation. The exceptions were, ironically, 1659 and 1660 when more people died of the operation.

Although surgery possibly saved Pepys's life and certainly spared him a good deal of pain, he was not entirely free of problems stemming from either the original disorder or the operation which had been performed to cure it. For the entire period covered by his diary, 1660–9, Pepys complained of a variety of related ills, ranging from pain and swelling of his 'cods', to difficulty in urination, to the actual passage of two stones in March 1665.[104] However, probably because of his fear of the pain he obviously had suffered before his operation, Pepys was unwilling to attribute any later symptoms to his earlier disease. Recurring tenderness and swelling of his testicles, combined with pain and difficulty in urination, he almost always attributed either to bruising or to taking cold.[105] Even when he actually passed two stones, he wrote 'I could feel them, and caused my water to be looked into, but without any pain to me in going out – which makes me think that it was not a fit of the stone at all'.[106] The following day he wrote 'I hope my disease of the stone may not return to me, but void itself in pissing'.[107]

This hope and the fear which accompanied it were never far from Pepys's mind. Indeed, he was even loath to use the words, 'the stone', instead referring to that disorder by implication. Thus, when he suffered from constant backache in June 1664, he wrote that he feared 'the worst'.[108] He was even apparently relieved, though mystified, when, in the following month, the physician Dr Burnett diagnosed an ulcer either in the kidneys or bladder.[109] He must have felt even better when in August Mr Holliard disagreed with this diagnosis, saying that the pain Pepys was suffering was 'nothing but cold in my legs breeding wind, and got only by my using to wear a gown'.[110]

Pepys suffered from another disorder which was probably unrelated to his urinary problems. This was the recurring colic, wind and constipation mentioned above. Although he complained of this disorder on and off throughout the 1660s, he suffered most acutely from it from September to December 1663. It gave him pain in his back and abdomen, and made it difficult for him to produce natural bowel movements. He also complained of pain in his cods and yard which resulted from 'straining to stool'.[111] As was the case with his urinary problems, Pepys worried a lot about this disorder, writing in October 1663, 'In no great pain, but do not think myself likely to be well till I have a freedom of stool and wind'.[112] Four days later he was able to report with pleasure that he had had his first natural bowel movement for five or six days.[113] Needless to say, he attributed none of his discomfort to the massive amount of physic he took during this illness.

Pepys had another relatively minor, though recurring, ailment. This was the swelling, redness and itching which attacked his whole body, mainly in cold weather. He first suffered from it in February 1663.[114] It not only made him feel ill, but also made him 'ashamed of myself to see myself so changed in my countenance'. Fortunately, on the first occasion, the 'itching and pimples' passed in two days. By the last time he experienced these symptoms, January 1665, Pepys was not particularly worried about them, writing 'and I find myself, as heretofore in cold weather, to begin to burn within and pimple and prick all over my body, my pores with cold being shut up'.[115]

Other diarists had illness profiles of their own, of course. Ralph Josselin's, Margaret Hoby's and Alice Thornton's will be discussed at length below. Some descriptions of symptoms are too brief and vague to be of use in compiling a medical biography. Other sources, like Dorothy Osborne's letters, Lady Margaret Clifford's diary and Roger Lowe's diary, are either too short, too intermittent, or too much devoted to other matters to yield much medical evidence.[116] Some diarists, such as John Evelyn, were remarkably healthy, suffering mainly from relatively minor common ailments.

Robert Hooke, whose physic-taking will be discussed at greater length below, presents a somewhat confusing picture. His multitudinous ailments can hardly be attributed to hypochondria. He was a chronically ailing child who, in his first seven years, ate only diary products and fruit, 'no flesh in the least agreeing with his weak constitution'.[117] As a teenager, Hooke was apprenticed to the portrait painter, Peter Lely, but had to leave this study because he could not stand the smell of paint.[118] Waller's description of his appearance as an adult suggests some form of physical illness or disability:

> As to his person he was but despicable, being very crooked, tho' I have heard from himself, and others, that he was straight till about 16 years of Age when he first grew awry, but frequent practicing, turning with a Turn-Lath, and the like incurvating Exercises, being but of a thin weak habit of body, which increased as he grew older, so as to be very remarkable at last: This made him but low of stature, tho' by his limbs he should have been moderately tall. He was always very pale and lean, and latterly nothing but skin and bone.[119]

However, Hooke almost never complained of specific illnesses, except for colds and minor stomach upsets. His most distressing symptoms were giddiness and sleeplessness, for which he dosed himself radically and experimented with various changes in diet. Indeed, one almost could argue that Hooke used his own body and its reactions as a kind of laboratory, testing a multitude of substances for their properties and the characteristics of his own responses to them over time. Thus, Hooke's contribution to this study will be very much in his role as patient rather than in his role as sufferer, although one cannot deny that he did suffer.[120]

Otherwise, Hooke's diary and the other sources consulted yield a good deal of miscellaneous information about the illness experiences of both the writers and the people who surrounded them. This information tends to support the evidence yielded by the London Bills of Mortality. For instance, the diarists mentioned a number of children who died young. Both John Evelyn and Sir Christopher Wren lost infants to convulsion fits.[121] Evelyn lost a 7-week-old baby to teeth and dropsy.[122] And both Evelyn and Ralph Josselin had children who were livergrown. Evelyn gave a useful description of this condition as it was diagnosed during an autopsy performed on the body of 5-year-old Richard:

> Being opened they found a membranous substance growing to the cavous part of the liver, somewhat near the edge of it for the compass of 3 inches, which ought not to be; for the liver is fixed only by three strong ligaments, all far distant from that part, insomuch as it could not move in that part; on which they confidently affirmed, the child was (as tis vulgarly called) liver-grown & thence that sickness & so frequent complaint of his side: & indeed both liver & spleen were exceedingly large.[123]

The spleen was apparently a disease most common among women and children.[124] The evidence of the diaries and correspondence consulted supports this observation. Lady Anne Clifford and Dorothy Osborne suffered from the spleen.[125] Lady Anne described her symptoms as a pain in her side; Dorothy Osborne's seem to have been mainly emotional and temperamental. Ralph Josselin's daughter Jane suffered from the same ailment.[126]

Only two of the diarists gave a personal account of undergoing a contagious disease. Alice Thornton and her family suffered multiple attacks of smallpox. John Evelyn contracted the disease while travelling in Switzerland in 1646.[127] His was a mild case, producing few spots and confining him to his chamber for only five weeks. However, it was both frightening and expensive. Evelyn paid his host forty-five pistoles of gold for lodging and nursing, his physician five pistoles for advice and medication.[128]

Although the other diarists escaped smallpox, at least during the periods in which they kept diaries, everyone knew someone who had had the disease. Several of Ralph Josselin's children caught it as teenagers, after becoming servants or apprentices in London.[129] And Hooke and Pepys frequently commented on the smallpox victims among their acquaintance.

Hooke's experience of the disease, although not personal, was intimate. A servant of his, Tom Gyles, died of smallpox after only three days of suffering.[130] Tom's attack was very acute. The day before he died he was both 'pissing blood' and bleeding at the nose and mouth – symptoms which his physicians interpreted as mortal.[131] Hooke's niece Grace also had a severe bout of smallpox while she was keeping house for him. She was ill for nearly three months during the summer of 1679.[132]

Although none of the diarists and correspondents or their

immediate family members suffered from plague, Samuel Pepys and John Evelyn wrote fascinating descriptions of plague-ridden London. These, along with Ralph Josselin's reflections on plague, will be incorporated into our discussion of ideas and attitudes regarding disease. The same use will be made of the diarists' references to syphilis. These diseases were powerful in name as well as in experience, affecting those they spared as well as those they attacked.

6

SUFFERERS AND PATIENTS: APPROACHES TO ILLNESS

The seventeenth-century English had two main approaches to illness, which, for the purposes of this study, will be called religious and secular. A subsidiary approach to illness, the magical approach, related to both secular and religious orientations, and will be described below. At the outset of this chapter, it should be emphasised that these three categories are employed largely because they provide a useful structure for discussion. Although they can be identified in seventeenth-century writing and behaviour, the categories are themselves somewhat anachronistic.

Secular and religious approaches to illness existed side by side. It was rare, if not unheard of, for any individual to be characterised by one approach to the exclusion of the other. The most secular people, Samuel Pepys for example, thanked God for their escapes from disease. Indeed, to divorce the divine from any aspect of human experience would have been an admission of atheism, a virtually incomprehensible position in seventeenth-century England. The pragmatic surgeon, Joseph Binns, whose career has been described above, acknowledged his debt to God by concluding the notes for a successful case with the words 'laus deo' or 'laus soli deo'.

By the same token, even the very religious, such as the Reverend Ralph Josselin, employed secular explanations and therapies in times of illness. Not to have done so would have been to disregard the gifts of God to mankind – to look a gift horse in the mouth, so to speak. None the less, the religious and secular approaches to illness can be distinguished in both the private papers (diaries and correspondence) and the published literature consulted. Medical behaviour depended to some extent upon the spiritual orientation of the sufferer.

The secular and religious approaches to illness did not necessarily operate in opposition to one another. For instance, it was generally agreed that God had the power both to inflict and to cure disease. It was also piously assumed that God had created certain medicinal substances and appointed certain healers (usually physicians) to help human beings battle illness.[1] This having been said, however, it should also be observed that the religious approach to illness favoured passive prayer and trust in God, while the secular approach was characterised by as active an attack as possible on the symptoms and causes of the illness.

Exemplifying the religious approach were the numerous books and pamphlets which might be called the literature of moral medicine. These works were intended for the use of laymen, who read them for both entertainment and instruction. Typical was Bishop Lancelot Andrewes's *A Sermon of the Pestilence*, which, although first preached in 1603, was published in 1636. While he paid lip-service to the knowledge and expertise of physicians, Andrewes argued that if the primary cause of illness – the wrath of God – be not dealt with, the other methods of dealing with it were bound to fail. In his own words,

> And as the Balm of Gilead, and the Physician there, may yield us help, when God's wrath is removed: so if it be not, no balm, no medicine will serve. Let us with the Woman in the Gospel [Mark 5, 26] spend all upon Physicians, we shall be never the better, till we come to Christ, and he cures us of our sins who is the only Physician of the diseases of the soul.

Andrewes's argument is well stated by the earlier secular writer, William Bullein, in his *A Dialogue against the Fever Pestilence*, published in 1578.[2] In this popular work the well-to-do Civis, after trying various remedies for his illness, realises he is dying. He says to his wife,

> Now my body is past cure, no Physic can prevail. . . . From henceforth . . . I shall be turned into a stinking carrion for worm's delight, dust, clay, rotten, most vile, forsaken of all men, poor without substance, naked without clothing, sown in dishonour, forgotten of my posterity, not known henceforth, vanish like a shadow, wither like a leaf, and fade as a flower.[3]

His wife wants to send for the physician, but Civis says,

> Help me into some house, whereas I might send for some man of God to be my heavenly Physician, teaching me the way to the Kingdom of Christ.[4]

Even works which were intended mainly to provide secular

information address quite seriously the religious issues involved. The well-known *The Anatomy of Melancholy*, by Robert Burton, first published in 1621, is one such book. Burton wrote that the general causes of illness were either supernatural or natural.

> Supernatural are from God and his angels, or, by God's permission, from the devil and his ministers. That God himself is a cause, for the punishment of sin, and satisfaction of his justice, many examples & testimonies of holy Scriptures make evident unto us.[5]

Although he advocated the consultation of physicians in cases of melancholy, Burton cautiously reminded readers that 'From Jove is our origin; we must first begin with prayer, and then use physick; not one without the other, but both together'.[6] He even suggested that physick might not work without prayer.[7]

The belief that God sent diseases in order to punish or educate human beings was pervasive. The many fast-days proclaimed by seventeenth-century parliaments were directed at propitiating divine wrath. God was capable of inflicting any sort of disaster. For instance, in January 1662 Pepys reported that Parliament had ordered a fast-day

> to pray for more seasonable weather – it having hitherto been some summer weather, that it is, both as to warmth and every other thing, just as if it were the middle of May or June, which doth threaten a plague (as all men think) to follow; for so it was almost the last winter, and the whole year after hath been a very sickly time, to this day.[8]

Any event out of the ordinary could be interpreted as an indication of divine displeasure. However, the most universally recognised weapon God employed was the plague.

It was generally agreed that plague was the result of human sin. Thus, the many pamphlets published during or immediately after plague years blamed mankind rather than God for the misery the epidemics produced. For instance, a pamphlet published in 1593 was entitled *An Approved Medicine Against the Deserved Plague.*[9] Its author wrote,

> And now my beloved, and important charge, I beseech you by the mercies of God, remember with me, there is no plague but for sin, and the Lion roareth not without his prey. We are now under this growing plague with others, let us repent effectually as others

> which truly seek the Lord, cast our sins from us, and draw the Lord's mercy to us.[10]

The tone of such writers did not change in the course of the following century. Richard Alleine's book, published in 1667, rejoiced in the lengthy title, *The Best of Remedies for the Worst of Maladies: or Spiritual Receipts and Antidotes for the Preservation of a Plague-Sick Sinfull Soul. Wherein is shown, sin is the Cause, and Repentence the Cure of the Pestilence. Seasonably published by a Lover of Peace and Truth: and one that desireth that all would (though the Lord's hand seems to be withdrawn, as to the late universally raging Pestilential Disease) forsake those Provoking sins, which call for Vengeance and Judgements on the Sons of Men.*

It is certainly not surprising that plague was identified as the Lord's preferred method of punishing collective sin. Although a great many remedies and preventatives existed for plague, nothing really helped. The disease was devastating in both the speed of its attack and the effects it produced. Not only did it kill, but also it completely disrupted social, economic and political life. The wealthy, including many in positions of authority and responsibility, fled before it. This group included both medical personnel and clergymen who might have been most useful in comforting and helping those who had to remain within striking distance of the plague. Shops were shut, church services forbidden, Parliament suspended.

Samuel Pepys wrote such excellent descriptions of plague-ridden London that they are worth quoting at length. In June 1665 he wrote,

> This day, much against my will, I did in Drury Lane see two or three houses marked with a red cross upon the doors and 'Lord have mercy upon us' writ there – which was a sad sight to me, being the first of that kind that to my remembrance I ever saw. It put me into an ill conception of myself and my smell, so that I was forced to buy some roll tobacco to smell to and chaw – which took away the apprehension.[11]

By early August he reported, 'The streets mighty empty all the way now, even in London, which is a sad sight'.[12] On 22 August he wrote,

> I went away and walked to Greenwich, in my way seeing a coffin with a dead body therein, dead of the plague, lying in an open close . . . which was carried out last night and the parish hath not appointed anybody to bury it – but only set a watch there day and night, that nobody should go thither or come thence, which is a

> most cruel thing – this disease making us more cruel to one another then we are [to] dogs.[13]

On 20 September:

> But Lord, what a sad time it is, to see no boats upon the River – and grass grow all up and down Whitehall-Court – and nobody but poor wretches in the streets.[14]

And finally, on 16 October:

> But Lord, how empty the streets are, and melancholy, so many poor sick people in the streets, full of sores, and so many sad stories overheard as I walk, everybody talking of this dead, and that man sick, and so many in this place, and so many in that. And they tell me that in Westminster there is never a physician, and but one apothecary left, all being dead – but that there are great hopes of a great decrease this week: God send it.[15]

The plague did not actually abate until mid-winter.

Pepys was unusual for one of his class and wide social contacts in that he stayed in London throughout the period of the epidemic. He sent his wife and servants to Woolwich, however, to put them beyond reach of contagion. Evelyn sent his family to Wotton to his brother's home. Like Pepys, he spent some time in London on official business, but did not concern himself as much as Pepys did with the havoc the plague was causing in the city. He seems mainly to have observed the misery when it was thrust upon him, writing in October 1665,

> I returned to London: I went through the whole City, having occasion to alight out of the Coach in several places about business of money, when I was environed with multitudes of poor pestiferous creatures, begging alms; the shops universally shut up, a dreadful prospect.[16]

Both Pepys and Evelyn obviously felt that the plague epidemic was a lottery. Both knew of people in high places who had died of the disease, and by no means felt confident about escaping it themselves. Evelyn reported that he had a fainting fit while dining with his brother, 'which much alarmed the family, as well it might, I coming so lately from infected places, but I bless God it went off'.[17] Pepys took several preventatives, including the tobacco mentioned above, Venice Treacle and plague water given him by Lady Carteret, hoping to ward off infection.[18] When his servant Will had to take to his bed with a headache, Pepys was in 'extraordinary fear'.[19]

However much Pepys and Evelyn feared the plague, others feared it more. Pepys's surgeon, Mr Holliard, and his minister, Mr Mills, both left London. Mr Mills had apparently left 'the parish before anybody went and now [stayed] till all are come home'.[20] Pepys's physician, Dr Burnett, might have gone as well, but Burnett was confined to his house early in the epidemic because one of his servants contracted plague. The physician died of the disease in August, shortly after his house was reopened.[21] London physicians left the city in great numbers and felt defensive about their behaviour later. Pepys reported that, at the first meeting of the Royal Society after the worst of the epidemic had ended, Dr Goddard (Robert Hooke's physician) defended the physicians' actions, 'saying that their particular patients were most gone out of town, and they left at liberty – and a great deal more, etc'.[22]

Fear of the 1665 plague was not confined to London and its vicinity. Ralph Josselin, although living in the relatively safe village of Earls Colne, Essex, was terrified of the plague. His fear, which will be discussed at length in another chapter, arose from his conviction that the plague was God's supreme punishment for sin.[23] Such collective punishment resulted from collective sin. To appease God's anger, collective repentance was required. Josselin felt that his village was very sinful, and that the total repentance both he and the Lord required was not forthcoming. He was amazed that, with the exception of one or two cases, the village was spared.[24]

Josselin's might be said to exemplify the religious approach to illness. Although he used conventional remedies for his many ailments, he almost never consulted healers. The only medicine he really trusted was prayer. Perhaps the reason he was less frightened of non-epidemic than he was of epidemic disorders was that he believed his prayers and those of his family would act as spiritual preventative medicine. Most certainly he believed that the illnesses and deaths of members of his family directly resulted from specific sins – usually his own. And even when 'secular' causes of ailments could be identified – cold weather producing a cold, for instance – Josselin might well have asked who sent the cold weather? The answer is obvious.

Josselin's faith supported him through long illnesses. These he could regard either as God's punishment or God's test of his faith. Even at one point in his life when he felt a bit out of touch with his heavenly Father – a feeling he described as a spiritual deadness – he never felt that re-establishment of contact was impossible. He simply continued to pray. His faith also helped him in times of bereavement. When his well-beloved daughter Mary lay dying at the age of 8, Josselin was able to write 'fear came on my heart very much, but she is not mine, but the Lord's'.[25] And even when a sick child did not die, Josselin frequently resigned him or her to God. He also saw the manifestations of certain diseases as symptomatic of the human spiritual condition, writing when his son Tom had smallpox, 'Tom's pox came out after a treacle posset. At night they began to run, oh that the inward filth and corruption of our heart might be drawn out'.[26]

For Josselin, all events were related to the providence of God. He wrote in 1658, 'One Dorothy Layer, being got with child by a weaver, afterwards was married to him, and delivered before her time, and died. God make such things to be warning to us'.[27] And in 1657 he wrote, rather smugly, 'it was no small mercy in my eyes that when agues and fevers as formerly the smallpox stepped in at many doors God preserved me and mine'.[28]

Josselin's viewpoint and medical behaviour certainly was reflected elsewhere in the population. The Lancashire mercer, Roger Lowe, was frequently called upon to pray with ailing neighbours who, like himself, were Presbyterians.[29] However, Josselin's dependence on prayer as the best physic was not typical even of other very religious people. The pious Lady Margaret Hoby, whose diary was written essentially as a spiritual record for the years 1599–1605, took physic, consulted healers, and even acted as an unlicensed general practitioner for people living in her remote area of Yorkshire. And Josselin's contemporary, the Reverend John Ward, served as both minister and physician in Stratford-upon-Avon from 1662 to 1681.[30] Thus, it must be emphasised that it is impossible to generalise about medical behaviour in the period, or even to assume a certain type of behaviour on the basis of knowledge of an individual's religious and occupational profile. Individual character, or humour, was, one suspects, a major factor determining behaviour in times of illness.

Distinctions made between 'religious' and 'superstitious' approaches to illness are invidious. Other terms must be found. None the less, since people living in seventeenth-century England themselves distinguished between 'lawful' religious practices and 'unlawful' practices smacking of witchcraft, demonianism, heresy or 'popishness', it would be improper to omit these practices, as they related to medicine, from our discussion.

None of the lay diaries or collections of correspondence examined in the course of this study described personal consultations of magical healers. However, these sources do yield evidence of practices at least related to magical beliefs. For instance, Samuel Pepys felt that his 'very perfect good health' in March 1665 was due to a combination of keeping his back cool, taking a turpentine pill every morning and carrying a hare's foot.[31] He also described the apparently usual practice of putting pigeons to the feet of a dying person.[32] Robert Hooke recorded numerous successful cures produced by unorthodox means. Perhaps most remarkable was the case in which Sir Christopher Wren cured his wife of a thrush 'by hanging a bag of live boglice around her neck'.[33] A patient of the London surgeon, Joseph Binns, did not find ease from a facial burn until she had stroked her scarred eyelid with 'a dead hand'.[34] And the physician Francis Herring wrote *A Modest Defence of the Caveat Given to the Wearers of impoisoned Amulets as preservatives from the plague* (1604), in which he advanced no objection to the wearing of amulets, provided that wearers did not neglect internal preventative medicines.

Certain medicinal substances routinely sold by apothecaries were valuable partly because of their inherent magical properties. One such substance was mummy – literally bits or powder of mummified human bodies. Pepys reported having seen a mummy in a merchant's warehouse:

> all the middle of the man or woman's body black and hard; I never saw any before, and therefore pleased me much, though an ill sight; and he did give me a little bit, and a bone of an arm I suppose.[35]

Another frequently used substance was human or animal excrement. The man-midwife Percival Willughby believed 'that an ass's hoof, or dung, put on coals, and the fume received under the labouring woman's clothes, will draw forth the child'.[36]

Such remedies, along with many others, were used by magical healers, in conjunction with rituals designed to relieve the sufferer.[37] Although not as frequently resorted to as the remedies themselves, these healers were apparently widely consulted. John Cotta, whose anti-quack writings have been referred to above, was thinking of magical practitioners in addition to other unauthorised healers when he maintained,

> So many and so infinitely do the numbers of barberous and unlearned counsellors of health at this time overspread all corners of this Kingdom, that their confused swarms do not only everywhere cover and eclipse the sun-shine of all true learning & understanding but generally darken and extinguish the very light of common sense and reason.[38]

And the licentiate in physic and surgery, Edward Poeton, wrote,

> So then, . . . it is not to be held a thing to be either new or strange that white witches should find so many friends and favourers (as now they do) in this last corrupt age of the world, in the which most men mind earthly things.[39]

Those who attacked magical healers did not usually argue that magical methods could not cure. Indeed, reserving their scepticism for those who knowingly pretended magical powers, most writers assumed that magic *could* cure. Robert Burton argued,

> Many famous cures are daily done in this kind, the Devil is an expert Physician . . . and God permits oftentimes these Witches and Magicians to produce such effects. . . . Such cures may be done, and, as Paracelsus stiffly maintains, they cannot otherwise be cured but by spells, seals, and spiritual physick.[40]

And Burton went on to state the case:

> It being assumed that they can effect such cures, the main question is whether it be lawful in a desperate case to crave their help, or a Wizard's advice. 'Tis a common practice of some men to go first to a witch, and then to a Physician; if one cannot, the other shall; if they cannot bend Heaven, they will try Hell. It matters not, saith Paracelsus, whether it be God or the Devil, Angels of unclean Spirits cure him, so that he be eased.[41]

However, regardless of the relief magical healers can bring,

> *Evil is not to be done that good may come of it.* Much better it were for such patients, that are so troubled, to endure a little misery in this life than to hazard their soul's health for ever, and . . . much better to die than be so cured.[42]

The belief that magic could cure was crucial. On the basis of this belief it was possible for people to consult and praise the white witch, wise-man or -woman, and cunning-man or -woman, while condemning the activities of witches practising harmful black magic. Thus, Poeton's character Gregory, speaking for all of 'the giddy headed vulgar', argues that, as cunning-folk get their skill from God, it is no sin to consult them.[43] Gregory and his living counterparts were willing to risk divine displeasure (if, as they doubted, God actually disapproved of white magic) in order to obtain cures.

In discussing 'magical' cures, it must not be forgotten that seventeenth-century sufferers made no artificial distinction between such remedies and the supposedly rational remedies listed in the *London Pharmacopoeia*.[44] As Keith Thomas points out, 'From the patient's point of view . . . , all medical prescriptions beyond his comprehension were in a sense magical, since they worked by occult means'.[45] Indeed, the same holds true today. How many in our 'enlightened' age can give a rational explanation of how aspirin relieves headaches? Thus, this categorisation of 'religious', 'magical' and 'secular' approaches to illness is employed merely for the sake of convenience. At best, it overemphasises a reality which existed; at worst, it gives a false impression by anachronistically exaggerating elements of belief and behaviour.

Virtually everyone in seventeenth-century England had a humoral view of the human body, health and illness. This generalisation covers those who employed magical healing techniques, those with an essentially religious approach to the causes and cures of illness, those adhering to academic orthodox medical theories and those espousing relatively new schools of medical thought, such as Paracelsians, Van Helmontians, iatro-chemists and iatro-mechanists.[46] Popular humoralism showed itself in many ways. It acted as a basis for describing physical appearance and behaviour. For instance, John Evelyn described his father as

> of a sanguine complexion, mix'd with a dash of choler. . . . He was for his life so exact and temperate, that I have heard he had never in all his life been surprised by excess, being ascetic and sparing.[47]

Humoralism was also evident in prophylactic and remedial therapeutics, which were directed at producing evacuation, whatever the intellectual orientations of the prescriber and the patient. Regardless of whether treatment actually cured disease, its importance cannot be underrated. Proper application of therapy might, for instance, prevent a relatively minor disorder from becoming worse. For instance, Evelyn was bled in the early stages of smallpox – a procedure usually not advised under those conditions. Evelyn's physician excused himself later by telling Evelyn that his blood 'was so burnt and vitious, as it would have proved the plague or spotted fever, had he proceeded by any other method'.[48]

Popular humoralism dovetailed nicely with popular astrology, which helped to explain variations in health and illness phenomena from person to person and time to time. Evelyn, for instance, was referring to his astrological profile when he noted the exact time of his birth – twenty past two a.m., Tuesday, 21 October 1620.[49] Astrology also was used to establish medical routines. It determined when medical herbs should be planted, harvested and prescribed. It also determined when particular individuals should undergo various types of treatment.[50] For example, astrology was responsible for the tradition of taking prophylactic physic in the spring.[51]

The humoral/astrological approach provided a satisfactory basis for the explanation and treatment of illness which was not successfully challenged on the popular level until the nineteenth century. It related the individual to the natural universe as well as co-ordinating the multitudinous parts of the human body into a comprehensive whole. It also opted out of religious controversy by allowing for the existence of the soul at the individual end of the spectrum and God as prime-mover at the universal end.

Thus, seventeenth-century sufferers could be far more confident about explaining their ailments than can their twentieth-century descendants. Pepys, for example, always knew the causes of his various aches and pains. More often than not, the culprit was cold. Thus, in November 1662 he developed 'some pain in making water, having taken cold this morning in staying too long barelegged to pare my corns'.[52] In September 1665, while visiting his wife in lodgings in Woolwich, where she was staying in order to avoid the plague, Pepys reported

> And so I to bed, and in the night was mightily troubled with a looseness (I suppose from some fresh damp Linen that I put on this night); and feeling for a chamber pot, there was none . . . ; so I was forced in this strange house to rise and shit in the chimney twice.[53]

According to Pepys, he was nearly always responsible for his own disorders. One might suppose that this gave rise to a good deal of guilt. However, it also allowed the hope that proper behaviour would produce health. In October 1663, when Pepys was recovering from a period of constipation and colic, he resolved upon a 'regiment of health' which he was sure would prevent recurrence:

> 1. To begin to keep myself warm as I can.
> 2. Strain as little as ever I can backwards, remembering that my pain [in penis and testicles] will come by and by, though in the very straining I do not feel it.
> 3. Either by physic forward or by clyster backward, or both ways, to get an easy and plentiful going to stool and breaking of wind.
> 4. To begin to suspect my health immediately when I begin to become costive and bound, and by all means to keep my body loose, and that to obtain presently after I find myself going to the contrary.[54]

This was but one of Pepys's good resolutions, taken to maintain or improve his health. He frequently vowed to give up drinking wine, to stop going to plays and, when his eyes began to fail, to stop reading by candle-light. However, Pepys was one of the best intentioned, but worst disciplined of men. Temptation always mastered him.

Robert Hooke also was confident about the causes of his own symptoms. For instance, he caught cold in August 1676 by wearing a new velvet coat and cloth breeches.[55] In December 1672 he complained of giddiness resulting partly from 'drinking milk and posset drink at night and partly from coldness of peruke'.[56] Like Pepys, Hooke made many resolutions designed to improve his health. His resolutions usually took the form of either deciding to take or give up a certain substance, such as chocolate, whey or tobacco, or resolving to give up all other employments in order to concentrate on his health.

The confidence Pepys, Hooke and other diarists displayed about the diagnoses and explanation of their own ailments resulted in the conviction that they, as individuals, were responsible for their illnesses in all senses of the word. In this they were quite typical. Seventeenth-century English men and women owned their own disorders. Even when they consulted healers, they reserved the option to accept, dictate or reject the therapies offered.

Their confidence was sometimes supported by the reading

of medical works. Indeed, much of the vernacular medical literature was specifically directed at lay-men. Many home-medicine and first aid handbooks were designed to help those who lived in remote areas or could not afford the services of physicians and surgeons.[57] Equally important were the many 'regiments of health', designed to help the reader prevent disease by establishing healthy living habits.[58] Other works, such as almanacks, cookbooks and gardening manuals, gave medical advice and recipes in addition to other information.

As Paul Slack points out in a recent article, one must be cautious in making assumptions about the extent to which these books were read or their ideas disseminated. He writes, 'Such works can scarcely have reached the illiterate poor, and the extent of the diffusion even among the literate may well be questioned'.[59] None the less, the hundreds of works giving medical information which were published in English make possible the tentative assumptions that there was a market for this sort of literature and that the ideas so vended influenced medical behaviour.

Certainly seventeenth-century diarists confirm this assumption. It is no surprise that Robert Hooke, who took an MD in 1691, read a number of medical works.[60] Lady Margaret Hoby had read Turner's *Herbal* and Bartholomew Vigo as part of her general education.[61] Grace Sherrington, born in 1552, read daily from her 'Herball and books of physick'.[62] And Ralph Josselin read two medical books in the year 1649.[63]

Seventeenth-century plays reveal both a considerable amount of medical knowledge and the assumption that their medical allusions and metaphors would be appreciated by their audiences. For instance, Beaumont and Fletcher lampooned both the practice of uroscopy and physicians who used it. Three physicians made three diagnoses from one flask of urine, thus:

1 Physician. A plurisie, I see it.
2 Physician. I rather hold it
For tumour cordis.
3 Physician. Do you mark the faeces?
'Tis a most pestilent contagious fever,
A surfeit, a plaguey surfeit; he must bleed.
1 Physician. By no means.
3 Physician. I say bleed.
1 Physician. I say 'tis dangerous;
The person being spent so much before-hand,

And nature drawn so low, clysters, cool clysters.
2 Physician. Now with your favours I should think a vomit:
For take away the cause, and the effect must follow,
The stomach's foul and fur'd, the pot's unflam'd yet.
3 Physician. No, no, we'll rectifie that part by mild means,
Nature so sunk must find no violence.[64]

People used the medical knowledge they gathered from their reading and from oral tradition to treat themselves, their family members, and their friends and acquaintances. Self-treatment was surely the most common type of medical therapy in seventeenth-century England. The diaries and collections of correspondence consulted are replete with examples of self-diagnosis. For instance, although most physicians no longer used uroscopy for the purposes of diagnosis by the mid-seventeenth century, many lay-men examined their own urine. Josselin, Pepys and Hooke all described characteristics of their 'water' in times of illness.[65]

People also prescribed for themselves. The remedies used were sometimes purchased at apothecaries' shops which, of course, laboured under no restrictions regarding prescription versus non-prescription drugs. In addition, many people, particularly women, made their own medicines. Dorothy Osborne dosed both herself and William Temple for colds with an unspecified medicine she had prepared herself:

> 'tis like the rest of my medicines, if it do no good 'twill be sure to do no harm, and 'twill be no great trouble to you to eat a little on't now and then, for the taste, as it is not Excellent, so 'tis not very ill.[66]

And Samuel Pepys usually tried to cure himself before consulting a healer. For instance, when he suffered from a combination of wind and difficulty in urination in July 1666, he took a clyster of sack and a coach ride, hoping to find relief.[67]

Undoubtedly Robert Hooke was the great seventeenth-century medicine-taker. Indeed, his diary gives the impression that Hooke considered many types of human activity, including eating, drinking, sleeping, dressing, exercise and orgasm, almost entirely in the light of their medical effects.

Thus, in examining his diary, it is difficult to determine where medicine-taking stopped and simple dining or snacking, for instance, began. As indicated above, aside from occasional colds, Hooke suffered from few of what his contemporaries would have recognised as diseases. Rather, he complained of recurring symptoms, including sleeplessness, indigestion, giddiness, loss of sense of smell, a noise in his head, an evil taste in his mouth and headaches. To prevent and cure these symptoms, he took a massive amount of medicine. Indeed, it is tempting to suggest, rather snidely, that most of his ailments were caused by Hooke's efforts to find health.

Hooke tended to give each new remedy a trial period. When he started writing his diary in August 1672, he had been drinking an iron and mercury preparation for a while. He then moved on to a steel drink. After that for a time he depended almost entirely on Dulwich water, taken from a natural spring at that location which was, 'at that time a pleasant hamlet 5 miles from London . . . , famous for its medicinal waters'.[68] He also used a preparation called Andrew's cordial for a long time, took Dr Goddard's tincture of centaury, swallowed Aldersgate cordial, drank senna and jalap in various liquids, took sal tartari and sal amoniac, and used a Mexican jalap called mechoacan. All of these remedies were expected to purge him. In addition, he took a variety of emetics. When these did not produce the desired vomits, he employed either a feather or a whalebone. To help him sleep, he took opiates. He bathed an aching shoulder with aqua vitae. He also was blistered, cupped and scarified by the healers he consulted.

In addition to taking medicine, Hooke deliberately experimented with substances not universally considered medicinal. For long periods he drank great quantities of chocolate, coffee, tea, whey, burnt claret and 'malago' wine. He smoked tobacco on and off. He ate stewed prunes and cherries. He also drank a diet drink recommended by a friend's wife, which he called 'Tillotson's ale'.

Hooke recorded the effects of both the measures he took to obtain health and the incidental behaviour which produced results. He frequently reported whether the food he ate digested well. Indeed, both the food he ate and the conditions under which he ate it were significant. Thus, on 19 March 1677, when his dinner digested well, Hooke wrote:

> I judge somewhat to be attributed to change of air, partly to a pleasant small beer, possibly to the warmer weather, possibly to my drinking ale with toast and cheese in the morning.[69]

Indeed, he was supremely confident in his interpretations of how various foods affected him. For instance, on one occasion rice pudding caused him to sleep badly.[70] Another time, he drank 'malago', which made him sick, then drank chocolate, which 'cleared his stomach'.[71]

Hooke was equally certain about the effects of the remedies he took. Most often, they 'wrought well'. Sometimes, they did not produce the desired purge or vomit and, by remaining in his stomach, caused discomfort. For instance, on 20 July 1673 he 'drank Dulwich', then 'slept ill, the water lying still in my belly, not so well next morning as last week'.[72]

Hooke's certainty about which substances caused which reactions gave rise to some complicated record-keeping. One powerful substance could produce many results. On 27 April 1674 Hooke 'took Dr. Thomson's vomit. It vomited twice. Purged 10 or 12 times. . . . Made me sleep ill, and made my arms paralytic with a great noise in my head. I had also some gnawing at the bottom of my belly'.[73] By the same token, several substances produced contrary results. On 16 February 1673 Hooke took Andrew's cordial, which purged him and

> brought much slime out of the guts and made me cheerful. Eat Dinner with good stomach and pannado at night but drinking posset upon it put me into a feverish sweat which made me sleep very unquiet and much disturbed my head and stomach. Taking sneezing tobacco about 3 in the morn clear my head much and made me cheerful afterwards I slept about 2 hours, but my head was disturbed when I waked.[74]

As one might expect, Hooke occasionally became infatuated with a new remedy. In midsummer 1675 he began to take spirit of sal amoniac. On 31 July he reported, 'In a new world with new medicine'.[75] The following day he wrote, 'This is certainly a great Discovery in physic. I hope that this will dissolve that viscous slime that hath so much tormented me in my stomach and guts'.[76] None the less, Hooke stopped taking 'SSA' soon thereafter, perhaps having discovered an unpleasant effect which he failed to record.

It is apparent that all of the medicines Hooke took failed to make him a healthy man. However, this failure did not cause Hooke to lose his faith in medicine. Indeed, the question of whether or not a remedy 'worked' was understood very differently by Hooke and his contemporaries than it would be by a twentieth-century sufferer. The seventeenth-century medicine-taker expected a preparation to show its strength by producing an immediate result – usually in the form of multiple bowel movements or vomits. Thus, the fact that a remedy 'wrought well' had nothing to do with whether or not it cured the sufferer's symptoms. Indeed, prophylactic medicine was expected to 'work' in the absence of illness.

In addition, medicine was not expected to make the taker feel good. While Hooke occasionally reported feeling relief after vomiting, for instance, the reader is reminded of the dubious pleasure of hitting yourself over the head with a hammer because it is so nice when you stop. Physic-taking confined the sufferer to his or her chamber until the effects of the physic had passed. Woe to the individual who left home prematurely; the public lavatory had yet to be invented. For instance, Samuel Pepys reported taking Lady Paulina Montagu, his patron's daughter, to a play in April 1662.

> In the middle of the play, my Lady Paulina, who had taken physic this morning, had need to go forth; and so I took the poor lady out and carried her to the Grange [a nearby inn], and there sent the maid of the house into a room to her, and she did what she had a mind to. And so back again to the play.[77]

In addition, most medicines tasted foul. Dorothy Osborne commented on the popular 'steel drink',

> I drink your [William Temple's] health every morning in a drench that would poison a horse, I believe, and 'tis the only way I have to persuade myself to take it, 'tis the infusion of steel, and makes me so horridly sick that every day at ten o'clock I am making my will, and taking leave of all my friends.[78]

Indeed, physic-taking could produce a worse effect than minor inconvenience. Ralph Josselin's only living children, Thomas and Jane, became 'sick even to death' when given prophylactic medicine in June 1650.[79]

None the less, the seventeenth-century English were enthusiastic medicine-takers. They patronised the shops of apothecaries, who grew prosperous and powerful because of their enthusiasm. They made their own remedies. They imported exotic substances from newly explored continents. And they eagerly took the products distilled by those relative newcomers to the medical scene, the chemists.

People also drank and bathed in the waters of the many natural springs around which fashionable spas had grown up. Hooke drank Dulwich and Epsom waters. The pleasure-loving Pepys visited Epsom and Bath, partly to take the waters and partly to amuse himself.[80] About one visit to Epsom, he wrote,

> I met many that I knew; and we drunk each of us two pots and so walked away – it being very pleasant to see how everybody turns up his tail, here one and there another, in a bush, and the Women in their Quarters the like.[81]

Mary Evelyn, Dorothy Osborne and Ralph Josselin also visited such spas.[82]

In addition to taking internal medicines, people underwent surgical procedures for both prophylactic and curative purposes. Phlebotomy was common, although some sufferers apparently thought more highly of it than others. John Evelyn was frequently let blood. For instance, in June 1651 he was let ten ounces of blood for a sore throat; in July of the same year he was let blood for haemorrhoids; in March 1652 he was let nine ounces of blood for 'a swelling in my throat and neck, which fore-ran the piles'.[83] Samuel Pepys was less attracted to phlebotomy, but occasionally underwent the procedure. In July 1668, for instance, he was let fourteen ounces of blood, 'towards curing my eyes'.[84]

Phlebotomy, like medicine-taking, was at best an unpleasant business. After Pepys was let sixteen ounces of blood in April 1662, his arm became so sore that he had to stay home from work the next day. At worst, blood-letting could be very dangerous. Joseph Binns reported several cases of phlebotomy which went disastrously wrong. At least two patients developed gangrene after being let blood from the arm.[85]

Other routine procedures could also be dangerous. Pepys and Hooke took many clysters without suffering any harm. However, Binns reported a case where the unskilful manoeuvring of a clyster pipe resulted in a patient's death.[86] Issues became infected, blisters burned.

Although many surgical procedures required a skilled hand, it should be emphasised that the patient (or consumer of medical services) was often in control of what sort of procedure was done and when it was administered. For instance, John Evelyn 'caused' an issue to be made in the neck of his 1-month-old son when the baby was suffering from convulsions.[87] Pepys sought out the surgeon, Mr Holliard, when he felt he should be let blood.[88] In this respect, surgeons and their assistants were in much the same category as the barbers whom people paid to draw aching teeth. Instead of acting as authorities, they were often employed as skilled craftsmen.

Medical decisions, then, were often made by the sufferer him- or herself. They were also made by parents for their children. We will discuss the Josselins' approach to childhood disorders below. Perhaps one reason for parental decisiveness in times of illness or accident was that no one else could be counted on for help. This was certainly the case when John Evelyn helped extract a bone from his 2-year-old son Richard's throat. The boy had choked while eating broth. The maid who had been looking after the child had fainted. There was 'no chirurgeon near'. Evelyn held 'its head down, incite[d] it to vomit. . . . It pleased God, that on the sudden effort & as it were struggling his last for life, he cast forth a bone . . . I gave the child some Lucotellus Balsame, for his throat was much excoriated'.[89]

In addition to self-treatment, people sought medical help from relatives, friends and neighbours. As indicated above, Lady Margaret Hoby acted as an informal, unpaid general practitioner for her neighbours and friends. Her midwifery and surgical skills were most frequently required. She attended the confinements of neighbours and relatives and dressed wounds. Indeed, in the year 1600, she made thirty-two references to 'dressing patients'. She sometimes had more than one patient at a time. For example, on 10 February 1600 she 'dressed her patients' in the morning, then 'dressed other poor folks' in the afternoon.[90]

Although most gentlewomen had neither the interest nor the time Lady Hoby expended on medical pursuits, proficiency in medical matters was expected of them. Lady Anne Clifford's mother had been 'a distiller of medicinal waters, a dabbler in alchemy, an expert in the properties of plants, flowers and herbs'.[91] Ralph Josselin's neighbour, Lady Honeywood, frequently offered medical advice and help to members of the Josselin family.[92] Jane Josselin returned the favour on one occasion by helping with the Honeywoods' sick child.[93] More frequently she treated the ailments of family members and attended the confinements of her daughters and neighbours.[94]

Samuel Pepys occasionally followed the medical advice given him by friends and other lay-people. When he suffered from itching, swelling and burning in February 1663, Sir J. Mennes

> would not have me take anything from the apothecary, but from

> him, his Venice Treakle being better than the others; which I did consent to and did anon take and fell into a great sweat; and about 10 or 11 o'clock came out of it, and shifted myself and slept pretty well . . . and in the morning, most of my disease, that is, itching and pimples, was gone.[95]

When Pepys had a bad attack of colic and wind in October 1663, Mennes and another colleague, Sir W. Batten, advised him to take juniper water, 'and Sir W. Batten sent to his lady for some for me'.[96]

Experience of a certain ailment gave the sufferer a certain expertise in it. For instance, when Dorothy Osborne had ague in April 1653, she wrote

> it is impossible I should keep it long for here is my eldest brother and my Cousin Molle and two or three more of them that have great understanding in Agues as People that have been long acquainted with them and they do so tutor and govern me that I am neither to eat drink nor sleep without their leave, and sure my obedience deserves they should cure me or else they are great tyrants to very little purpose.[97]

However, a person need not have suffered a disorder to be interested in its treatment.

Robert Hooke seems to have collected bits of medical advice and recipes the way some people collect stamps. Some of the advice was obviously not intended for him. For instance, he recorded one Mr Middleton's remedy for rattlesnake bite.[98] However, more often the advice concerned ailments Hooke suffered from himself. For instance, Mrs Tillotson gave him the recipe for a 'physic ale' which he drank with apparently good results for quite a while.[99] He did not try the recipe told him by a woman who cured vertigo with 'stone horse dung'.[100]

In addition to self-treatment and treatment given by friends and acquaintances, the diarists consulted healers. Some of these were unlicensed. Hooke, for instance, drank 'Mountebank's drink', presumably purchased from a mountebank.[101] Most of the healers referred to, however, were recognised physicians and surgeons.

Ralph Josselin consulted physicians and surgeons most rarely of all the diarists referred to in this study.[102] He summoned a physician to a child's death-bed only once.[103] He consulted physicians and surgeons fewer than ten times during the forty-year period covered by his diary.

Samuel Pepys, John Evelyn and Robert Hooke, on the other hand, routinely consulted physicians and surgeons. However, their medical behaviour was not necessarily as 'modern' as it appears to be. Evelyn seems to have used the services of healers rather as he employed servants. He praised the good ones he consulted and despised those who were apparently more inept. He very often directed the activities of his medical attendants and does not seem to have paid them very well.[104] Beginning in the late 1650s, most of his physicians were acquaintances of his; after 1660, fellow members of the Royal Society. However, Evelyn still consulted *with* them, possibly considering his own medical judgment to be as reliable as theirs.

His confidence and superiority stemmed partly from his university education and elevated socio-economic status, partly from his own medical interests and observations. During his travels on the continent in the 1640s, Evelyn visited several hospitals, herb gardens and medical schools.[105] In the 'Hospital of the Charity' in Paris, he saw five people cut for the stone on the same day.[106] And in 1672 he observed the amputation of a sailor's gangrened leg.[107] He apparently also watched the autopsy which was performed on his 5-year-old son.[108]

Like Evelyn, both Pepys and Hooke had interest in and knowledge of medical subjects which ranged beyond those of their contemporaries. As indicated above, Pepys attended lectures at Surgeon's Hall and Hooke eventually took an MD. Both men numbered many surgeons and physicians among their acquaintance. The medical men they consulted were also friends of theirs.[109] Thus, their consultation of licensed healers may be viewed as being similar to their uncritical acceptance of medical advice from 'lay' friends. Only once did Pepys refer to his own attitude toward his medical attendants. This was at least partly in fun. When in September 1665 he drank some 'strong drink', he wrote that he was

> fain to allow myself [this pleasure], by advice of all and not contrary to my oath, my physician being dead and chyrurgeon out of the way whose advice I am obliged to take.[110]

Indeed, on the one occasion when Pepys consulted both his physician, Dr Burnett, and his surgeon, Mr Holliard, about the same condition, his healers disagreed about the diagnosis. Burnett felt that Pepys's back pain and difficulty in urination was due to an ulcer in his bladder or kidneys.[111] Holliard first diagnosed it as a return of Pepys's old complaint of the stone.[112] However, later he decided that it was merely wind, and that Pepys had no ulcers.[113]

A similar, but more disturbing, disagreement occurred when Pepys's brother Tom lay dying. Tom's 'doctor, Mr. Powell' diagnosed the pox. Samuel called another physician, Dr Wiverly, who denied that Tom had syphilis. To relieve his own mind, Samuel and Dr Wiverly 'searched my brother again at his privities, where he was as clean as ever he was born'. Wiverly told Powell that 'he should cease to report any such thing', and Samuel Pepys 'threatened him that I would have satisfaction if I heard any more such discourse'.[114] Such was the evil reputation attached to syphilis that Samuel wrote, 'The shame of this very thing, I confess, troubles me as much as anything'.[115]

It is not surprising that Pepys, Hooke and others 'shopped around' for medical advice. The quality of medical care varied. Pepys was fortunate in coming into contact with two skilful practitioners – Mr Holliard, who had removed his bladder stone in 1658 and was still treating him eleven years later; and Dr Williams, who twice successfully treated Elizabeth Pepys for her genital abscesses.[116] Pepys's experience with Dr Burnett was less rewarding. Perhaps it is significant that he did not consult another physician in the four years between Burnett's death and the close of his diary. His respect for physicians was certainly not increased by his observation of their behaviour during the 1665 plague.

Although Hooke consulted the physicians, Goddard and Cox, and the surgeon, Gidly, he seems mainly to have patronised apothecaries' shops. He compared the products of various apothecaries and made his own evaluations of them. For instance, on 30 May 1674 he bought two vomits, one each from the apothecaries Witchcot and Child.[117] Child's vomit, taken 31 May, 'wrought well' at the time, but did him 'much harm' the following day. Witchcot's vomit, taken 5 August, made him worse.[118] Hooke attached no more weight to the medicines prescribed by his physicians than he did to remedies recommended by acquaintances or purchased from apothecaries' shops. His approach to medication was truly Baconian.

Indeed, one can say about both Hooke and Pepys that each was essentially empirical about medical treatment. A good result was more important than fashion or the dictates of medical authorities. It is not possible to make the same observation about the other diarists and correspondents. As we have seen, Dorothy Osborne carried on taking the steel drink, upon the advice of her physician, even though it tasted nasty and made her sick. She hoped it would do her good. And Lady Margaret Hoby mainly took prophylactic physic, which made her feel unwell.[119] The remedies she took when ill did not usually do her much good. The young mercer, Roger Lowe, was rarely ill. When he did develop an ailment, it is unclear whether he ever consulted healers or took medicine.[120]

It is difficult to obtain much information about seventeenth-century attitudes towards healers from diaries and correspondence. A better source is the large body of popular literature referring to medicine, published during the period. A few of these works were semi-serious prose attacks on the medical status quo. A few were poems.[121] The majority were plays, performed and published to entertain. While it is hard to know how seriously to take the opinions expressed in such literature, examination of it is valuable because it helps to balance what the healers said about themselves.[122] Medical historians have always been too eager to accept licensed physicians and surgeons of the past at their own valuation.[123]

How representative were the attitudes expressed in popular literature? Some authors, Gideon Harvey for example, were eccentrics whose opinions reflected only their own bitter experiences with the medical establishment. However, there do appear to have been both serious criticism of various types of medical practitioners and the mirror image of these attacks – stereotyped caricatures of healers. Whatever may have been the individual opinions of the laymen to whom healers tried to sell their services, the images of these healers as portrayed by dramatists and the popular press were as much a part of general mental furniture as are the 'doctor jokes' current today.

The physician was frequently attacked. His academic education and Latin conversation were beyond the understanding of most prospective patients. His rich dress and haughty manners were resented. The relatively high fees he charged were disapproved of. Disagreements between physicians were pointed to as evidence of the basic inexactness of their art and the amount of hocus-pocus that found its way into diagnosis and treatment. In the 1680s Gideon Harvey made fun of the physicians'

> great learning, vast skill, gravity, formality, conceited caps, valpony gowns, anatomical theatre, circulation library, coach and horses.[124]

One hundred years earlier, Pedro Mexia had criticised medical theories, writing that it was more important to know the cure than the cause of a disease:

> And why should I more believe Hippocrates (who affirmeth the substance of the matter to be in the spirits) than Erisistratus, who attributed it to the turning backward of the blood and the arteries. And why should I credit more these than others, who assigned other principles?[125]

Mexia also accused physicians of using increasingly complicated and exotic medicines in order 'to give a more comely visage to their new science that none may know the secrets thereof' and 'to deceive and bewitch the people'.[126] He even suggested that physicians used these means to murder their patients.

Gideon Harvey was still more savage about therapeutic techniques used by all licensed healers, writing that the patient

> is falsely convicted of this or that Felony on himself; and, most commonly, if his crime or Disease be great, is sentenced to die, and to be executed by tying a Halter about his arm, and afterward to be stabbed in it with a Lancet, to draw off so much blood, until he be Herring-dead. Another way of execution they use, is to impale the sufferer with a machine of Box or ivory, being in nothing different from a clyster-pipe; and this to be used so oft, until it comes out at his mouth; or, if this fails, to order such la Voisine drenches to be poured down his throat, which may do them the good service to stifle the sufferer's . . . vital flame in a few days.[127]

However, it should be recalled that these procedures and prescriptions were actually demanded by sufferers and sometimes used without the sanction of a healer. Thus, Harvey was criticising the approach of lay-men to illness as well as the approach of healers.

The dramatists, like the writers of polemics, disagreed about the value of physicians and physic. Shakespeare tended to favour academically trained physicians. Concerning Gerard de Narbon, he wrote that his

> skill was almost as great as his honesty; had it stretched so far, would have made nature immortal, and death should have play for lack of work. Would, for the King's sake, he were living! I think it would be the death of the King's disease.[128]

Most other dramatists thought less highly of physicians. Ben Jonson wrote:

Mosca He has no faith in physic: he does think
Most of your doctors are the greater danger
And worse diseases, to escape. I often have
Heard him protest, that your physicians
Should never be his heir
. . . .
No, sir, not their fees
He cannot brook: he says they flay a man,
Before they kill him.[129]

And Beaumont and Fletcher lampooned the many remedies physicians prescribed. In this case, the sufferer had insomnia.

1. Courtier. What cures has he?
Bawdber. Armies of those we call physicians, some with glisters,
Some with lettice-caps, some posset drinks some pills,
Twenty consulting here about a drench,
As many here to blood him.
Then comes a Don of Spaine, and he prescribes
More cooling opium than would kill a Turke,
Or quench a whore ith dogdayes: after him . . .
An English doctor, with a bunch of pot herbs;
And he cries out endiffe and suckory,
With a few mallow roots and butter milk,
And talks of oil made of a churchmans charity,
Yet still he wakes.[130]

The endless controversy over medical theories was also ridiculed.

1. Doctor. Why I, for if he be a chemist, his opinion and ours must needs differ, and consequently not agree in consultation.
2. Doctor. I am, sir, of your opinion, for I think it infra dignitatem to hold consultation with mountebanks. . . .
3. Doctor. Pardon me gentlemen, I have known some chemical physicians learned and rational men; and though not strict adherers to the Galenical method, produced with great reason, and good success, which, I take it, answers all we can say or do.
2. Doctor. I profess I think it as bad as murder to cure out of the methodical way. Oh what satisfaction 'tis to have a patient die according to all the rules of art.[131]

The dramatists were gentler with surgeons, mainly lampooning their connection with syphilis. George Chapman wrote:

Pock: My name is Pock sir; a practitioner in surgery.
Darioto: Pock the surgeon, y'are welcome sir, I know a doctor of your name master Pock.
Pock: My name has made many doctors sir.
Rinaldo: Indeed tis a worshipful name.
Valerio: Mary is it, and of an ancient descent.
Pock: Faith sir I could fetch my pedigree far, if I were so disposed.
Rinaldo: Out of France at least.
Pock: And if I stood on my arms as others do.
Darioto: No do not Pock, let others stand on their arms, and thou a thy legs as long as thou canst.
Pock: Though I live by my bare practice, yet I could show good cards for my gentility.[132]

Apothecaries were mentioned chiefly as the servants and henchmen of physicians. When they were ridiculed, it was for avarice and for the plethora of harmful and useless remedies they sold.

Unauthorised healers were even more vulnerable to attack than were the physicians. We have dealt with the serious criticisms of them launched by the anti-quack writers above. Needless to say, dramatists found them irresistible. Thomas Heywood's *Wise Woman of Hogsdon* has been quoted above.[133] Shakespeare's weird sisters were more interested in black magic than in white, although their concoction sounds like many of the medical recipes current at the time.[134] However, the character Pinch – described in *The Comedy of Errors* – was a caricature of the travelling mountebank.

Antipholus of Ephesus: Along with them
They brought one Pinch, a hungry, lean-fac'd villain,
A mere anatomy, a mountebank,
A threadbare juggler, and a fortune-teller,
A needy, hollow-ey'd, sharp-looking wretch,
A living dead man. This pernicious slave,
Forsooth, took on him as a conjurer,
And gazing in mine eyes, feeling my pulse,
And with no face, as 'twere, outfacing me,
Cries out I was possess'd.[135]

A lighter treatment of the same theme was presented in *The Skilful Mountebank* . . . published in 1638. Similar in form to the do-it-yourself medical works popular during the period, it offered humorous cures for a number of disorders. For instance, for melancholy, it prescribed a joke and a warm bed with a virgin in it, along with the following cordial:

> The stones of a goat, the guts of crabs, the brains of sparrows, monkey's marrow, pith of oxens, with the yolks of 5 new layd eggs, laid by an hen of the Game.

The book ends with a song sung by the mountebank himself:

> Are any fools that would be wise?
> Are any falling that would rise?
> Is any such that would be poore,
> Ile purge his substance in an hour:
> Is any bound that would be free?
> Ile do 't, let him repair to me.
> I come to cure what e'er you feel,
> Within, without, from head to heel.

Like authorised healers, unlicensed practitioners had their defenders. Pedro Mexia took a leaf from the physicians' own book when he created a pedigree for unlearned practice, writing that early men

> cured one another for charity, and not for interest, and they cured with herbs and vertuous simples experimented, and not with venemous compositions that now are used, which you know not what they be.[136]

Mexia favoured experience over theory. However, he hedged a bit, saying that there were good physicians as well as bad, and that the good should be allowed to get on with their work.

The portrait painted of healers and medicine by seventeenth-century popular writers is both detailed and confusing. It indicates the great extent to which both writers and their audiences were familiar with medical matters. It also shows the diversity of opinion on medical topics. It indicates, for instance, that the physicians were justified in feeling insecure about the trust and support they received from the general public. It also suggests that although people took a lot of medicine, they were cynical about the salutary results the medicine would produce. In addition, the popular literature reinforces the notion that the seventeenth-century medical marketplace was perceived as such by both healers and sufferers. Sufferers came, willing to buy, but suspicious of being cheated. Healers came, anxious to sell, eager to convince potential buyers of their worth.

The above discussion has concentrated upon seventeenth-century medical variety. It has described the disorders people suffered from and the ways they dealt with these disorders. It has indicated the diversity of approaches to illness which existed. At this point in our study, then, it is appropriate to turn to an in-depth analysis of the medical experiences of one seventeenth-century family – to move discussion from the general to the particular.

7

IN SICKNESS AND IN HEALTH: THE JOSSELINS' EXPERIENCE

I INTRODUCTION

The extent to which diaries reflect general experience is frequently, and deservedly, questioned. The seventeenth-century diarists whose writings have survived were members of the middle and upper classes. Furthermore, diarists and autobiographers are unusual in any age, feeling a need most people never feel to commit thoughts and experiences to paper. Their attitudes and behaviour can be taken as representative, neither of general experience, nor of the experience of others at their social level.

None the less, such records of unique, personal experience are invaluable to the historians, providing, as they literally do, a voice from the grave which can make the past live as no other source can. And the fact that the experiences they describe may not be representative is, perhaps, insignificant, since each individual's experience is, to a large extent, unique, whether or not he or she describes it in a diary. One cannot quantify pain, fear, grief, confidence or comfort.

In any case, this chapter is not concerned with general experience. It will concentrate on the health and illness of one family, seen through the eyes of the head of that family, Reverend Ralph Josselin. Josselin was born 25 January 1616, and died in August 1683. His diary, preceded by a brief autobiography and annual notes, covers the period between the autumn of 1643 and July 1683.[1]

From late 1640 until his death, Josselin was the vicar of Earls Colne in Essex. In the course of his life there, he became a prosperous landowner, one of the ten wealthiest men in his village.[2] He and his wife, born Jane Constable, produced ten live-born children, five of whom were living at the time of Josselin's death. Although the Josselins were middle class by any definition of that vague term, they socialised with people of higher status living in the vicinity, including two gentry families, the Harlakendens and the Honeywoods. They kept one maid-servant to help with the housework, hired nurses for short periods after childbirth and, in later years, employed a man-servant.

Ralph Josselin's diary is an unusually good source of information on medical matters. He was interested enough in medicine and disease to have read at least two works on the subject.[3] In addition to his intellectual interest, he appears to have been unusually preoccupied by his own ailments, describing symptoms of both major and minor disorders in loving detail, always fearing the worst. Fortunately for the historian, he was also concerned about the ailments of his wife, children, servants, friends, neighbours, relations and colleagues. Thus, the diary provides medical information about quite a large number of people, something which is not equally true about otherwise 'rich' diaries of the period. The length of the Josselin diary is also an advantage. Unlike some diarists, Josselin was consistently conscientious about making his entries. Thus we have a nearly daily record of the family's illnesses, accidents and childbearing during a period of approximately forty years.

The Josselins underwent a variety of disorders during this time. These will be discussed within three major categories: the discomforts and dangers relating to childbearing, children's accidents and diseases, and adult disorders, including Ralph Josselin's own. Needless to say, there are overlaps between categories. All of the members of the family suffered from some ailments, such as colds, the 'scab' and stomach upsets. Josselin and some of his children seem to have been particularly prone to eye disorders. And he and at least three of his children suffered from worms. Thus, something should be said to justify this categorisation.

The first heading, dealing with pregnancy and childbirth, needs no explanation. Neither, perhaps, does the last, which will cover adult ailments, excluding those discussed within the first category. A separate category has been set aside for the diseases and accidents of children, because of the high level of infant and child mortality, both within the Josselin family and within the seventeenth-century English population at large.[4] Diseases which provoked minor upsets in adults might kill a child. With good reason, the first two years of life were regarded as particularly dangerous by Josselin and his contemporaries.[5] Certain ailments, such as those associated with teething, mainly affected children in that age group. Weaning, which in the case of the Josselin children occurred between 12 and 19 months, was regarded as a perilous process.[6] Children were also particularly endangered by accidents. The Josselin children fell downstairs and into fires, set their clothing and household linen afire, and were kicked by horses.[7] For all of these reasons, their disorders deserve separate discussion.

II DISORDERS

Pregnancy and Childbirth

Jane and Ralph Josselin took seriously the biblical injunction to be fruitful and multiply. They married relatively young; Jane was just under and Ralph just over 20 years old. In their first twenty-two years of marriage, Jane had at least fifteen pregnancies producing ten live-born children and at least five miscarriages. She probably breast-fed all of her children.[8]

The Josselins were delighted when they felt certain of Jane's first pregnancy, some ten months after their wedding. Ralph's diary entry for July 1641 attests to their 'great joy and comfort' concerning her condition. He was not as communicative about the news of her subsequent pregnancies, although he was never happy about her miscarriages, regardless of the size of his family. On one occasion in June 1656, when four of the seven children which by then had been born to the couple were living, he wrote, 'This morning my wife thought she miscarried, lord a miscarrying womb is a sad affliction'.[9]

Jane's feelings when anticipating yet another pregnancy were not recorded, but they certainly must have been mixed. She did not carry her babies easily. She was sick and uncomfortable throughout her pregnancies, and dreaded her deliveries for months before the baby was due. She suffered from nausea, faintness, weakness and pain in her back, false labour, after-pains and pain in her breasts, in addition to sometimes long, usually painful, and always frightening deliveries.[10] Indeed, Ralph recognised his wife's unusually uncomfortable pregnancies, writing on 30 October 1653, 'My poor wife very ill, she breedeth with difficulty,' and later in the same pregnancy, on 11 December, 'my wife very ill, and weakly in her childing'.[11] Surely Jane must have echoed his prayer at the beginning of that pregnancy, 'the lord bear up her head under the difficulties of her condition'.[12]

None the less, Jane apparently accepted her obstetrical fate with equanimity and interest. She had, for example, a considerable degree of success in predicting the sex of her unborn children very early in her pregnancies. Ralph reported her predictions for five babies. The first four were accurate. The fifth guess she muddled by changing her mind: on 15 May 1657 she reported being pregnant with a girl. By 31 May she was sure she carried a boy. Mary was born on 14 January 1658. Jane should have stood by her first hunch. None the less, Ralph was right when, in recording her prediction of the sex of their third child, he wrote, 'She useth not to be mistaken'.[13]

Jane's fears about her deliveries were understandable and, probably, very common. The hazards of childbirth in seventeenth-century England were immense. Complications, such as an unusual presentation of the baby, or the mother's inability to expel the child once it was in the birth canal, were often fatal to both mother and child. Even normal deliveries were fraught with danger. Haemorrhages could not be stopped. Infection after birth was common. Tears could not be effectually repaired. Neither midwives nor the occasionally called surgeons could do much to help the labouring women who came into their hands. Both could hurt a great deal – the midwives with well-meant but ill-judged interference intended to speed up labour and delivery; the surgeons with their clumsy instruments used, mainly, to extract dead children when all other means of delivering them had failed.[14]

Jane Josselin's fears had been shared and written about in the 1620s by a woman with the oddly coincidental name of Elizabeth Joceline. Elizabeth was so convinced that childbirth would kill her that 'when she first felt herself quick with child (as then travelling with death itself) she secretly took order for the buying of a new winding sheet'.[15] Elizabeth was certain she was carrying a girl. She wrote her book in order to provide religious instruction for the child, doomed to grow up without a mother. All of Elizabeth's predictions came true. She died of fever nine days after giving birth to a daughter. Her book found a sympathetic readership. It was first published in 1624, two years after the author's death, and was republished six times between 1684 and 1894.

Like Elizabeth, Jane Josselin took her fears to God. On one occasion she prayed with neighbour women when she felt the child quicken.[16] On another, she and Ralph prayed together the night before her labour began, because Jane 'was oppressed with fears that she should not do well on this child'.[17] With the next pregnancy as well Jane was 'under great fears she shall not do well of this child'.[18] It is not surprising that Jane should have been particularly frightened during this pregnancy. In the preceding year, 1646, two neighbour women had died in childbed, one after an excruciating labour lasting for two weeks.[19]

Even years of fortunate experience did not lay Jane's fears to rest. When in August 1661 she thought she might be pregnant, Ralph wrote, 'I see she apprehends a breeding again with fear, the blessing of a fruitful womb is by weakness of nature her fear'.[20]

Childbirth in seventeenth-century England was a social occasion. Indeed, the church required that at least two or three 'honest women' in addition to the midwife be present to witness the birth for legal reasons. The invitation of several 'gossips' to a birth was also required by social convention. Acquaintances who did not receive an expected invitation might justifiably take offence.[21] When Jane was delivered of her third child at nearly midnight on 25 November 1645, the midwife and 'almost all' of the women Ralph had summoned were present.[22] When her fourth child was born, the midwife was not there, and she was attended by 'only' five neighbour women.[23] In her turn, Jane attended the confinements of her neighbours and her daughters.[24] In one case, Ralph reported that she saved the life of a labouring woman.[25]

Jane Josselin was fortunate in that all of her labours and deliveries appear to have been quite straightforward. This is not to say that they were easy. Ralph reported Jane's experience of 'sharp pains' or unusually long difficult labours during the births of their third, eighth, ninth and tenth children.[26] In two cases she gave birth without a midwife present.[27] Even when a midwife was there, her presence was not always regarded as an unmixed blessing. After the birth of her eighth child, Jane criticised the midwife for not having done 'her part'. Not only was this labour unusually 'sharp', but also the baby appeared to be dead at birth. Josselin attributed its revival to the intervention of God.[28]

After the birth was over, the mother's health was a subject of special concern for a few weeks at least. The risks of fever and breast infections were very real indeed. Jane was again fortunate. She suffered from sore breasts after the birth of her first child, which were healed 'with use of means'.[29] When her fourth child died at 10 days old, Jane became 'weak and faint with the turning of her milk'.[30] Otherwise, there was no apparent cause for concern. Jane left her bed within three weeks, and left the house between one and two months after her deliveries.

Because Ralph Josselin was so conscientious about recording details of the symptoms and illnesses of the members of his family, it is possible to compare Jane's health during her childbearing years (1642–63) and during the last twenty years of her marriage (1663–83). During the first twenty-one years of their married life, Ralph reported 131 instances of Jane being unwell. Of these, seventy-three cases were clearly related to pregnancy and childbirth. Fifty-eight cases recorded a plethora of symptoms ranging from toothache, to ague, to being 'sickly with toiling over' a dying child.[31] Some of these miscellaneous disorders may have actually arisen from gynaecological or obstetrical problems. For instance, in July 1656 Jane suffered from symptoms which she first diagnosed as the 'falling down of the mother' (prolapse of the uterus) and later, with relief, as piles.[32] This episode occurred a month after she thought she miscarried.[33]

Once Jane's reproductive years were over, she apparently became much healthier. In the last twenty years of the Josselins' marriage (1663 to Ralph's death in 1683), Ralph reported that Jane was unwell only seventeen times. This significant improvement might be explained in a number of ways. It is possible that for a short period of time Ralph lost interest in recording his family's symptoms. Certainly the years between 1665 and 1672 are remarkably poor in their references to illness. However, it is more likely that the Josselins were fairly healthy during those years. It is also possible that after November 1672, when Ralph was first troubled with the leg ailment which probably killed him, he ceased to mention any but the most dramatic illnesses of family members, concentrating, as the elderly and sick may be excused for doing, on his own problems.[34] However, this is also unlikely, for he did mention a cold Jane had in November 1680.[35] Indeed, Jane's health was of great concern to Ralph for purely selfish reasons. He frequently echoed the prayer he made when she was ill with a pregnancy in 1648, 'Blessed be God, oh continue her a comfort to me and mine'.[36] The prospect of being left alone to care for a large house and family would have been grim indeed. Thus it seems that Jane's health did improve considerably once she finished childbearing. Certainly she outlived her husband and was apparently healthy at the time of his death.

Children's Accidents and Diseases

In seventeenth-century England, as in most 'developing' societies, childhood was an especially dangerous period of life. As we have seen, the London Bills of Mortality included special categories for infants and 'chrisom' children – infancy seeming to be in itself a sufficient explanation of the cause of death.[37] Certain illnesses, such as being livergrown, ailments associated with teething, and rickets were peculiar to the early years. Other ailments, like 'the scab' and worms, although they affected adults as well, were most common and dangerous among children.

Of the five Josselin children who died before their father, three were under the age of 8. One baby, the first Ralph, died at 10 days. The second Ralph died at 13 months. Mary, the first-born, died aged 8 years, 1 month. Each of the three died under circumstances which would have been tragically familiar to Ralph Josselin's peers.

The first baby Ralph was born on 11 February 1648. He was the Josselin's fourth child; the elder three were living when he was born. Josselin himself was very ill with ague at the time of his birth. He first mentioned the baby's illness on 17 February, when he wrote that the child 'was ill, full of phlegm', and that they sent for the physician. This was, quite remarkably, the only occasion when Josselin mentioned having summoned a physician to the bedside of any member of his family! At this point Jane Josselin had already 'persuaded herself that it would die[,] it was a very sick child indeed', and Ralph himself 'took my leave of it at night, not much expecting to see it alive'.[38] On 20 February Ralph wrote

> This night again my son very ill, he did not cry so much as the night before, whether the cause was want of strength I know not: he had a little froth in his mouth continually, in the morning there came some red mattery stuff out of his mouth, which made us apprehend his throat might be sore.[39]

By this time the baby was being fed breast-milk, and had been dosed with syrup of roses.[40] He died on the 21st, the Josselins having 'looked on it as a dying child, 3 or 4 days'.[41]

The second baby Ralph and Mary died within six days of each other. Indeed, the late May and early June of 1650 was a disastrous period for the Josselins, since they lost a close friend, Mrs Mary Church, the same day that baby Ralph died.

The second Ralph was born 5 May 1649. His father mentioned that he was treated for wind on 13 May. He was reasonably well thereafter until the end of November when his father wrote that he was ill, 'but I hope it was only breeding teeth'.[42] On 1 December the baby 'pined and grew very tedious these cold nights to his poor mother'.[43] On 21

December Jane took the child to Lady Honeywood's, who 'fears he is in a consumption, but indeed he is troubled with the rickets'.[44] The lady suggested that the boy be treated with an issue, but Jane decided against this therapy. On 27 January 1650 the baby was still ill. On 5 February he 'was very sick as if he would have died, he vomited, and something stirred in the bottom of his stomach, which he endeavoured to bring up but could not'.[45] On 18 February his eyes were 'wonderful ill as if he should be blind'.[46] By 10 March the child's eyes were better, but he had broken out 'in very many angry pimples and the rheum continues'.[47] On 27 March the child was still ill, and his parents resolved to wean him from the breast.[48] On 21 April 'My little boy continueth ill, and sore, and forward'.[49] By 7 May the Josselins had concluded that little Ralph was 'liver-grown, there is no passage between his short ribs, which is a sign thereof'.[50] By late May 8-year-old Mary was dying, so attention was somewhat diverted from the ever-ailing Ralph. However, on 26 May Josselin wrote that 'my little son in all peoples eyes is a dying child'; and die he did on 2 June, his father commenting that 'his life was continual sorrow and trouble, happy he who is at rest in the lord'.[51]

Mary Josselin was born 12 April 1642. Her first major illness was a severe cold she had at about the age of 3, during which she spat blood. She had ague at 5 and, along with her brother and sister, a skin disorder on her scalp at the age of 6. She had trouble with her eyes at the same time as her infant brother Ralph in early 1650. With these exceptions, she was an unusually healthy child until a month before her death. On 28 April her father mentioned that she was 'ill but not down sick'.[52] On 5 May she was still ill. By 12 May Ralph wrote, 'my dear Mary, very ill, she is heavy, and joyless as it were, god in mercy restore her and spare her life'.[53] On 21 May he wrote, 'the last night Mary talked idly, she began to sweat'.[54]

The Josselins suspected that she suffered from worms, and on 22 May Ralph went to the priory requesting a medicine for that disorder. Upon his return home he was told 'she had had a stool, and 3 great dead worms'. The same day they gave her a clyster which 'wrought very well'.[55] On 24 May Mary 'void six worms more'.[56] On the 25th Ralph had some hope that Mary would survive, but by the next morning 'all our hopes of Mary's life was gone, to the Lord I resigned her'.[57] She died on 27 May, and was buried the following day.

Although they mourned the losses of all three children, Jane and Ralph were especially grief-stricken over Mary's death. On 4 August, more than two months after Mary died, Jane was 'very faint and ill'. Ralph wrote, 'I apprehend she disquiets herself in grief for Mary as the occasion of it'.[58] While the two boys had been sickly infants, not expected to live, Mary had actually survived the perilous early years and showed great promise. Ralph wrote of her, 'She was a child of ten thousand, full of wisdom, woman-like gravity, knowledge, sweet expre[ssions of god, apt in her learning,] tender hearted and loving, an [obed]ient child'.[59]

The townspeople of Earls Colne reflected the different reactions of the parents. While 'many of my neighbours' attended the first baby Ralph's funeral, 'most of the town' came to Mary's, including the wives of two of the foremost citizens, Mrs Margaret Harlakenden (her husband was the richest man in town) and Mrs Mabel Elliston, who laid her in her grave.[60]

Of course, childhood illnesses and accidents were not always fatal. Many of the Josselin children were ill when they were cutting teeth.[61] They suffered from numerous skin ailments, ranging from pimples, to shingles, rashes on their scalps, the itch and boils.[62] They also were subject to worms. The first Mary had worms when she was nearly 3 and John was 'full of worms' at the age of 4.[63] Ralph senior and several of the children had the 'rheum' in their eyes, and other eye ailments.[64] The second Ralph and Jane were supposed to have had rickets which, in Jane's case, may have been associated with weaning.[65]

The children also suffered from ailments which today are commonly viewed as childhood diseases. In July 1649 one of Ralph's two sons (probably 5-year-old Thomas) developed 'great swellings' under both his ears – possibly mumps.[66] In March 1656 John, Jane and Ann developed 'colds nigh chincolds', Josselin describing their 'fierce and troublesome cough that is too hard for means that we can use'.[67] This sounds like whooping cough. In July 1658 4-year-old Ann and the Josselins' maid had the measles.[68] And in August 1652, when he was 18, Thomas also had the measles.[69]

Although Josselin and his wife apparently escaped the ravages of smallpox, their children were not so fortunate. Thomas, John, Ann and Elizabeth each caught the disease as teenagers, while living in London.[70] Only 15-year-old Thomas, who contracted smallpox only two weeks after being sent to London as an apprentice, returned home to be nursed. The others remained in London, sending word of their condition home to their anxious parents. Despite the seriousness of the disease and the fear it inspired, these adolescents survived it without any permanent handicap worthy of remark.

Like their father, the Josselin children suffered from frequent colds and occasional bouts of ague. On a number of occasions, the whole family came down with colds at the same time.[71] Colds were usually regarded as unpleasant but inevitable, worthy of comment but not of fear. However, in children they were sometimes regarded as dangerous. When 3-year-old Mary suffered from a 'great cold' during which she 'strained and spit much blood', her parents sought help for her from Lady Honeywood. Ralph was worried about her to the extent that he prayed that 'the Lord will preserve her'.[72] Colds were even more dangerous in infants. When 10-month-old Thomas developed a cold in the night which seemed 'ready even to stop him up', Jane Josselin was so frightened 'that she was even at death's door'.[73] Agues could be even more severe. The intermittent hot and cold fits were very unpleasant and the disease was very debilitating, often lasting for months. When she was only about 8 months old, Elizabeth picked up an ague which lasted from early February until mid-April.[74] None the less, Ralph Josselin apparently feared the consequences of an ague only once, and that, perhaps understandably, was when he suffered a bad case of it himself in February 1648.[75]

The Josselins and their friends were also involved in accidents. Like many of his contemporaries, Josselin recorded his family's brushes with disaster as marks of God's providence. Thus he wrote on 7 October 1644, 'I found god had graciously kept my daughter Mary who was struck with a Horse her apron rent off with his nails, and her handkerchief rent and yet she had no hurt'.[76] Mary was 2½ at the time. While adults also had accidents, children were most at risk because they were only beginning to learn how to deal with their environment.

Fire was particularly dangerous. The Josselin house had six hearths. In February 1648 Jane, then just over 2, fell into the fire without hurt. A year later she fell into a fire and hurt her hands.[77] The second Mary also burnt her hands in an open fire at just under 3 years of age.[78] On 27 October 1658 4-year-old Anne both fell into a 'great fire' and tumbled down the entry stairs. At the end of the day she was unhurt.[79] Candles were as hazardous as open fires. In January 1669 11-year-old Mary's neckcloth caught fire on a candle, 'and she blew it, which increased the flame, my maid damped it and I with both hands over it quenched it'.[80] On 27 September 1672 10-year-old

Becky 'fired a bed mat with a candle. My wife run up into chamber and quenched it'.[81]

Then as now, children frequently fell and hurt themselves. In July 1650 6-year-old Thomas fell down the school stairs and hurt his cheek.[82] In November 1653 2-year-old John broke a bone in his foot by falling at the street threshold.[83] The following year John fell down the school stairs (which must indeed have been dangerous!) but received no hurt.[84] In addition, children were injured by the adults looking after them. When the second Mary was 2½, her arm was pulled out of joint 'by a snatch of our maid Alice'.[85]

The Josselin children also endangered each other. In February 1648 2-year-old Jane 'dagged a pair of scissors in Thom: eyebrow', fortunately not much injuring him.[86] And in 1654 Jane, then nearly 9, dropped 2-month-old Ann into a bowl of milk. The baby was unhurt.[87] Equally the children saved each other from harm. In December 1644 2-year-old Mary held 1-year-old Thomas out of the fire, crying until their father came to help.[88] Indeed, in view of the dangers which surrounded them, the Josselin children were remarkably fortunate in escaping both accidental injury and death from epidemic diseases. This good fortune certainly supported Ralph Josselin's belief in the special providence of God towards him and his.

Adult Disorders

Although Ralph Josselin conscientiously reported the illnesses of his family, friends and neighbours, he was most interested in his own ailments. He was not a true hypochondriac; his illnesses cannot be regarded as 'imaginary'. However, he was unusually preoccupied with his symptoms, major and minor – so much so that his wife lost patience with him at one point. In January 1672 Josselin began to suffer from the pain, swelling and ulceration in his left leg which remained with him until his death over eleven years later. He wrote, at that time, 'I am sensible I bear my infirmities about me, but my wife taxes me for great impatience, when I fear there is a provoking carelessness in her etc. and impatience too much, that bears nothing but expects I must bear all'.[89] The reader of the diary cannot help but sympathise with both Ralph and Jane. Certainly Ralph spent most of his life handicapped by minor, annoying ailments. However, one imagines that his exhaustive (and exhausting) descriptions of his sensations found their way into breakfast-table conversation, as well as into the pages of his diary.

Ralph noted the state of his health in both daily entries and in weekly summaries, written on Sundays. In addition, he frequently made marginal notes which, as often as not, referred to an acute or chronic disorder.[90] Like his contemporaries, he was involved in determining the diagnoses and prognoses of his own illnesses, and helped decide the therapeutic 'means' to be used.

Josselin suffered from frequent, long-lasting colds which he described in great detail. He mentioned colds in the throat, poses (the term he used to refer to head colds), rheums, 'stuffing' and 'wheezing' (mostly at night), chest colds, 'stopping' in the chest and aguish colds.[91] Out of some 317 mentions of his own illnesses, 114 referred to colds. He also gave full descriptions of the onset and various stages of his colds. For instance, he wrote in June 1646, 'I was now in taking of cold sensible of it most in my throat, a roughness and kind of soreness at the upper part next my mouth and especially on the left side'.[92] During another cold in December 1646, he wrote 'my cold begun to thicken, and to stuff and wheeze exceedingly'.[93] His conjectures about why he 'caught' cold sound much like those we hear today. For instance, he came down with a pose and chest cold as a result of wearing thin stockings in October 1677.[94]

Although Josselin very occasionally took medicine for his colds, his attitude towards them was far more fatalistic than towards his other ailments.[95] For one thing, despite the discomfort they caused him, Josselin's colds never appeared to him to be very serious illnesses, unlike other ailments such as severe agues or the chronic leg problem (variously diagnosed as scurvy and dropsy) which tormented his final years. For another thing, Josselin's colds dragged on so long that to have allowed himself to take up a sick role during them would have been financially and professionally disastrous.

This is not to say that Josselin always regarded colds as minor ailments. As we have seen, children's colds sometimes concerned him greatly.[96] However, Ralph's own colds, though annoying, were considered minor problems and even served as rather gratifying tests of faith and fortitude. For instance, he wrote in September 1647, 'This week I was somewhat troubled with a pose, but though rheums and pose haunt me I praise God, they do not cast me down'.[97]

Josselin was prey to a host of minor symptoms which annoyed more than worried him. During his early years at Earls Colne he frequently mentioned rheums in his eyes.[98] He also developed a sore tongue, pain in his chest which he concluded was wind, and occasional soreness in his bones.[99] At one point he also developed swellings in both sides of his groin which mercifully abated within a week.[100] Some of the sensations he experienced were downright mysterious – for example, the 'coldness or moistness in the crown of his head' which he felt on 14 January 1649.[101] In addition to these problems, Josselin was a bad traveller. Frequently even short journeys left him feeling ill. Sometimes he experienced nausea and vomiting; sometimes he felt aguish and sore.[102] In one case, while returning from London, he was overcome with wind and had to be treated in the home of an acquaintance.[103]

Like their contemporaries, Josselin and his family were occasionally 'ill in their stomachs'. However, the humoral theory dominant in the period, which regarded evacuation as beneficial, helped them to bear their discomforts. For instance, when Ralph suffered from diarrhoea in April 1646, he 'conceived it a mercy'.[104] Again, in December 1648 he wrote, 'After above 30 hours illness in my stomach I fell into a great looseness which I conceive did me much good'.[105] When 5-year-old Ann had an 'each day ague' in August 1659, the fact that she vomited and sweat gave her parents hope.[106] In some cases the evacuation was indeed a blessing. This was true in August 1656, when Ralph suffered from worms, and in November 1672, when he vomited after a surfeit of oysters.[107]

Also in company with their contemporaries, the Josselins were plagued by toothache. In one case Ralph's gums began to swell in March 1655. He suffered through the month of April, and finally had the offending tooth drawn in May. The tooth itself 'was corrupted, and the flesh within it, most loathsome'.[108] Two days after the tooth was drawn, Josselin 'pulled out a piece of bone by the place where my tooth stood . . . it was firm, but I conceive begun to rot, it was putrified round about, it must needs have been dangerous if God had not directed me to draw my tooth'.[109] On 23 June another small piece of bone emerged from the tooth socket, after which Josselin's face finally healed.[110] On a number of other occasions he suffered from painfully swollen gums.[111] In July 1646 Jane had a toothache 'which brought her as it were to death's door'.[112] In this case, the pain went away, so the tooth was not pulled.

Almost every member of the Josselin family had ague at one time or another, in most cases more than once. These attacks ranged from single fits to life-threatening illnesses such as the ague Ralph had in February 1648. During this illness, Josselin wrote that his friends were very worried about him – despite the fact that his wife gave birth to a son who died during Ralph's convalescence. At one point, a week after his fits had begun, Josselin wrote a will.[113] His illness actually ended within fourteen days of its onset, but it frightened him considerably. Some attacks lasted a good deal longer than this. Jane Josselin (senior) developed a quartan ague in October 1668, which lasted until mid-March of the following year and was so serious that her adult daughter Jane was summoned home to look after her.[114]

In addition to the ailments mentioned above, Josselin suffered from two long-term illnesses worthy of mention. The first was an inflammation of his navel which troubled him between September 1648 and mid-April 1652.[115] This was a discouraging illness because his navel would appear to heal, then would become sore and moist all over again, despite the various treatments Ralph tried on it. Although never incapacitated by the discomfort his navel caused him, he was worried about it. In March 1649 he wrote that he had 'heard of one that after 2 years illness was killed with a rawness in his navel, but God shall heal me of this infirmity'.[116] However, as time passed, he grew less concerned, writing in August 1651, 'my navel was a little but not much ill, it hath not been dressed near a year'.[117]

The second long-term illness Josselin suffered from was the swelling and ulceration of his left leg which incapacitated and probably eventually killed him. The first hint of a problem came in November 1672, when Ralph had a 'sciatica pain' in his hip.[118] This passed by the end of the following month, when he reported being able 'to take many steps without stick or stay'.[119] However, by 27 February 1673, 'or sooner, some red spots appeared on my lame thigh, which they conceived the scurvy'.[120] From that time on, the diary is a catalogue of pain, swelling, different treatments applied, fears and disappointed hopes. As the old sores healed the swelling broke open in new places. By early 1683, after ten years of misery, Josselin was a very ill man indeed. His leg was swollen and painful. His belly also swelled. He was very short of breath. He developed a 'great and dangerous cough' and double vision.[121] Despite his infirmities, he continued to preach.[122] However, he must have feared that death was near, for he wrote on 1 June, 'I saw my countenance much changed . . . I did no[t think] I gathered strength nor lost any, but in the use of means continued in the same way. However I stay [myself] on my good god, that this sickness doth not issue in death, but in a trial to do me much good'.[123] This forlorn hope was never realised. Josselin died two months later, at the age of 67.

Josselin described his own last illness, and those of his children who died in childhood, in some detail. It is interesting that he does not give descriptions of the deaths of two adult children, Thomas and Ann, in the summer of 1673. Alan Macfarlane suggests that Thomas may have died of consumption.[124] However, Josselin himself wrote nothing to support this diagnosis, reporting only that 29-year-old Thomas had come home ill on 22 March 1673, and that he died on 15 June, having suffered very little.[125] We do not know when Ann returned to Earls Colne from London, but Josselin wrote that she was ill on 17 June.[126] On 20 July she was 'ill and deaf and thereby uncheerful'.[127] She died on 31 July, aged 19. Josselin wrote 'God hath taken 5 of 10. Lord let it be enough, and spare that we may recover strength'.[128]

As we have said, Ralph Josselin was most concerned about his own ailments and those of his family members. Josselin's 'family' included his servants. Since the smooth operation of his domestic life depended upon the labour of at least one maid-servant, the health of his servants was important to him.[129] Thus he reported the ill-health of servants in his diary, although he never went into much detail about their ailments. For instance, when his maid Jean went home to her mother's 'very sick, urina nigra', he prayed 'God restore her to her health'.[130] In another case, 'our maid wonderful out of quiet with a sore finger, so that she especially had little rest'.[131] The ill-health of a servant could certainly inconvenience the household. When Josselin's maid was very ill in March 1650, his wife was 'toiled above measure'.[132] A servant's illness could also endanger the family, as in January 1649, when Ralph feared that his maid had smallpox.[133] In turn, the family's ailments could endanger the servant, as in August 1658, when the Josselins' maid caught the measles from 4-year-old Ann, and had to return home.[134]

Josselin was less forthcoming about the illnesses of neighbours and friends. Although it was his duty as a clergyman to visit the sick, he did not report doing so very often. Sometimes he was summoned to sick-beds, as in the case of 'a sick man one Guy Penhache who was much troubled in mind upon his life: he had strong temptations from Satan'.[135] In other cases, the sick person was his friend, as when in June 1646 he visited Mr Thomas Harlakenden who was suddenly ill.[136] Jane Josselin was more involved with sick friends and neighbours, often taking the role of nurse in their illnesses and confinements.[137]

Although Ralph Josselin was not as active in visiting the sick as his sociable contemporary, Samuel Pepys, he was interested in the ills which beset others. He was particularly fascinated by the deaths of other ministers. On 1 September 1644 he reported that 'Mr. Pilgrim Minister of Wormingford fell down dead in his pulpit'.[138] He heard of the deaths of two ministers (including the apparent successor to Mr Pilgrim's living) on 28 August 1646.[139] And on 18 June 1657 he 'heard of Mr. Whiting's death minister of Lexden, who putting his finger into a man's mouth whose throat was ill with a squinsey, and non compos mentis, he bit it vehemently on which it gangrened, and killed him about 8 days after'.[140]

Perhaps similar to his interest in the calamities befalling other ministers was his preoccupation with the providence of God in afflicting those who broke heavenly rules. His satisfaction is apparent in his story of 'one John Chrismas a miller in our town whose parents were godly and one in a way of doing well, but his heart boding him to tipple and game, and his wife being sharp to him, he got what he could together, and left her, his brother brought him home, but about a week after he was sick of the pox and died, a warning not to go out of God's way'.[141] Josselin was even more smug in the following report: 'I observe a providence. A man I was hiring one Peakes son, declined me to go to a Quaker I know not his motives, there he fell sick of the small pox, and his mother keep[ing] him came home and died, the Lord watch over me and mine for good'.[142]

In addition to their physical ills, Josselin and his contemporaries were prey to a host of mental disorders. Some were essentially spiritual in nature. Josselin himself apparently suffered from a severe depression during the spring and summer of 1652, writing frequently of a deadness of heart which he felt powerless to combat.[143] However, in Josselin's world the distinction between mental and physical ills was cloudy at best. His friend, Mr R. H. (Richard Harlakenden?), had a spiritual crisis which Josselin felt should be treated with physical means. He wrote, 'Mr. R. H. in great agony of heart sent down for me, weeping, apprehending himself lost for ever. I feared his head most. Got a physician who let him blood, advised him to alter his course of diet[,] he promised it. I lay with him that night. God gave him rest, and I hope in time perfect health.'[144] Another Harlakenden, William, died in 1675, after suffering from madness for a time. His insanity was actually cured by a physical complaint. Josselin wrote, 'an illness in his feet from his running abroad brought the madness out of his head, but he recovered no great use of his reason spiritual or natural, only on discourse, he savoured of both'.[145] Unhealthy mental states brought on physical illness. When Josselin's daughter, Jane, had a relapse of ague, he wrote, 'my wife thinketh with fear and grief to see her mother so tormented as she was with a felon on her finger'.[146] And when Jane Josselin senior became faint and ill two months after the death of her daughter Mary, Ralph felt her disorder was caused by grief.[147]

Like their children, seventeenth-century adults were victims of accidents. The Josselins were fortunate in this respect. Although Ralph reports quite a few 'near misses', only a few of the accidents he and Jane were involved in resulted in injury. Thus on 27 October 1649, 'I was cutting wood the axe slipt and cut the leather at the toe of my shoe almost through without any hurt'.[148] In May 1651 Jane, who was pregnant at the time, fell from her horse, but was not hurt.[149] Sometimes they did hurt themselves, as when Ralph hurt his eye 'very dangerously' and when Jane fell and bruised her eye.[150] However, their neighbours fared much worse. Josselin reported a case where 'One Robert Davy of my town a butcher cutting out of meat, his son in law Kendall stood beside him, was stricken with the cleaver upon the forehead dangerously, beat out his eye etc'.[151] In another case, 'One Mr. Talbot [was] killed in our town by a fall down his stairs at new-house in Coln'.[152]

Despite these examples, the overall impression given by the Josselin diary is that people had less to fear from accidents in seventeenth-century rural England than they do in our gadget-ridden age, regardless of our supposed safety consciousness. A far greater threat posed by the environment was disease – both infectious and non-infectious. The above discussion has concentrated on the ills people suffered from. The next section will describe what Josselin and his social circle did about their ailments.

III 'MEANS' AND HEALERS

Although Ralph Josselin's diary is replete with details about symptoms (particularly Ralph's own), it is much less informative about the treatments used and healers consulted. Indeed, considering the seventeenth-century fondness for remedies (a predilection we share with the people of that time), the diary is tantalizing in what it does not say. In all, Josselin reported approximately 762 cases of illness or injury happening to himself, his family members, his friends, acquaintances and neighbours. In only seventy-nine cases did he mention the treatments applied. And in only twenty-one cases did he even suggest consultation of a healer. What do these numbers mean? It is possible, but unlikely, that most symptoms went untreated. It is more likely that Josselin simply did not always mention the treatments applied. Concerning the consultation of healers, the diary is probably a bit more reliable. Such consultations, except when they involved the midwife or the local bone-setter, required either a journey or formal correspondence. In either case, it would have been uncharacteristic of Josselin to fail to note an incident which cost him either effort or money or both.

Like many of his contemporaries, Josselin was fairly knowledgeable about medical matters. In 1649 he read two medical works – Leonard Lessius' *Hygiasticon, or the Right Course of Preserving Life and Health unto Extreme Old Age* (1634) and Daniel Sennertus' *Institutionum Medicinae* (many Latin and English editions). He routinely examined his own urine during times of illness, interpreting its characteristics in order to determine the prognosis of the disease. For instance, when recovering from a severe ague attack in early March 1648, he wrote, 'my water broke very ragged and a little red sediment[,] it argued as I conceive a remainder of ill humours in me and that nature was concocting and expelling them'.[153] His comment upon the maid Joan's 'urina nigra' mentioned above suggests that he may have examined the urine of other members of his household as well.[154] Josselin also commented upon other bodily excretions. As already indicated, he subscribed to the humoral view of the body and its processes. Thus when he took two ounces of syrup of roses during his 1648 ague, he wrote that it 'wrought very kindly with me, gave me 9 stools brought away much choler'.[155] When he suffered with a 'pose' in November 1646, he hoped it would 'purge out my rheumes', thus helping to end the cold he had had since August.[156]

Together with his wife, Ralph Josselin diagnosed the ailments of his children. They decided that their baby daughter Jane had rickets, that the second Ralph was livergrown, and that 6-year-old Jane had the spleen.[157] When Jane and Thomas were 'shrieking' in their sleep in October 1650, Ralph felt they probably had worms.[158] Having diagnosed a disease, Ralph and Jane treated it themselves or sought out treatment they felt would be appropriate, feeling free to reject both new diagnoses and suggested treatments. Thus, when Jane took 7-

month-old Ralph to Lady Honeywood's to consult with her about his problems, the diary reported the interview as follows:

> my lady fears he is in a consumption, but indeed he is troubled with the rickets, my lady adviseth an issue to which my wife hath no mind god in mercy bless other means that are used.[159]

Indeed, the main authority on medical matters in the Josselin household was not Ralph, but Jane. Ralph did not indicate whether or not she had read medical works, but he mentioned her role as nurse and medical consultant during many illnesses of family members, friends and neighbours. Jane made at least two of the medicines she used – a distillation of roses and hyssop syrup.[160] She dosed members of her family, acted as a surgeon when their burns, cuts and ulcers needed dressing, and helped out during her neighbours' and daughters' confinements.[161] She nursed her husband and children when they were ill, sometimes becoming ill herself in the process.[162] Indeed, nursing was so important a part of her expected role that Ralph was quite annoyed when she withheld this service, as was the case on 16 November 1676, when 'my wife on some discontent which I know not, would not assist me in dressing my poor leg'.[163] Jane was also summoned to the sick-beds of friends and neighbours. When her dear friend Mary Church hurt her leg in April 1647, Jane applied leeches to it.[164] When Lady Honeywood's child was ill in August 1648, Jane went to Markshall (the Honeywoods' home) to help out.[165] Jane also treated herself, dosing herself with 'pills' for wind and tobacco for toothache in one instance.[166]

The Josselins relied mainly on herbal remedies and 'simples', rather than the compound medicines favoured by apothecaries and physicians. When Ralph was stung by a bee in September 1644, he applied honey to the bite.[167] He used 'violet cake' for an aguish feeling in March 1645, syrup of roses for ague in February 1648, and a mixture of plantain water and loose sugar as a dressing for his sore navel in November 1648.[168] Similarly the Josselins dressed baby Ralph's sore eyes with rose ointment and plantain water, and treated Tom with treacle posset when he had the smallpox.[169]

Very occasionally more complex remedies were tried. In April 1649 Ralph treated a cold both with mithridate, which he must have purchased, and with a 'Stibium vomit prepared at Cogshall', presumably by an apothecary.[170] During his final illness, he took Daffy's elixir, Talbor's pills and a medicine prescribed by the London physician Dr Cox, with whom Josselin corresponded.[171] In an attempt to cure his leg, Josselin also made a trip to Tunbridge Wells, drinking the waters there between 13 July and 1 August 1675. He also had an 'issue made on me in order to the cure of my leg' in June 1675.[172] However, even during those last ten years of torment, Ralph relied mainly on simple, herbal remedies, both as dressings and as internal medicines. He poulticed his leg with red rose leaves and milk, with bread, with burdock leaves, clote leaves and green tobacco leaves.[173] He ate nutmeg, took hartshorn drops and drank 'Mrs. Spicer's ale'.[174]

A question which is often asked is 'did these remedies work?' Certainly modern herbalists and homeopaths rely on substances which would have been familiar to the Josselins. However, the purpose of this study is not to determine by controlled experiments whether herbal or 'old-fashioned' remedies actually ameliorate symptoms like those the Josselins suffered from, but to explore the Josselins' experiences as related in Ralph's diary. As indicated above, the question of whether or not a medicine 'worked' was understood differently by Ralph Josselin from the way it would be by a modern patient.[175] For him, a remedy could 'work' without curing the patient. This was the case when his daughter Mary, five days before her death, was given a clyster which 'wrought very well'.[176] Indeed, medicine was expected to make the patient feel sick. When Josselin's two children, Thomas and Jane, were given physic in June 1650 (presumably in a state of health), they 'were sick even to death, so that our hearts trembled, fearing the issue, but the lord in mercy to us quickly blew it over, and they revived and are now well'.[177]

Of course, the Josselins hoped that medicine taken during times of illness would help to produce a cure. In May 1683, when Ralph was desperate for relief from his multiple ailments, he wrote to Dr Cox in London for prescriptions. He reported, 'Cox sent me his old receits: the Apothecary made [me] pay dear'.[178] Several days later he wrote, 'I took my physic from Dr. Cox . . . my wife apprehends it doth me no good, but I cannot be fully of that mind'.[179] Some remedies were more definite in their effects. When Jane senior had wind and toothache in July 1646, pills 'wrought very kindly and carried the wind sensibly out of her side' while tobacco gave her 'much ease' from her toothache.[180] And when Ralph returned from travelling, aguish and sore, Jane's 'careful use of means', together with her tenderness and God's goodness, cured him.[181]

In most cases Ralph and Jane Josselin relied upon their own medical knowledge and skill to treat their own ailments and those of their children. However, they occasionally asked for the help of other people – friends, nurses, part-time healers and full-time medical 'professionals'. Lady Honeywood apparently acted as an informal general practitioner, advising the Josselins when their children were ill, and even looking after Ralph senior for over a month when his left leg first began to trouble him.[182] About this visit Ralph wrote on 27 January 1673, 'Went to Markshall. My L. Honeywood sent her coach for me. There I stayed to March 10 in which time my Lady was my nurse and physician and I hope for much good'.[183] As we have seen, Jane Josselin was able to return Lady Honeywood's favour, helping out at Markshall when a Honeywood child was ill. The Josselins also asked the Harlakendens at the priory for medical help, getting from them a medicine for worms during Mary's final illness.[184] Neighbours other than the local gentry also helped the Josselins during their illnesses. When Ralph suffered from a particularly severe ague fit on 13 February 1648, '2 hours before day . . . some neighbours came in'.[185] And when Jane became faint and ill with grief in August 1650, Ralph 'sent for neighbours'.[186]

In addition to this informal help from lay-people, the Josselins also consulted two local women who apparently acted as bone-setters. When John Josselin 'had a fall about the street threshold which made him limp', the 'shut-bone in his instep' was set by 'Spooner's wife'.[187] When the second Mary's arm was pulled out of joint by the maid, 'Mrs. Withers came and set it', splinting Jane senior's instep at the same time (for what injury we are not told).[188]

When Jane Josselin gave birth she was routinely attended by the midwife and a number of neighbour women. In at least one case a nurse was present. Twice Jane's labours were so quick that the midwife could not be summoned.[189] As Ralph wrote on one of these occasions, 'when god commands deliverance there is nothing hinders it'.[190]

In three recorded cases the Josselins hired a nurse to help out for the first few weeks after a baby was born, when Jane was still in bed. The nurse stayed for about a month after their third child was born, and stayed for five days after the death of the first Ralph.[191] She stayed only two weeks after the birth of their eighth child, but this was because she had promised her services to another woman.[192] Ralph thought no less of her for this, calling her 'an honest harmless quiet woman'. The nurse was apparently summoned about a week before the child was expected. For instance, although in the last mentioned case where the nurse left when the baby was 2 weeks old, Josselin indicated that she left on the twentieth day of her stay.

The Josselins almost never consulted physicians and surgeons. Despite the fact that five Josselin children died between February 1648 and July 1673, only once was a physician called to a child's death-bed. Oddly enough, this one occasion was four days before the death of the first Ralph, then only 6 days old.[193] One wonders whether the physician also saw Ralph senior, then ill of ague, since the baby was prescribed syrup of roses – the same medicine his father had taken three days earlier.

Otherwise the only member of the Josselin family to consult physicians, surgeons and apothecaries was, as far as we know, Ralph senior. This he did on only one recorded occasion in his early life, during a quotidian ague.[194] He did not see a physician thereafter until 1675, when he had already suffered with his swollen and ulcerated left leg for two years. During his long final illness, Josselin consulted the physicians Dr Talbor and Dr Cox.[195] He apparently visited Dr Talbor in person, while he merely corresponded with Dr Cox. During the same illness he also consulted two surgeons – the first unnamed, the second a Mrs Doughtie.[196] He also used the services of an apothecary to make up Dr Cox's prescriptions.[197]

It would be incorrect to suggest that Josselin 'did not believe in' physicians. In one case already cited, the instance when Mr R. H. suffered an emotional crisis, Josselin sent for a physician himself, feeling that medical intervention was necessary. Indeed, Josselin had a personal friend who was a physician. Dr and Mrs Colier and their daughter arrived from London on 1 August 1664, and stayed with the Josselins until 19 August. During their visit, John Josselin developed a violent fever: Josselin wrote, 'it was a great mercy Dr. Colier was with us'.[198] None the less, it seems obvious that the Josselins only rarely felt that the services of a physician were necessary, even in the most extreme cases. Since Ralph never wrote about his feelings about physicians, one can only speculate about the reasons for his behaviour.

Possibly the Josselins avoided licensed medical practitioners because of the expense involved in consulting them. Despite Ralph's comparatively high socio-economic standing in Earls Colne, he mentioned cash-flow problems on several occasions, and certainly as a man with a large family, he felt the need to be careful about expenditure.[199] Perhaps there were so few physicians and surgeons in the vicinity that the Josselins felt it impractical to rely upon them even during crises. However, the most likely explanation of the Josselins' behaviour is that neither healers nor remedies were of ultimate importance in determining the outcome of an illness. Whatever happened was God's will.

Josselin rarely mentioned health or illness without mentioning God. In this, as indicated above, he was a man of his time. It might be tempting to argue that Josselin, the vicar, was merely paying pious lip-service to convention. After all, he did resort to physical remedies as well as prayer. However, the diary leaves no doubt that Josselin's faith was real and, from his point of view, rewarded. For instance, when Josselin was troubled with an ague in 1643, his physician told him he would have one more harsh fit, 'but on Friday night seeking God for my health that if it pleased him I might go on in my calling, I was strangely persuaded I should have no more fits neither had I'.[200] As this example demonstrates, although Josselin occasionally consulted healers and used medicines, hoping that these would help, he placed far more confidence in the Divine Physician.

Josselin truly felt that the best remedy was prayer and the best preventative medicine was a sinless life. As Alan Macfarlane points out, Josselin held himself responsible for both his own ailments and those of his children.[201] This belief is taken to its logical extreme in Josselin's assumption that God had punished him for his fondness for playing chess by killing the infant Ralph.[202] Josselin's feelings of guilt and responsibility drove him to ever-stronger devotion to God: after all, his family and friends were, in effect, hostages for his good behaviour.

Fortunately for Josselin, the divine pendulum swung both ways. His preoccupation with providence as it affected himself and his neighbours has been mentioned above. Believing that evil-doers were surely and swiftly punished, he was often relieved and grateful when potential disasters failed to harm him and his. For instance, on 31 March 1648 on a trip to Colchester, 'my horse threw me as I returned home, but through the good providence of God, I had no hurt at all'.[203] However, only good behaviour and prayer could predispose God in Man's favour, and even those sometimes failed. Because of his limited capabilities, Man could not always know how he had sinned in order to bring calamity upon himself. Thus, when both his wife and daughter were ill, Josselin wrote, 'It's hard to find out the particular cause of our troubles, but what good we omit, or ill we do that is hinted to us, it's safe to reform, to thee oh . . . lord we come in Christ for thy healing in body and spirit'.[204] Therefore, Josselin and his family were perpetually at work to propitiate their stern heavenly father. They prayed as individuals, in family groups and with friends and neighbours to heal sickness, survive childbirth, avoid epidemics and, in one case, help a parishioner while he was being cut for the stone in London.[205]

Ralph Josselin's theological view of illness dovetailed nicely with his humoral orientation. Both approaches saw ill-health as a personal, particular manifestation stemming from divine displeasure, or an imbalance of the individual's humoral make-up. Thus, each individual's ailment was different from those of others, requiring individual understanding for its cure. Thus a cold could be caused either by the sufferer's sin or by his having had wet feet. In either case, it could be dealt with by a combination of physical 'means' and prayer. Without divine sanction, it could not be cured. In the case of epidemics, of course, collective sin and 'distempered and infected air' worked together to produce a calamity in the face of which humanity could only bow its collective head.[206] Perhaps this is why Josselin so feared epidemic diseases such as smallpox and plague. His own good behaviour and repentance might not be enough to save him and his family from such infections. Consider his reflections in August 1644, when the plague, 'that arrow of death', was at Colchester. 'What a mercy of God is it to respite our town Lord spare it, and let not our sins, our covetousness and pride of the poor in the plenty of their Dutch work cause thee to be angry with us'.[207] How fearful, to have to depend upon the relative virtue of all of one's fellow townspeople!

IV SICKNESS BEHAVIOUR AND ATTITUDES

Despite the numerous references to ill-health contained in the diary, neither Ralph Josselin nor members of his family often took up a 'sick' role. While they frequently complained and sometimes took medicines, their behaviour was analogous to that of modern people whose livelihoods would be threatened by too frequently 'calling in sick'. This is not surprising. When Ralph fell sick, he had either to find a local clergyman willing to preach to his congregation or to leave his flock without spiritual comfort. As noted above, even when he became a near invalid in his last years, he managed to preach on Sunday. Certainly his living was by no means so secure that he could afford to neglect his duties. Particularly after the

Restoration, Josselin remained in Earls Colne on sufferance.[208] A long illness might have helped to persuade the already suspicious authorities that the Nonconformist Josselin had to go.

Jane Josselin also could not afford to take to her bed when she felt unwell. Although she had a maid-servant to help with housework and childcare, her task was a heavy one. Her house was relatively large, her family at most times numbering seven or eight (including husband and servant as well as children). In addition to helping with the cooking, cleaning and farm-work she nursed her husband, children and servant when they were ill, and also helped friends and neighbours, as indicated above. She was needed. Thus, although her pregnancies were uncomfortable and she frequently complained of aches and pains when she was not pregnant, she neither took up a sick role nor was regarded as sick by her husband unless her illness actually incapacitated her.

The diary does not always indicate when one of the Josselins was confined to bed. Jane senior spent about three weeks in bed after each childbirth. Ralph was confined to bed for about two weeks with a severe ague attack in February 1648. Thomas spent at least two weeks in bed with smallpox in June 1659. Mary spent between two and three weeks in bed with her attack of worms before she died in May 1650.

During acute bouts of illness, the Josselins were treated differently from the way they were during periods of minor discomfort. They were visited by friends and neighbours, remedies were actively sought and, in at least Ralph senior's case, the sufferer's urine was examined. Family members took care of one another. We have already seen that Jane or her daughters were expected to dress Ralph's diseased leg. When Jane senior was seriously ill with a quartan ague in the autumn of 1668, her adult daughter Jane came home to tend her. And when Elizabeth was reported to be fatally ill in London in March 1682, Jane senior hurried to be with her.

The process of arising from a sick-bed was gradual and apparently conformed to certain expected conventions. Ralph reported when Thomas was able to sit up and when he first came downstairs during his recovery from the smallpox.[209] He mentioned when his wife arose from her bed and when she first left the house – usually to go to church – after giving birth.[210]

Conversely Josselin occasionally commented when an illness did not confine the sufferer to bed or keep him or her from daily employments. On 28 April 1650, in one of his many weekly reports of his family's health, he wrote, 'Mary, and my wife, ill but not down sick'.[211] And when Ralph had a cold, 'pose' and pain in the right side of his head in September 1646, he wrote 'yet praise be god I continued able to do my work'.[212]

Unfortunately the diary does not mention special food or clothing used during times of sickness. It says virtually nothing about the expected sick role and treatment of young children. Yet it certainly gives the impression that the Josselins had definite expectations of themselves and others during periods of acute illness. Sick people were expected to act sick – to stay in bed, be waited on and (possibly) take medicine. People well enough to be out of bed were entitled to complain about discomfort but were expected to carry on with their normal duties as far as possible. The major exception to this rule, then and now, was chronic illness. Although Ralph was able to preach during the last ten years of his life, he behaved in other respects like a sick person, trying many remedies, consulting several healers, and expecting special services and consideration from family members.

As we have seen, the Josselins suffered from and died of a variety of illnesses. However, the ailments they had, with minor exceptions, were not the ones Ralph most feared. For instance, although his daughter Mary died of worms, he did not appear to be particularly concerned when he or others of his children suffered from that complaint. After her death, he even mentioned his relief that her disease had not been infectious.[213] Yet he was terrified of epidemic diseases, particularly smallpox and plague. He mentioned his apprehension about smallpox no fewer than twenty-one times in the course of some thirty years. His fear remained even after several of his children had contracted the disease and recovered from it. Whenever smallpox was in Earls Colne, Josselin mentioned the fact, and often gave details of those who died from it.[214] Always nervous about it, his fear apparently reached a peak during a particularly virulent outbreak of the disease in 1651. When both Thomas and John developed rashes in early 1652, Josselin was certain they had the smallpox.

Although plague was a less frequent visitor to the vicinity, Josselin feared it terribly. During the great plague year 1665–6, he recorded figures from the London Bills of Mortality weekly. His comments on Earls Colne's virtual escape from infection ranged from the complacent 'God good in our preservation', to the frantic 'when will Colne lay it to heart', to the mystified 'and yet Colne, sinful Colne spared'.[215]

Josselin's fears were based on both medical and religious concerns. Plague and smallpox were particularly deadly diseases. Although there were many remedies which promised to prevent or cure the plague, it was generally regarded as incurable. And, while physicians argued the merits of 'hot' or 'cooling' regimens in the treatment of smallpox, the disease mutilated those it did not kill and was, therefore, particularly horrific.[216]

More frightening than the failure of medicine to deal with epidemics was their sudden and mysterious onset. Josselin was convinced that epidemics, like all other diseases and misfortunes, were God's punishment for sin. Seeing epidemics as a threat, Josselin yet felt he could do very little to keep them away. He could merely pray and watch their progress with horrified fascination. He also may have seen epidemics as possible heralds of the end of the world. For instance, he described the late summer of 1647 as a time

> of great sickness and illness, agues abounding more than in all my remembrance, last year and this also, fevers spotted rise in the county, whether it arise from a distempered and infected air I know not, but fruit rots on the trees as last year though more, and many cattle die of the murrain, this portends something.[217]

Whatever the reasons, epidemic diseases were for Ralph Josselin what cancer is for many modern Westerners. The mysterious terrors of their very names made the shivering and burning of ague fits seem desirable by comparison.

V CONCLUSIONS

The Josselins' experience of ill-health can by no means be assumed to be typical for mid-seventeenth-century England. For instance, Ralph Josselin's near contemporary, Samuel Pepys, was both more secular in his attitude toward disease, and more likely to consult a licensed physician or surgeon than was the vicar. The conclusions we can draw must therefore refer only to the Josselins themselves.

Ralph Josselin was unwell, or at least uncomfortable, most of the time. It is no wonder that he at one time reflected that 'this life is a bundle of sorrows'.[218] The nearly continual colds which plagued him and his family, their unpleasant eye and skin disorders, and the endless discomforts of Jane's pregnancies, surely encouraged the feeling that ill health was a normal state of affairs. Indeed, Josselin commented on good health whenever he could in his weekly reports, thus giving the impression that such a state of affairs was at least worthy of remark.[219]

Although the Josselins occasionally consulted healers and more frequently used medicines, they did not expect to be cured by such measures. Rather, they hoped for some help through them, but were not disappointed when remedies and healers failed. Their ultimate trust was in God, and they did not expect to feel completely well in any case.

For the Josselins, as for their contemporaries, death was familiar and expected. It could come at any time, as the result of any accident or illness. Thus, it was natural to think of death for oneself or one's loved ones in almost any situation. For instance, nine days after giving birth, Jane was 'very ill, as if she would have even died, [and] she uttered as formerly these words thou and I must part'.[220] When 2-month-old John became ill, his father expected death and 'cried to my God with tears for him and he heard presently he sweetly revived'.[221]

However, for Ralph Josselin the expectation of death did not reduce the value of the loved one. If anything, his wife and children were precious to him partly because his fear of losing them was quite real. Certainly Josselin did not fail to become emotionally attached to his children because of the likelihood that they would not survive. His grief for 8-year-old Mary produced the most moving passage in the diary, and his desolation is apparent in his reflections on the deaths of Thomas and Ann in the summer of 1675: 'god hath taken 5 of 10. lord let it be enough, and spare that we may recover strength'.[222]

And, in the same vein, despite Lawrence Stone's argument, naming a child after a deceased sibling did not, for the Josselin family, indicate 'a lack of sense that the child was a unique being, with its own name'.[223] There were probably two different reasons for the two examples of this practice in the Josselin family. In one case, two infants born within fifteen months of each other were named Ralph after their father. In this case the re-use of the name indicates, not disregard for the individuality of the first baby (though he died at only 10 days old), but a special value placed upon the name itself. In the second case, the Josselins' eighth child was named Mary nearly eight years after the death of her older sister of that name. In this case, it is fair to assume that the name was meant as a memorial to the deceased older child rather than as a negation of her individuality.

Despite expectation of death, the Josselins were relatively fortunate in surviving the hazards of their time. Ralph himself lived to be 67. His wife, only ten months younger than he, survived him, as did five of his children, the eldest of whom was nearly 38 and all of whom were over 19 at the time of his death. Considering Lawrence Stone's findings, that in 1650 40 per cent of squires and above left no son; that nearly 40 per cent of children born in 1650 died before the age of 15; and that peers born in 1625 could expect to live until only about 31, Ralph Josselin and his family did very well indeed.[224]

8

THE CHARACTER OF A GOOD WOMAN: WOMEN AND ILLNESS

I INTRODUCTION

In this chapter we will see the experience of sufferer and healer combined. Women, like men, endured the multifarious ills of seventeenth-century life. However, as indicated above, their traditional role demanded that they also act as healers. Such a demand was not unique to seventeenth-century England. One anthropological study states

> No matter how we may wish to interpret a prehistoric gynomorphic world and women's ritual roles in it, it is clear that feminine ritual domains and roles today usually centre on midwifery, participation in possession cults, and healing. Women participate in rituals of healing nearly everywhere, for in most cultures such ritual roles are both achieved and ascribed.[1]

The stereotypes of the female witch, midwife, nurse and traditional healer remain a familiar part of our own cultural heritage.

The evidence suggests that by the seventeenth century both the scope of activities of female healers and the respect generally accorded them was in decline. Muriel Joy Hughes's excellent study of *Women Healers in Medieval Life and Literature* gives details of both literary characters and female medical practitioners known in medieval Europe.[2] Her work shows that women acted as both amateur and paid healers and that some women received medical educations comparable to those of their male colleagues. Although few medical faculties opened their doors to women, those at Florence and Naples apparently did in this period.[3] Some medieval female healers were both respectable and famous.[4]

Alice Clark, whose *Working Life of Women in the Seventeenth Century* remains the standard authority on the subject, maintained that the gradual exclusion of women from many

L I B E R

LIBER QVARTVS.

DE VARIETATIBVS NON NA-
turalis partus, & earundem curis.

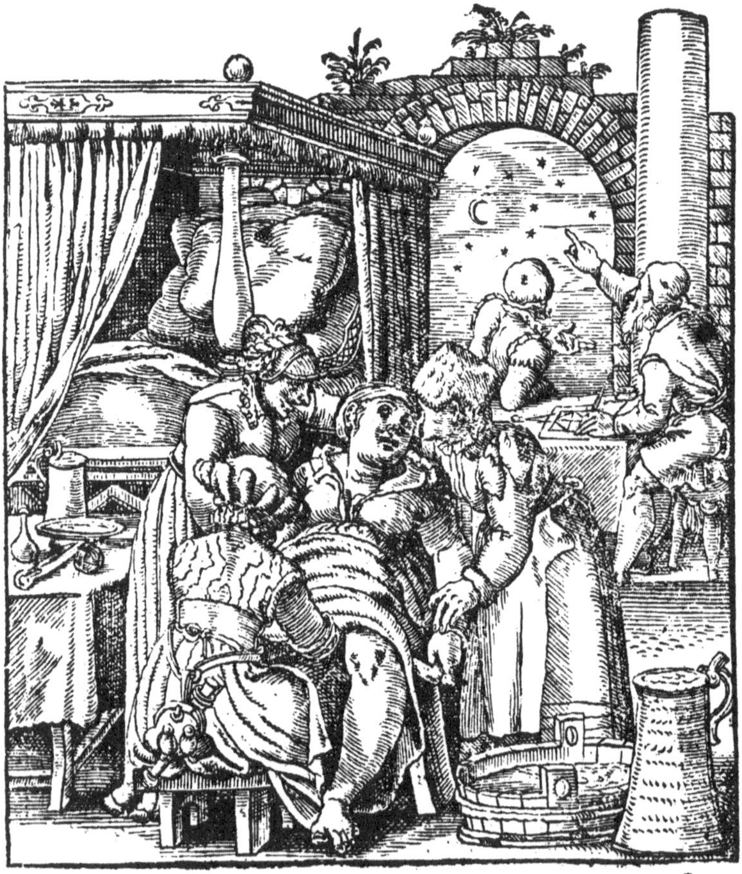

Quan-

A late sixteenth-century birth scene. While the midwife delivers the baby, the mother's friends comfort and encourage her, and the physician casts the new-born's horoscope. (J. Rueff, *De conceptu et generatione hominis*, 1580.)

paid occupations was an aspect of the growth of capitalism and industrialisation. She wrote,

> It has been shown that when social organisation rested upon the basis of the family, as it chiefly did up to the close of the Middle Ages, many of the services which are now ranked as professional were thought to be specially suited to the genius of women, and were accorded to them in the natural division of labour in the family.[5]

In the seventeenth century such services as school teaching and healing had established themselves in the marketplace. Removed from the domestic sphere, they became less and less appropriate for women.

Although many women did practise as paid healers in seventeenth-century England, their activities were frowned upon by male practitioners and most conventional avenues for medical and surgical education were closed to them. English universities would not admit them. Neither would the Royal College of Physicians. While the London Company of Barbersurgeons admitted women to the 'freedom', these practitioners were denied the privileges of full membership.[6] And the Charter of the Company of Barbersurgeons at Salisbury (1614) specifically excluded women.[7]

Such discrimination was directly related to commonly held views regarding the basic nature of women. These views were partly determined by theology. Judaic and Christian scholars saw women as the daughters of Eve, inherently sinful and evil. The only way a woman might possibly escape such categorisation was by denying her femaleness and becoming a nun. According to St Jerome,

> As long as a woman is for birth and children, she is different from man as body is from soul. But if she wishes to serve Christ more than the world, then she will cease to be a woman and will be called man.[8]

Classical and medieval theories of female physiology supported the theological line. Some writers, with Aristotle, saw women as inversions of men, imperfect and corrupt; the mere uncreative vessels of male seed. Some took Galen's slightly more positive view that women were unique in design, like men possessing the creative 'semen' necessary to produce a child.[9] However, none of the medical writers argued that women were equal to men. They assumed that women were peculiarly vulnerable to disease because of their physiology and often took a female patient's menstrual and childbearing history into account in diagnosing and treating her, regardless of the ailment she complained of. Menstruation, the common denominator of female experience and identity, while necessary to the mature woman's health, was also the mark of her inferiority. Menstrual blood itself was regarded as venomous, sometimes hurting women as it flowed, and posing danger to anything or anyone coming into contact with it.[10] Menstruating women soured wine and caused plants to die. A book published in 1506 warned that sexual intercourse during menstruation would be fatal to the man.[11]

In addition, women were viewed as sexually insatiable. Lack of orgasm, like amenorrhoea, could cause illness. The physician Nicolas Fontaine wrote in 1652, 'Wives are more healthful than widows or virgins, because they are refreshed with the man's seed, and ejaculate their own'.[12] For men, however, retention of semen increased physical and moral strength.[13] The man's sexual urge was controllable; the woman's was not.

Thus, female physiology reinforced the view that women were both inferior and dangerous. Such views permeated social life and were manifested in various ways. Perhaps the most extreme was in the scholarship concerning witchcraft. The *Malleus Maleficarum* (1486), for two centuries the chief handbook for witch-hunters, is imbued with male fears about female physiology and sexuality.[14] Although authorities on the subject agreed that men as well as women could be witches, the *Malleus* argued that 'Women are chiefly addicted to Evil Superstitions'.[15] Such women copulated with devils. They also came to innocent men as they slept and sexually assaulted them in a kind of demonic rape. Witches could make men impotent. They also performed a form of magical castration, working 'some Prestidigitory Illusion so that the Male Organ appears to be entirely removed and separate from the Body'.[16] Women deprived of normal sexual activities were most likely to become witches, partly because Satan offered himself to them as a sexual partner.

Witches, both male and female, were involved with the causing and curing of illness. Traditional healers, such as white witches, cunning-folk and wise-men and -women, were particularly vulnerable to the attacks of witch-hunters. Indeed, the feminists Ehrenreich and English see the European witchcraze as essentially a male conspiracy to remove women from their prominent place in the practice of medicine.[17] While this overstates the case, persecution of witches did much to discourage the open practice of traditional medicine.

Of course, most women were not witches. However, their bodies handicapped them both socially and morally. Medical writers took a cooler tone than did witch-hunters. None the less, in their works

> woman is considered to be inferior to man in that the physiological effects of her cold and moist humours throw doubt on her control of her emotions and her rationality; furthermore, her less robust physique predisposes her . . . to a more protected and less prominent role in the household and in society. Although apparently not bound by the authority of the divine institution of matrimony, doctors nonetheless produce a 'natural' justification for woman's relegation to the home and exclusion from public office, and provide thereby, as well as coherence with a central tenet of theology, an important foundation on which arguments in ethics, politics and law are based.[18]

Writers of sermons and works on household management conventionally advised husbands that it was their duty to control their wives. Man, as the rational half of creation, was required to direct and organise irrational woman.

None the less, women were felt to possess natural aptitudes which were basically good. Healing, if done within the proper sphere, was one of these. Timothy Rogers, whose handbook was published in 1697, wrote that the good woman was one who

> distributes among the indigent, money and books, and clothes and physick, as their several circumstances may require.

She relieved

> her poor neighbours in sudden distress, when a doctor is not at hand, or when they have no money to buy what may be necessary for them; and the charitableness of her physick is often attended by some cure or other that is remarkable. God gives a *peculiar blessing* to the practice of those women who have no other design in this matter, but the doing good: that neither prescribe where they may have the advice of the learned, nor at any time give or recommend any thing to try experiments, but what they are assured from former trials is safe and innocent; and if it do not help cannot hurt.[19]

Such a description of female duties obviously was intended for women of middling and upper status. That many gentlewomen conformed to this ideal is evident. We have seen that Lady Margaret Hoby, Lady Honeywood and Jane Josselin, among others, gave medical treatment to relatives, friends and neighbours. In addition, examples are cited of poor women who cured and gave medical advice.[20] Along with household duties, gardening, bearing and caring for children and looking after men, healing was a natural manifestation of the feminine duty to nurture and sympathise.

As an amateur activity, healing remained respectable. In the early eighteenth century Cotton Mather wrote,

> It is time to fix my three elder daughters in the opficial and beneficial mysteries, wherein they should be well instructed; that they may do good unto others. . . . For Katy, I determine knowledge in physic and the preparation and dispensation of noble medicines. For Nibby and Nancy, I will consult their inclinations. . . . To accomplish my little daughters for housekeeping, I would have them at least once a week, to prepare some new thing, either for Diet or Medicine.[21]

More than a century earlier, Lady Mildmay, born Grace Sherrington, wrote that the cousin who had brought her up included medical studies in her general education:

> And when she did see me idly disposed she would set me to cypher with my pen, and to cast up and prove great sums and accounts, and sometimes to set me to write a supposed letter to this or that body concerning such and such things, and other times let me read in Dr. Turner's Herbal and Bartholomew Vigo, and other times set me to sing psalms, and other times set me to some curious [needle] work.[22]

This lady's daughter wrote of her that she 'spent a great part of her days in the search and practice [of] man's body drugs, preparations of medicines, and signs of disease'.[23]

Even the anti-quack writers, despite their doubts about women's fitness for learned endeavours, were uncharacteristically taciturn about the activities of gentlewoman healers.[24] These women were not only respectable, but also necessary. Even learned physicians accepted and used recipes culled from gentlewomen of their acquaintance.[25] Such ladies continued to heal long after the end of the seventeenth century.

Less generally respected, but certainly as useful, were the women who acted as paid healers. Lowliest in status were sick-nurses. Alice Clark reminds us that not all nurses were amateurs. Hospitals employed them and expected them to conform to convent-like rules. Parish account books record payment of nurses who attended the poor. Private families also hired nurses.[26]

The archetypal female healer was the midwife.[27] However, women also became surgeons and apothecaries. This sometimes happened as the result of a family connection. For instance, the sister of the great seventeenth-century oculist, Dr Turberville, practised in London after his death. Sometimes the family connection is either unknown or non-existent, as is the case with the female bone-setters and surgeon consulted by Ralph Josselin.[28]

It should be emphasised here that the services performed by paid female medical practitioners were identical to those performed by amateurs. Women routinely prepared and administered medicines, delivered babies, gave enemas, applied leeches and dressed wounds. As long as they remained unpaid, the worst crime male healers accused them of was interference.

Thus, women were intimately involved with all the health incidents of humanity – illness, injury, childbearing, old age and death. Female bodies, with their recurring cycles of menstruation, pregnancy, childbirth, lactation and menopause, tied women both personally and socially to the physical processes of life. Their roles as sufferers and healers were interwoven; within the domestic sphere, women were the medical authorities of seventeenth-century England.

II CASE STUDIES

In order to give a personal dimension to our exploration of the female experience of illness, we will examine a diary and an autobiography written by seventeenth-century women. The same difficulties attend the use of these materials as are associated with the use of similar records kept by men. The writers are invariably of middling or upper social status. Thus, one cannot assume that their attitudes and experiences are representative of those of the general population. This is particularly true for women, since fewer women than men have left any sort of personal account. In addition, the search for information relating to medical matters inevitably distorts our perception of the writer's general preoccupations. None the less, this study has thus far concentrated upon the experiences, attitudes and behaviour of male healers and sufferers. It is time to hear from the ladies.

Diaries and autobiographies, although equally useful to the medical historian, yield different sorts of information about the writer's illness experience. Diaries tell us of the day-to-day ailments, major and minor, suffered by the writer and her social circle; they also reveal much about attitudes toward pain and disease. Autobiographies, on the other hand, may say little about daily aches and pains. However, because their subject matter is selected from the writer's past, they can indicate much about the importance matters of health and illness had for her. In this section we will explore and compare the medical experiences of two women, the diarist Lady Margaret Hoby, and the autobiographer Mrs Alice Thornton.

Lady Margaret Hoby

Margaret Dakins was born in Linton, Yorkshire, to the prosperous landowner Arthur and his wife Thomasine in February 1571.[29] As their only child and heir, Margaret's future prospects were taken seriously; she was educated in the 'sternly Puritan' household of Catherine, Countess of Huntingdon. There she met her first husband, Walter Devereux, second son of the Earl of Essex. She was married in 1589 at the age of 18. As her husband was only 20, one might have expected the marriage to last for many years. However, he was killed in 1591, while taking part in his brother Robert's mission to assist Henry IV of France in the siege of Rouen.[30] Margaret and her fortune were again eagerly sought after in the marriage market. Within two months of Devereux's death, she married Thomas Sidney, favourite nephew of the Countess of Huntingdon. However, this marriage did not last much longer than her first. Sidney died in July 1595, and Margaret was again a widow.

Within a week of her husband's death, Margaret was approached by Sir Thomas Posthumus Hoby who, with the help of his redoubtable mother, Lady Russell, had sought her hand after Walter Devereux's death.[31] Hoby, whose personal attractions were apparently not great, pressed his suit eagerly.[32] However, it seems that business, rather than love, won the lady for him. Hoby and his powerful connections helped Margaret in a law suit she was involved in concerning land which both she and the new Earl of Huntingdon claimed.[33] She became Lady Hoby in August 1596, and took up residence in Hackness, Yorkshire. There she lived during the years 1599–1605, when she wrote her diary. There she died in 1633 after a long and virtuous life.

Margaret Hoby was a very wealthy woman. Her property was worth £1,500 a year when she died. She had no children, but committed herself and her fortune to the conventional lifestyle of the Puritan gentry of her time and to a variety of good works. She was very religious. After her death, Sir Thomas acted upon her wishes by having a chapel built in Harewood Dale 'for divine service for the good of the souls and bodies of the inhabitants' dwelling in the vicinity.[34] However, her spiritual concerns certainly extended beyond death-bed bequests. During her life she spent much of her time in prayer and devotional reading and conversation. So important was religion to her that she intended her diary as a kind of spiritual account-book, giving details of her devotional exercises and her emotional responses to them.

Despite the fact that hers was a spiritual diary, much may be learned from it about Margaret's illnesses, her healing activities and her attitudes concerning medical matters. It is noteworthy, however, that her diary is relatively poor in details regarding symptoms and treatment. It also mentions few disease names. Thus, while Margaret and Thomas were frequently unwell, we are rarely told what ailed them.

Such vagueness and brevity does not indicate ignorance on the writer's part. As we have seen, Lady Hoby was an active amateur healer who practised both physic and surgery. She grew medicinal herbs, and made many remedies.[35] We know little about her medical education. However, some of it at least came from her reading. As part of her normal routine, she 'read of the herbal'.[36] By the age of 28 she had a reputation as a healer which attracted patients from a large area surrounding her home. Thus, her taciturnity about the ailments she suffered and dealt with requires another explanation.

Matters of health and illness were sufficiently important to Margaret to warrant frequent mentions in her diary. However, they, along with other temporal matters, took a definite back seat to the spiritual concerns which dominated her life. Her entry for 13 January 1600 is quite typical:

> In the morning I, being not well, was driven, to the discomfort of my heart, with short prayer and preparation to go to church: after I came home I dined and, though I were not well, I went again to church where I heard a good sermon. . . . After, I passed the afternoon with little reading because of my sickness.[37]

Illness, as an obstacle to spiritual exercise, was to be either ignored or dealt with as quickly as possible. Intrinsically it was not of sufficient importance to warrant detailed description. Only as a sign of God's displeasure was it significant. Thus, in September 1599 she wrote,

> I was at public prayers very sick: the Lord pardon the sin for which I was so punished, it being the will of God often to punish one sin with another, for I had little profit by that prayer, by reason of my sickness.[38]

Illness was one of God's tools for educating and chastising humans. Only in this context was it truly worth mentioning in a spiritual diary.

A similar observation may be made about Margaret's healing activities. Entries are characteristically extremely brief. Most often she merely recorded having 'dressed' her 'patients'.[39] Even these single words tell us that she was rendering surgical services to people who viewed her as a healer and whom she viewed as clients. However, they tell us almost nothing about the disorders her patients suffered from. Surely her references to her healing activities were made because they redounded to her credit in the spiritual balance sheet she kept concerning herself and other people.

Like many of her contemporaries, including Ralph Josselin and Alice Thornton, Margaret Hoby believed in providence. Her God rewarded the good and punished the evil in this world as in the next. Illness and injury were never random. Thus, on 26 December 1601,

> Was young Farley slain by his father's man, one that the young man had before threatened to kill and, for that end, prosecuting him: the man, having a pike staff in his hand, run him into the eye and so into the brain: he never spoke after: this Judgment is worth noting, this young man being extraordinary prophane, as once causing a horse to be brought into the Church of God, and there christening him with a name, which horrible blasphemy the Lord did not leave unavenged, even in this world, for example t'others.[40]

Unlike Josselin, she rarely viewed her own ailments as punishment for specific sins. However, she credited God with both causing and curing them. Illness, like all other experience, was grist for her spiritual mill: she wrote after recovering from a pain in her shoulder, 'afflictions draw one nearer to God'.[41]

The personal medical history which can be extracted from Margaret's diary is brief, undetailed and undramatic. She was, after all, only 28 when she began writing it. She reported no major illness between 1599 and 1605. Indeed, she was blessed with comparatively good health, which she occasionally mentioned.[42] She did not suffer the repeated colds which tormented other diarists such as Josselin and Pepys. Neither did she report having had ague, although on one occasion Sir Thomas thought he was coming down with that disorder.[43] She noted no menstrual disorders; and, despite the fact that dynastic considerations probably made children desirable, she never mentioned her childlessness as either a physical or a spiritual problem.

This is not to say that she was never ill. Her repeated bouts of toothache sometimes made her so ill that she could not go to church.[44] She also suffered from two fits of the stone in 1601.[45] In addition, she complained of several colds, a cough, headache, pain in her spleen and pain in her shoulder.[46] However, usually she was simply 'unwell'. She reported feeling ill most frequently in the years 1600 and 1601, noting twenty-five complaints in 1600 and twenty in 1601. After that, her reporting of illness dropped dramatically. She mentioned being unwell only once in 1602 and 1603, three times in 1604 and twice in 1605. However, this was more likely the result of her gradual loss of interest in keeping a diary than a reflection of perfect health.

Although she was convinced that God caused illnesses, she did not expect Him to cure them without human aid. None the less, she believed that the hand of the healer was guided by the Lord. She wrote,

> I may truly conclude it is the Lord, and not the physician, who both ordains the medicine for our health and ordereth the ministering of it for the good of his children, closing and unclosing the judgements of men at his pleasure: therefore let everyone physician and patient call upon the Lord for a blessing.[47]

Like her contemporaries, Margaret dosed herself, was treated by friends and consulted healers. She rarely specified the kinds of remedies she took, reporting only the use of 'means'. Only infrequently did she note that a medicine had done her good. In September 1599 'means' cured her of a sickness. And in May 1605 she took 'something' which relieved a pain in her shoulder which came 'by reason of the cold'.[48] She reported only once that remedies had not helped. When she had a toothache on 28 February 1600, she 'was forced to use diverse medicines that did little profit'.[49] On other occasions we can only assume that the treatments applied had the effects she expected.

Both Margaret and Thomas Hoby took prophylactic physic. In April 1600 they travelled to York where they visited friends, heard sermons and consulted healers. Margaret saw two physicians, Dr Benet and Mr Lister, and was probably treated by a surgeon as well. It is likely that she was healthy at the time and that the trip was made primarily for medical reasons. She arrived in the city on 8 April, visited Dr Benet on the 10th, saw 'her physician' again on the 12th, took physic the 14th, 15th and 16th, was let blood on the 18th and took a clyster on the 19th. It is not surprising that she reported feeling unwell on the 20th and 21st.[50] Indeed, the physic she took on the 16th made her so ill she could not pray. Such a medical journey was quite typical for those of the Hobys' social status in the seventeenth century. Many people routinely took physic in the spring; and York, as the nearest population centre, provided a concentration of healers not available in the countryside.

During the period in which her diary was written, Margaret's physician was Mr Lister. She consulted him regularly after an initial interview in September 1599, when she noted that she had 'talked with a physician which, I hope, the Lord hath provided for me in stead of Dr. Brewer'.[51] Brewer had died suddenly about a month previously after having taken 'a medicine he ministered to himself to cause him to sleep'.[52] Lister became a friend of the family, visiting and dining with the Hobys in times of health as well as illness.[53] During a visit to York, when Sir Thomas was taking physic, Margaret 'talked awhile with Mr. Lister, and walked abroad and did see his lodgings' one morning. That evening Lister came to supper. The following morning, Margaret 'talked awhile with Mr. Lister of some of my griefs'.[54]

In addition to Mr Lister, Margaret consulted other healers, paying one, Stephen Tewble, a £7 fee.[55] She was also treated by lay-women of her acquaintance. When she suffered from a cold in London in December 1600, she took a medicine made by 'my lady of Limbrick'.[56]

Friends gave moral as well as medical support in times of illness. During the same cold mentioned above, Margaret stayed in her chamber and was 'visited by Mrs. Thornborow every day'.[57] Indeed, Margaret noted visits during illness and physic-taking as a matter of routine. When Thomas kept his chamber after taking physic in September 1600, he was 'visited by Mrs. Thornborow, Mrs. Blackcollor, and other[s]'.[58]

Margaret returned the favour, visiting the sick-rooms of relations and friends.[59]

However, Margaret's help to the ailing was more often medical than social. It is hard to tell whether her healing activities were more extensive or expert than those rendered by other gentlewomen of the time. None the less, it is certain that she viewed healing as an important duty. Between January and April 1600 she noted that she 'dressed' her 'patients' no fewer than thirty-two times. She appears to have held informal clinics in her home, to which those in need of her services came. For example, on 2 February 1600 she wrote, 'After I had prayed I dressed the sores that came to me'. In another entry she reported that she had 'dressed a poor boy's leg that came to me'.[60] Occasionally she attended her patients twice a day.[61]

She rarely described the problems she dealt with. Many appear to have been wounds. For instance, the serving-man Blakeborn cut his foot with a hatchet on 17 April 1600. Margaret dressed the wound that day and those following until at least the 27th.[62] She also dealt with other 'surgical' problems, giving a 'poor woman of Caton salve for her arm' on one occasion and making 'a salve for a sore breast' on another.[63] Her attempt to find a passage for the waste products of a baby born without an anus have been described above.[64]

In addition, Margaret prepared and prescribed internal remedies. She recorded having made an oil and having prepared a 'purgation for my cousin Ison's woman'.[65] She also attended confinements, although she never reported having delivered a baby herself.[66]

The great majority of her patients were nameless 'poor' people. Thus she provides an interesting contrast to Jane Josselin who treated friends and neighbours regardless of their economic and social circumstances. Margaret Hoby's healing activities smack of *noblesse oblige*. She gave medical treatment as charity – partly because she was skilful, partly because God approved. As a gentlewoman healer, she was conventional; as a Puritan, she aspired to salvation in all she did.

Margaret Hoby's experience of illness serves as a reminder of the dangers of basing historical generalisations on assumptions regarding the behaviour of people whose circumstances conform to predetermined categories. For instance, because she lived in the early years of the century in a remote rural area, was deeply religious and acted as an amateur healer, one might expect her to depend upon self-treatment and God's will in preference to the services of physicians. However, as we have seen, she regularly consulted physicians even when she was not ill, even making special journeys to York to do so. The previous chapter demonstrates that despite certain similarities, she and Ralph Josselin differed markedly in this respect. Both were intensely religious; both comparatively well educated. Both lived in rural communities. Both numbered physicians among their friends. Yet Margaret Hoby was routinely treated by physicians and Ralph Josselin was not. Perhaps the explanation lies in the differences in the circumstances of the two diarists. Josselin, although prosperous, was by no means wealthy. He had a large family to provide for. His village was his social world; he travelled little and lived on the fringes of gentry social circles very much as the neighbourhood vicar. On the other hand, Margaret Hoby was both wealthy and childless. She travelled often to York and London, a respected member of the gentry circuit of town and country houses. In consulting healers as she did, one suspects that she was simply acting in a conventional manner. Certainly her behaviour in this respect is similar to that of Alice Thornton and Lady Anne Halkett, despite their different religious views. Members of the gentry and nobility employed healers as they employed servants – to provide a specific service which they did not wish to do for themselves.

Alice Thornton

Alice Thornton's autobiography tells the tale of a gentlewoman whose status was in decline. She was born in February 1627, to Christopher and Alice Wandesford, wealthy landowners then residing in Kirklington near Ripon. Her father's cousin and patron was the Earl of Strafford. Due to that powerful connection, Christopher Wandesford became Lord Deputy to Ireland, 'acquiring a noble position and estate'.[67] Thus, Alice spent the years between 1632 and 1642 in Ireland, there living among the loyalist gentry and nobility. Her father died of a fever in 1640, and the family finally left Ireland after narrowly escaping harm in the Irish rebellion of 1641. The Wandesfords spent the years of the Civil War, at first wandering around England, then living at Hipswell, Alice's mother's jointure. Although her father's Irish property provided no income for them, enough was available of the English property to maintain their genteel life-style, despite the troubles and expenses inflicted on them by the war.[68]

In 1651 Alice married William Thornton of East Newton in Ryedale. According to the editor of her autobiography, the

Thornton family 'had occupied a fair position among the minor gentry of the North Riding of Yorkshire' for more than three centuries.[69] Greater matches had apparently been proposed to Alice. However, her mother favoured Thornton's suit, and his income (£600 a year) combined with Alice's portion (£500 from the English estate and £1,000 promised from the Irish) appeared to promise a 'handsome competency'.[70]

Alice was a dutiful rather than a joyful bride. She wrote of her engagement,

> Nor could I, without much reluctance, draw my thoughts to the change of my single life, knowing too much of the cares of this world sufficiently without the addition of such incident to the married estate.[71]

Some of her doubts concerned Thornton's religious convictions. His family had converted from Roman Catholicism to Presbyterianism in about 1600. Alice, having been 'educated in the faith of God, and the profession of the true protestant Church of England' could not bear to think of her children being brought up to be Presbyterians. However, Thornton assured her that he was 'for a moderated episcopacy, and kingly government' and that, if she would marry him their children might be educated as she wished.[72] This reservation having been satisfied, Alice accepted his proposal. However, her misgivings went with her to the altar. After the service, she became very ill with 'a great vomiting and sickness at my heart, which lasted eight hours'. This 'condition was extremely bewailed by my husband and mother and my friends, and looked upon as a sad omen to my future comfort'. Alice wrote with hindsight,

> Thus was the first entrance of my married life, which began in sickness, and continued in much afflictions, and ended in great sorrows and mournings. So that which was to others accounted the happiest estate were embittered to me at the first entrance, and was a caution of what trouble I might expect in it.[73]

Despite the bleakness with which she approached her marriage, Alice devoted herself to William Thornton until his death from palsy in 1668. Together they produced nine children, only three of whom survived infancy. None the less, her editor wrote that William was 'a weak, improvident man', who reduced rather than increased the income he had had at their marriage, eventually dying a bankrupt. In addition, Alice was 'unfortunate enough to be deprived of the greater part of her own inheritance'.[74] After her husband died, the widow lived on in the house the couple had had buily shortly after their marriage. She occupied herself with legal business concerning her property, fighting the slanders directed at her by enemies, and religious exercises. And, to record the events of her life and vindicate herself, she wrote her autobiography which she finished in 1669.

Because an autobiography is written from memories of the sometimes distant past, the process of selection involved in its composition reveals much about the general preoccupations of the writer. Alice Thornton was interested in the honour of her family (the Wandesfords), the events of the Irish Rebellion and Civil War, estate business and her own good name. In addition, she was concerned about matters of health and illness. She gave details of all of her own major illnesses and those of her husband and children. She described the last illnesses and death-bed scenes of a number of close relatives. She also recorded narrow escapes from injury and death as marks of the providence of God. Thus, her autobiography provides a wealth of information for the medical historian.[75] It is not as rich a source as diaries written to record the events of daily life, such as those kept by Ralph Josselin and Samuel Pepys. However, it is arguably as useful as the spiritual diary kept by Margaret Hoby because of its attention to detail. And, because it describes the writer's childhood ailments and those of other children in the household, it gives us information about more than one generation's experience of illness and healing.

Alice's preoccupation with the health incidents related to the bearing and rearing of children is understandable, considering her adult experience. She wrote that her own mother had 'brought me forth in great peril of her life, she being weak upon the birth of all her children, having had seven in all, four sons and three daughters'. Alice was 'both a strong and healthful child all along, never having had either the rickets or any other disease' – a fact which she attributed to having been nursed by the same healthy careful wet-nurse who had fed her elder brother.[76] This wet-nurse had 'fresh' milk for Alice, having 'had a child betwixt the nursing my brother and myself'. In this Alice was apparently more fortunate than were some of her own children.

Her daughter, Katherine, for instance, died aged 1 year, 6 months and 21 days, having 'been long in the rickets and consumption, gotten at first by an ague, and much gone in the rickets, which I conceive was caused by ill milk at two nurses'.[77] There is a suggestion that Alice's first living child also suffered from rickets.[78]

Alice's autobiography is a good source for information concerning breast-feeding. Her eldest child, Alice, was nearly overlain by her nurse when she was a new-born.

> One night my mother was writing pretty late, and she heard my dear child make a groaning troublesomely, and stepping immediately to nurse's bed side she saw the nurse fallen asleep, with her breast in the child's mouth, and lying over the child; at which she, being affrighted, pulled the nurse suddenly off from her, and so preserved my dear child from being smothered.[79]

Her experience of wet-nurses certainly suggested to Alice that she should breast-feed her children for their own good. She fed her son Robert until he was 3 years old.[80]

The most serious children's disorders Alice described were rickets, measles, convulsions and smallpox. When she was staying with her Aunt Norton, her father's sister, at about the age of 4,

> It pleased God to bring me into a very dangerous weakness and sickness, upon an accident of a surfeit, by eating some beef which was not well boiled; this causing an extreme vomiting, whose violence drove me into great fever, and that into the measles, and both brought me so low and weak that my aunt and . . . our maid almost despaired of my life.[81]

This description has been quoted at length because it demonstrates the common belief that one disorder could easily change into another, given the appropriate circumstances.[82]

Although the London Bills of Mortality indicate that convulsions claimed the lives of many children in the seventeenth century, in Alice Thornton's experience only one child suffered from this disorder. Her daughter Alice (or Naly, as she was called) had recurring seizures beginning when she was 1 year old. In the first instance, Naly

> being asleep in one cradle and the young infant [Katherine] in another, she fell into a most desperate fit, of the convulsions . . . her breath stopped, grew black in her face, which sore frighted her maid Jane Flower. She took her up immediately, and with the help of the midwife, Jane Rimer, to open her teeth and to bring her to life again. But still, afterwards, no sooner that she was out

> of one fit but fell into another fit, and the remedies could be by my dear mother and Aunt Norton could scarce keep her alive, she having at least twenty fits; all friends expecting when she should have died.[83]

In another instance, the 6-year-old Naly was taken to see a procession celebrating the Restoration. Having 'never seen any such things as soldiers, or guns, or drums, or noises, and shouting', she became distraught and 'fell into most dreadful fits of convulsions there, while she was at Richmond, in Mr. Smithson's shop'.[84] Again, all feared she would die.

Smallpox, in Alice's experience, was most dangerous to children. Like John Symcotts, Alice reported having had this disease more than once. She and her brother Christopher contracted smallpox in 1631 while living in London. Their father sent them to Kent, presumably to rid his house of the infection, and the two children, aged 4 and 6 respectively, 'lodged at one Mr. Baxter's, being kindly used with much care in that house'. Alice's case was mild and she recovered quickly.[85] Eleven years later, during their flight from Ireland, the Wandesford children found themselves in the midst of a smallpox epidemic. This time it was Alice's brother John who became ill first, having 'taken them of one of my cousin William Wandesford's sons'. John had a bad case which left him 'very much disfigured, having been a very beautiful child, and of a sweet complexion'. Alice's mother warned her to stay away from John's sick-room, obviously not assuming that previous experience of the disease would provide immunity. Alice obeyed, but she sent messages to her ailing brother tied around a little dog's neck,

> which, being taken into his bed, brought the infection of the disease upon myself, as also the sight of him after his recovery; being struck with fear seeing him so sadly used and all over very red, I immediately fell very ill, and from that time grew worse till I grew so dangerously ill and inwardly sick, that I was in much peril of my life, by their not coming well out but kept in at my heart.

She was treated by her mother, physicians and 'others', but had no ease until God 'pleased to hear out petitions for my life and to spare me in much mercy, and caused them to come well forth'.[86] As we shall see in Alice's descriptions of her own children's bouts with smallpox, the question of whether the spots 'struck' in or out was of much moment in the prognosis for any case.

Alice and John survived this epidemic. They were fortunate compared to Frank Kelly, a 9-year-old Irish boy whom their father had taken into his household 'for charity'. This child became very ill, was 'miserably sore and could not swallow; his sight was eaten out'. He died after fourteen days of torment, notwithstanding the efforts of Alice's mother, a 'doctor' and 'two watchers'. His death-bed conduct was exemplary, pious and selfless. Alice's account of it, like John Evelyn's descriptions of the deaths of his mother and 5-year-old son, create a picture of the ideal seventeenth-century English death. Alice wrote,

> All the time of this boy's sickness he was so full of sweet expressions and heavenly minded, with much acts of religion, that it was a great comfort to my mother, and all about him, with abundance of patience and gratitude to God and my mother for all they had done for him. . . . This poor boy . . . still prayed for me; when he heard I was in danger of death, desired with tears that God would be pleased to spare my life, and to bless me, that I might live to do much good to others, as to him, and that he might rather be taken away and I spared.

Such reports gave the dear departed the status of secular saints in the memories of those who survived them. They also enabled the healthy to make a much needed mental distinction between the beautiful spirit and disgusting body of one suffering from such a 'loathsome disease'.[87] In an age when the desperately ill were not segregated from the rest of the community, a 'good' death was doubly important to those being reminded of their own mortality.[88]

Alice's own children suffered from smallpox. One infant, William, died of the scourge at only 1 week old. In this drastic case the pocks 'struck in', taking the form generally recognised as the most deadly.[89] Indeed, the 'hot' regimen in treating smallpox favoured by most physicians, which included keeping the patient warm in bed and prescribing cordials, was specifically designed to force the spots outward. Another of Alice's new-borns, Christopher, may have died of the disease at 3 weeks.[90] Katherine had smallpox at the age of 10. Her illness began

> with a violent and extreme pain in the back and head, with such scrikes and torments that she was deprived of reason, wanting sleep, nor could she eat anything.

After three days the spots appeared, but due to her

'unguidableness struck in again'. After medication, they came out again and 'she was all over her face in one scurf, they running into each other'. She was bedridden for a month, afterwards healing well, but she 'lost by this sickness her fair hair on her head, and that beautiful complexion God had given'. Two months later, 5-year-old Robert contracted the disease, running through the now familiar pattern of general illness, concern about whether the spots would strike inwards, loss of sight, then a crisis, after which recovery followed quickly. However, Naly came down with smallpox just as Robert was recovering. She had a hard time, like Katherine losing her hair and complexion.[91] The experience of the Wandesfords and Thorntons makes clear just how common and deadly smallpox was in the mid-seventeenth century. It also demonstrates that the scarring left by the disease was not a handicap in the marriage market. In that practical age, social status and economic circumstances were far more important than a pretty face.

The Thorntons, like the Josselin children, encountered numerous accidents as well as illnesses. Alice herself suffered two serious injuries in childhood. At the age of 3 she stumbled in a passageway and struck her forehead against a stone. The wound was so severe that 'the skin of the brain was seen'. This hurt was healed by her mother.[92] The other injury occurred when she was 11. Unlike the accidents befalling the Josselin children, this came as the result of a game. Young Alice, along with other ladies, was 'using the custom to swing by the arms for recreation', an exercise regarded as particularly healthful for children. Alice was being swung vigorously by a young French page and let go of his hands, falling on her face on the floor. She landed

> with such a violent force with all my weight on my chin-bone upward, that both the chin and chap-bones was almost broke in sunder, and put the bone out of its place, and did raise a great lump as big as an egg under my chin and throat, which suddenly astonished me, and took away my breath in so much as I was nigh death.

Again, her mother was able to cure her.[93] In another play injury, Alice's daughter Naly received a 'wound in her belly'.

> My two children was playing . . . in the parlor window and Kate [then 5] being full of sport and play did climb into the window, and leaping down fell upon her sister Alice and thrust her upon

> the corner of the same with a great force and strength she had, and her sister cried out with pain and soreness which had grievously hurt the inner rind of her belly so sore till I was afraid she had broken it.

With hindsight, Alice praised 'the name of my God for ever that she was not wounded so as to break her bowels, it being in so dangerous [a] place and hazard in her bearing of children'.[94] For a girl with a reasonable marriage portion, such a handicap might ruin her future.

Solitary play was dangerous as well. At the age of 3 Kate 'was playing with pins, and putting them in her mouth. . . . At last she got a pin cross in her throat' which Alice removed with her finger. However, the situation was quite extreme, for Kate was 'as black as could be, and the blood set in her face with it'.[95] We are reminded of John Evelyn's son choking on a bone.[96] Kate, who was apparently a bit of a handful, while

> playing with her cousins in Newton barn and swing cross by a rope, she got so high a fall . . . that she was taken up dead, being black and without breath for a long time . . . ; and it was half an hour before any signs of life appeared. . . . [She] knew nothing of the fall a long time; it had done her much harm in her head, with great pains.[97]

Alice's descriptions of children's accidents make the reader wonder whether the Josselin diary might not have contained many more notes of the special providence of God regarding children's narrow escapes from death or serious injury had it been written by Jane, the main caretaker of the children, rather than Ralph.

Of course, adults suffered injuries as well as children. Alice's brother George drowned while attempting to cross a river on horseback.[98] Alice nearly lost the sight in one eye when it was pecked by a pet chicken.[99] She also tripped and fell when she was six months pregnant and worried that she might miscarry.[100] As it happened, the baby 'stayed in the birth, and came cross with his feet first' – a problem which Alice attributed to her fall. The infant died after less than an hour of life. In addition, she fell downstairs when pregnant with her son Robert, but the child was unharmed.[101]

The aspect of Alice Thornton's medical history which has received most attention from historians is her experience of childbirth and breast-feeding. Lawrence Stone was principally interested in the Thornton family's high infant mortality and

Dorothy McLaren in that mortality as it related to breast-feeding and wet-nursing.[102] Alice was certainly less fortunate concerning the survival of the babies she bore than was Jane Josselin. Five of Jane's ten live-born infants survived, as opposed to three of Alice's nine.[103]

Alice's own experience motivated her to feed her later babies herself. Her first living child, Naly, was nearly overlain by her wet-nurse, as we have seen. She fed Elizabeth for a short time, but the child died at 18 months of rickets and consumption caused 'by ill milk at two nurses'.[104] It is unlikely that Alice fed her third daughter, Katherine, herself, since the next baby was born only eighteen months after Katherine's birth. That infant died only half an hour after birth, so his death could not have been the result of bad nursing. However, Alice resolved to take no chances with the next baby. She wrote of William that he was

> in good health, sucking his poor mother, to whom my good God had given the blessing of the breast as well as the womb, of that child to whom it was no little satisfaction, while I enjoyed his life; and the joy of it maked me recruit faster, for his sake, that I might do my duty to him as a mother.[105]

Alice found breast-feeding personally satisfying; however, it failed to save William, who died of smallpox aged 1 week. None the less, after this experience, Alice continued to nurse her babies. She fed Robert until he was 3, weaning him only two weeks before giving birth to Joyce, whom she also breast-fed. Joyce died at 4 months of a 'cold which struck in many red spots all over her body and face'. Alice was still suckling her at this time. Her last child, Christopher, took readily to the breast and 'he thrived very well and grew strong, being a lovely babe'. However, this infant also contracted smallpox, dying at just under 3 weeks of age.[106]

As we have seen, Alice tried to give her younger five children the best possible start in life by breast-feeding them. This was uncommon for women of her social status. However, life in seventeenth-century England was fraught with deadly perils for those at any age. Infants were most at risk. Despite the evils of wet-nursing, only one of the six babies Alice lost died because of it. Disease and the hazards of pregnancy and birth accounted for the other five.

Alice's pregnancies were all uncomfortable, although she always felt healthier when she was carrying boys.[107] She was pleased when she conceived seven weeks after her marriage.

However, she was unwell until the child quickened, had a severe nosebleed when about four months pregnant and developed a 'putrid fever' at nearly eight months after journeying to her mother's house at Hipswell, where she planned to bear the baby. This illness was very dangerous, but her 'old doctor', Mr Mahum, 'could do little towards the cure, because of being with child'. Alice wanted to be let blood, a procedure generally frowned upon for pregnant women. This treatment was finally ordered by another physician, Dr Wittie, after an argument with Mr Mahum. Six days later, Alice's labour began. At this point, she had not felt the baby move for several days. The labour lasted for about twenty-four hours, the infant dying before it could be baptised. Alice suffered from the effects of her illness for a long time after the birth. She had a 'terrible shaking ague' for three months, which gave her two fits a day. Her hair and nails fell out and her teeth grew loose and black. Finally, 'upon great and many means used and all remedies', she recovered.[108]

This was not the only eventful and hazardous pregnancy and birth Alice underwent. As indicated above, she had several falls while pregnant which she feared would cause her to miscarry or would harm the baby. Indeed, concerning the pregnancy with her son Robert, she wrote that she had had 'five great trials and hazards of miscarriage'. The first was an illness she suffered; the second, 'a fright which came on me by surprise of the sight of a penknife which was nigh to have hurt me'. This shock caused the child to be born with 'a mark of a deep bloody colour upon the child's heart'. The third and fourth 'hazards of miscarriage' resulted from business troubles; the fifth was a fall down stairs.[109] Alice's fears reveal how perilous the world seemed to pregnant women in the seventeenth century. The bearing of children was important for both estate and personal reasons to women of her class. Sons were particularly precious. When William died, Alice was terribly grieved, and reported that her husband was sorely 'afflicted for his loss, and being a son he takes it more heavily, because I have not a son to live'.[110] With the threat of miscarriage ever-present, it is no wonder that Alice felt triumphant when she carried a baby full term and produced it alive.

Alice's labours were long and her deliveries difficult. For example, with her fifth child she experienced contractions for three days before 'sharp travail' began on Wednesday, 9 December. Her pains were so strong that the midwife felt she would deliver soon. However, the position of the baby was such that he could not be born. This

> condition continued till Thursday morning between two and three o'clock, at which time I was on the rack in bearing my child with such exquisite torment, as if each limb were divided from other, for the space of two hours; when at length, being speechless and breathless, I was, by the infinite providence of God, in great mercy delivered.

This birth was so traumatic for the baby that he lived only half an hour after it.[111]

Not all of Alice's labours were this difficult. However, they all weakened her terribly; and her troubles were not over once the baby was born. After several of her deliveries Alice lost a great deal of blood. In the first instance Alice was frightened by her daughter Naly's attack of convulsions after she had delivered Elizabeth. She experienced 'so great floods that I was spent, and my breath lost, my strength departed from me, and I could not speak for faintings'.[112] Sometimes in her weakened condition after childbirth, Alice fell prey to only tangentially related ailments. For instance, after the birth of her fifth child, she suffered 'the bleeding of the hemords every day for half a year together', along with lameness in her left knee. At the same time, her physician felt that she was 'deeply gone in a consumption, and if it continued longer I should be barren'.[113] And her three months of illness after the birth of her first child has been described above.

Despite the hazards of childbearing, Alice very much wanted children. As we have seen, she was very happy when she became pregnant shortly after her wedding, worried about miscarriages while she carried her babies, enjoyed feeding them once they were born and watched over them carefully as they grew. However, she was very aware of the dangers of childbirth. This awareness began before she ever had children herself. At the age of 19 Alice was present when her only sister, Catherine Danby, died after giving birth to her sixteenth child. Catherine had suffered more than her share of obstetrical troubles: she had miscarried six babies 'when she was above half gone with them . . . upon frights by fire in her chamber, falls, and such like accidents happening'. She was ill while carrying her last child. This, combined with 'the horrid rudeness of the soldiers and Scots quartered then amongst them', caused her to fall into labour prematurely. The 'child came double into the world, with such extremity that she

[Catherine] was exceedingly tormented with pains, so that she was deprived of . . . sleep for fourteen days . . . neither could she eat'. After one month of fever she died, having disposed of her worldly responsibilities and committed herself to God.[114] For Alice, Catherine's illness and death surely served as a warning of what married life had in store for her.

Alice did not voice her fears about carrying and bearing children until after the birth and survival of her son Robert. About her pregnancy with her eighth child, Joyce, she wrote that

> It pleased God to give me a new hope of comfort of bearing Mr. Thornton another child, although these are accompanied with thorny cares and troubles, and more to me than others.

When her delivery approached, she 'being terrified with my last extremity, could have little hopes to be preserved in this' without the help of God. She prepared for her ordeal by making recommendations for the education of her three living children and disposing of her own estate. Her labour was 'sharp and perilous', and she felt she only narrowly escaped with her life.[115] Thus, when she became pregnant again, she wrote

> and if it had been good in the eyes of my God I should much rather . . . not to have been in this condition. But it is not a Christian's part to choose anything of this nature, but what shall be the will of our heavenly Father, be it never so contrary to our own desires.

She was so tormented by her labour that her daughter Naly, 'with fear and grief for me, fell so sick . . . that she was in much danger of death'.[116]

As indicated in the previous chapter's discussion of Jane Josselin's experience, Alice's fears concerning her deliveries were certainly not unique.[117] Indeed, it would have been surprising if women did not fear something which was likely to bring them close to death. However, the bearing and rearing of children was viewed by both sexes as the divinely appointed duty of women – the only excuse for their creation. Women rarely attained more social importance than when they were giving birth. That God and the world of men approved of their condition was surely some comfort to such women as Jane and Alice.

In addition to the ills surrounding pregnancy and childbirth,

Alice and her relations suffered a multitude of ailments. Her mother had recurring bouts of the stone. Her brother Christopher had fits of the spleen. Her husband became a chronic sufferer from palsy in 1665, three years before his death. Her cousin died of pleurisy.[118]

An important cause of disease, in Alice's experience, was surfeit. As we have seen, she came down with measles after a surfeit upon improperly prepared beef. Her cousin Edmund Norton died after eating melons which were 'too cold for him'. Naly had a choking fit in her sleep after a surfeit upon turbot.[119] The dangers of surfeit reveal the importance of moderate and careful diet for subscribers to the humoral view of illness. Eating too much or the wrong kind of food might cause a serious imbalance in the body's humours.

Another frequent cause of illness was emotional upset. William Thornton developed an ague as a result of 'sadness and discontent' occasioned by the money matters surrounding his marriage. We have seen that Naly became ill with worry when Alice was in labour with her last child. However, Alice herself was the principal sufferer from this kind of disorder. It would not be an exaggeration to say that Alice's usual reaction to the illnesses of her family members was to become ill herself. She had to be sent home from Catherine Danby's death-bed because she had become very weak. Her excessive bleeding after giving birth to her third child resulted from worry about Naly's convulsions. Alice was pregnant and ill with business worries when her daughter Katherine contracted smallpox. She became so distressed about the child's illness and so disturbed by her 'crying night and day, that I was forced to be removed . . . into the scarlet chamber, for want of rest'. Upon receiving the news of her husband's first attack of palsy, she

> was brought into a violent passion of grief and sorrow, with fits of sounding [swooning], which I never knew before; and prevailed so exceedingly that I immediately went sick to bed, being so weak upon that occasion that all gave me for dead, so that it was an impossibility to carry me alive to see my dear husband.

And when he suffered a later attack, she took to her bed again.[120]

Other sorts of upsets made her ill as well. Her illness on her wedding day may well have been due to her doubts about marrying at all. Business troubles weakened her. And her anger at the slanders directed at her by Mrs Anne Danby caused her to fall 'into a very great and dangerous condition of sickness, weakness of body, and afflicted mind'. Indeed, it is likely that illness was a refuge for Alice, however uncomfortable it made her. In bed, she was cared for and could muster her strength for her return to the cares of the world.[121]

Like Margaret Hoby, Alice Thornton routinely consulted physicians. Most important of these was Dr Wittie or Witty of Hull, who first attended her during her first pregnancy. It is probable that Alice obtained the services of this physician along with her married name, for she recorded that Wittie had treated William Thornton before their wedding. In any case, the physician treated the Thorntons at least until William's death, often travelling long distances to do so. While she was living with her mother at Hipswell, Alice was treated by Mr Matrum or Mahum, who also attended her during the illness surrounding her first delivery. And another physician, Alice's brother-in-law Timothy Portington, treated the Thorntons during the period 1666 to 1669.[122] On a number of occasions these healers consulted together over the condition of their patient, sometimes disagreeing about the proper course of treatment.

From these healers the Thorntons received the conventional therapy of the time. They were purged, vomited and let blood. Like their contemporaries, they sometimes suffered the consequences of 'heroic' physic. Alice's mother-in-law died as the result of taking an antimony vomit which caused 'a flux of blood by siege, as it was supposed to have a vein broken inwardly'. And both Naly and Alice's nephew contracted smallpox after taking physic to prevent the disease.[123]

The relationships between Alice and her relatives and the healers they consulted were generally good. Alice and William deferred to Dr Wittie's judgment and were content with his therapies for many years. However, there is more than a suggestion that they, like their contemporaries, suggested many of the treatments administered to them. As we have seen, when Alice fell ill during her first pregnancy, she felt that only phlebotomy would cure her, despite Mr Mahum's objections. One may even suppose that she called upon the services of Dr Wittie because she assumed he would support her. Clearly the human frailties of physicians were recognised. Alice's mother was annoyed when her husband lay dying because when she 'desired the physicians to give her a true state of his condition, whom she perceived grew weaker . . . , they would not deal truly, nor acknowledge his desperate case'. Both she and the dying man realised the truth of the matter when the physicians prescribed 'pigeons cut' to be 'laid to the soles of the feet' – a measure which Christopher recognised as 'the last remedy'.[124]

Despite their consultation of learned healers, it is clear that the Wandesfords and Thorntons conformed to the contemporary pattern of self- and lay-treatment. After both of the serious injuries Alice had during her childhood, Alice's mother nursed and healed her. Her mother also treated her, her brother John and Frank Kelly when they had smallpox.[125] Alice followed this pattern by treating her own children when they fell ill. Her knowledge of children's disorders and medicines is revealed in her description of baby William's illness. The baby

> began to be very angry and forward; so that I perceived him not to be well, upon which I gave him Gascoyne powder and cordial, lest it should be the red gum in children, usual at that time, to strike it out of his heart at morning after his dressing.[126]

She also rendered first aid to her servants, on one occasion removing a piece of goose pinnion from her maid's throat when it was choking her.[127] However, unlike Margaret Hoby and Jane Josselin, Alice does not appear to have acted as an amateur healer to her friends and neighbours. Her attention was fully absorbed by her own health problems and those of her family.

Alice's approach to illness was quite conventional. Concern about surfeit and cold reveal a basically humoral orientation. Convictions about the mutability of diseases depending upon the circumstances and the blending of emotional and physical disorders are common in the diaries and autobiographies consulted. As far as one can tell, the remedies she and her relatives used were also quite usual. Blood-letting, clysters, vomits, visits to spas and various herbal preparations are mentioned. Only remarkable is her religious orientation to disease and injury.

Scholars such as Alan Macfarlane have analysed the providential views of such Puritan sufferers as Ralph Josselin. The unspoken assumption is that people of other religious persuasions had a different orientation to disaster.[128] However, the royalist and Anglican Alice Thornton, like Ralph Josselin, listed her family's providential escapes from disaster.[129] She clearly felt that God caused and cured illness. Thus, although 'secular' therapies were used, for instance, when her daughter Naly had smallpox, Alice wrote of her recovery,

> But oh that our hearts were enlarged in thankfulness to the great Lord our God for the preservation of this my eldest child, whose special deliverance must not be forgotten, to give glory to the great God of Israel, which had pity upon myself, husband, and three children, by restoring their lives when they were all so nigh many deaths.[130]

Each page of Alice's autobiography reveals her deep religious faith. While she did not, like Margaret Hoby, spend her days in formal spiritual exercise, hearing sermons and talking to religious advisers, she was none the less guided in her behaviour and general attitudes by her religion. This fact, then, raises the issue of how different Puritans were from their High Church contemporaries.[131] Certainly English medical behaviour appears to have been determined more by social and sexual status than by religious conviction, despite the rather distracting example provided by Ralph Josselin.

III CONCLUSION

The title of this chapter, 'The Character of a Good Woman: Women and Illness', is appropriate because all of the women whose writings have been consulted self-consciously aspired to be, and to have the reputation for being, good. Indeed, unlike their male counterparts, female diarists and autobiographers wrote their personal accounts partly in order to demonstrate or protest their goodness. Female virtue was achieved by sound religious convictions and dutiful behaviour. A woman's duty involved both suffering (particularly childbearing) and healing. Her nature and her social utility were combined in the medical arena. So important was her medical role in determining her goodness that it sometimes was mentioned in the catalogue of virtues appearing in epitaphs of the period. Lady Grace Mildmay's monument recalls a

> most devout, unspotedly chaste Maid, Wife, and Widow, compassionate in Heart, and charitably helpful with Physic, Clothes, Nourishment, or Counsel to any in Misery. She was most careful and wise in managing worldly estate so as her life was a blessing to hers and in her death she blessed them, which happened July 27th, 1620.[132]

Thus, chastity, charity (including healing) and good management characterised the ideal seventeenth-century gentlewoman. These attributes certainly belonged to Lady Margaret Hoby and Mrs Alice Thornton. They also described others.

For instance, Lady Anne Halkett wrote her autobiography both to describe the dramatic events of her youth (mainly having to do with the Civil War) and to vindicate her own behaviour.[133] Like Alice Thornton, she was both royalist and highly connected. Hers was a busy life, occupied for many years in flitting between a number of gentry households in England and Scotland. At one point, she became engaged to a married man, and her chief preoccupation for some years was to extricate her good name intact from this predicament. She also was embroiled in several petty household scandals. Throughout these events, she protested her piety and devotion to duty. And, despite her full schedule, she acted as an amateur healer. Along with 'Ar.Ro.', probably a surgeon, she treated at least sixty soldiers injured in the battle of Dunbar. And when staying in Fife, she helped 'the sick and wounded persons [who] came to me'.[134] She attended confinements and treated herself when she became ill.[135]

Even Anne's ailments, like Alice Thornton's, testified to her virtue. On several occasions she took to her bed as a result of emotional upsets associated with her unfortunate engagement. And when she came down with bloody flux in 1653, her illness was the result of toil and want of sleep.[136] By the same token, her escapes from accidental injury were marks of the favour of God.[137]

The experiences of a number of women have been considered in this study. Some, like Jane Josselin and Elizabeth Pepys, are known to us only through the diaries of their husbands. Others, like Lady Anne Clifford and Dorothy Osborne, have left such brief records that their medical experiences can be only hazily conceptualised. Seen as a group, they are a motley crew. They range from gentry to middling status; from Roman Catholic to Puritan religious orientations. They were married and unmarried; childless and the mothers of many. Some were young at the time the records were written; some far older. However, there are many similarities. None of these women suffered from true poverty; some, indeed, were very wealthy. All were literate. All were pious. Many were good business women, deeply involved in the management of and litigation regarding their estates. All were knowledgeable in medical matters, treating themselves and others. And, of course, all were women living in a male-dominated society.

In which respects did the male and female experiences of illness and medicine differ in the period under discussion? With the obvious exception of obstetrical and gynaecological conditions and certain urological problems affecting men, the sexes suffered from the same ailments. Both sexes also engaged in self-treatment and amateur healing.

None the less, the duties of most lay-men took them far from medical spheres. When they offered medical advice, it was because of personal experience or special interest. When they suffered, their disorders came as a result of individual or collective sin, or an imbalance of humours. Neither their ailments nor their healing activities were specifically attributable to their sex.

Women, on the other hand, had a special relationship with illness and healing by virtue of their sex. Their physiology made them particularly vulnerable to disease. Their experience of menstruation, pregnancy, childbirth, breast-feeding and menopause identified, unified and segregated them. Their particular talents for nurturing and healing were seen as inherent in their female nature. Regardless of their social status, their medical advice and services were accepted by men from all social and occupational groups. They were the nurses, pharmacists and 'natural' medical authorities of seventeenth-century England.

9

CONCLUSION: THE EXPERIENCE OF ILLNESS

Before embarking upon a discussion of the experience of illness, it would be appropriate to say something about that elusive and indefinite state of being – the experience of health. Health is notoriously difficult to define, yet most people have a notion of what it means for them. For instance, Joseph Binns regarded a patient as 'well' when the condition for which he was treating him or her had either totally disappeared or had so stabilised as to cause no inconvenience or handicap.[1]

Seventeenth-century diarists frequently thanked God for their health. Sometimes this gratitude was expressed at regular intervals. Ralph Josselin gave a summary of his family's health every Sunday. Although weeks during which no one had been ill were rare indeed, he always specially remarked them.[2] Samuel Pepys was most likely to comment on his overall physical state on 26 March, when he celebrated his having been successfully cut for the stone. For instance, in 1665 he noted that he was in 'very perfect good health and have long been'.[3]

For both the diarists and the medical practitioners, good health could apparently be defined as the absence of illness. It was something to be maintained by sensible living habits and something to be sought after in times of illness. Humorally speaking, health was balance. Religiously speaking, health was the great gift of God. However one thought of it, health was a rare possession. Too many ailments hovered around for the owner to keep it long.

Thus far, this study has considered the experience of illness largely from the point of view of the individual sufferer. We have been concerned with his or her sensations, fears and medical choices. To some extent, this concentration is fair. Although one can sympathise, or even empathise, with a sufferer's complaints, much of illness is a lonely business. Each person experiences discomfort idiosyncratically. Illness experience, therefore, is determined by individual physiological and psychological factors as much as it is by the surrounding culture which provides the medical options for dealing with it.

However, illness affects many people beside the sufferer. In seventeenth-century England it involved friends, relations, neighbours, servants, masters and healers. Epidemic diseases affected whole communities. This concluding chapter will address itself, then, to the social experience of illness. It will attempt to draw together the miscellany of source material consulted in the preceding chapters in order to widen our viewpoint on seventeenth-century illness.

Illness experience varied depending upon the disorder. Minor ailments, such as colds, were least disruptive to both the sufferer and his or her social circle. However, even colds set the sufferer apart from the surrounding 'healthy' population. The sufferer complained. He or she sometimes went to bed. Occasionally remedies were taken. These were either obtained from apothecaries' shops or prepared within the home. Friends, relatives and servants sympathised and sometimes administered medication. Wives, daughters and maids prepared remedies, soothed rumpled bed-linen, offered fresh nightclothes and were awakened during the night to comfort the sufferer.

Disorders which confined the sufferer to bed for more than a day or two were far more disruptive. Even when the sick person's life was not felt to be in serious danger – in normal childbirth, for instance, or in ordinary ague attacks – the household reorganised itself around the sufferer. Sometimes nurses were hired. As we have seen, the Josselins hired a special nurse to help out during Jane's confinements. Pepys hired a nurse to look after his brother Tom when he was seriously ill.[4] And Pepys's relief that no nurse would have to be engaged to care for his wife during the treatment of her genital fistula has been noted.[5]

Even when nurses were not hired, a great deal of support was demanded from those surrounding the person who had taken up a sick role. It should be emphasised that this role change was often a matter of choice. Then as now, people frequently carried on as usual, despite unpleasant symptoms. Taking to bed was and is the signal for alterations in the behaviour of the sufferer and those around him or her.[6] Thus, the Josselins summoned neighbours in the middle of the night on more than one occasion.[7] Roger Lowe was called upon, both to pray with ailing neighbours and to make their wills.[8]

The Pepyses sometimes slept apart when one or both of them were ill.

Joseph Binns's casebook implies a great deal about the special services demanded of servants and/or housewives during long periods of illness. Fractured legs, for instance, required lengthy bedrest. Patients had to be lifted from their beds – often to pallets on the floor, so that beds could be made. Presumably patients in this condition used bedpans, which had to be carried and emptied. Linen fouled by excrement, sweat, vomit or wound drainage required changing and laundering.

The more serious the disorder, the more extraordinary the demands placed on those surrounding the sufferer. Robert Hooke's servant, Tom Gyles, became ill 9 September 1677, with what was at first diagnosed as the measles. By 11 September he was suffering acutely from smallpox. That day he received two visits from three different medical practitioners. (The surgeon, Mr Gidly, came twice.) He was watched all night. On 12 September Hooke himself visited Mr Gidly at 5 am because Tom was so ill. Gidly sent him to 'old Dr. King', who felt that Tom's illness was mortal. This opinion was confirmed by Dr Mapletoft and Dr Diodati, who met with Hooke at 9 am. Tom died just after noon.[9]

Other masters were likewise concerned with their servants' illnesses. Pepys allowed his 'boy' Will to lie on his own bed when the servant had a severe headache during the 1665 plague.[10] And the Pepyses also contemplated sending a maid-servant, Sarah, to the country for a change of air when Sarah had an attack of ague.[11] The Josselins' concern about their servants' illnesses has been discussed above.

It is tempting to see the above examples of masters caring for servants during times of illnesses as evidence of the patriarchal relationship which was piously advocated by seventeenth-century moralists and which has been referred to nostalgically by those wishing to see in pre-industrial England a golden age.[12] However, such a conclusion would be both romantic and incorrect. A major reason for employers' concern about servants' health was the inconvenience a servant's illness caused within the household.[13] For instance, Pepys wrote in 1660, 'This day or two my maid Jane hath been lame, that we cannot tell what to do for want of her'.[14] Further, as we shall see, if a servant contracted an illness which might endanger the employer's family, that servant was speedily removed from the household in a way an ailing family member would not have been, despite the conventional inclusion of the servants as part of the master's 'family'.

Whether or not a sufferer went to bed, he or she sometimes decided to become a patient, that is to consult a healer. In many cases the healer visited the patient in his or her own home. Sometimes visits were made daily or even more often. Occasionally the healer was able to send a servant or apprentice to do routine dressing changes or administer emergency first aid.[15] But healers frequently travelled long distances at inconvenient times and in bad weather in order to attend patients. Often, more than one healer was involved in caring for a single patient. Indeed, the Barbersurgeons' Company required that patients in danger of death be examined by several surgeons to make certain that the treatment applied was proper and sufficient. Joseph Binns participated in a number of cases where he was invited to consult by the attending physician or surgeon.[16] Such consultations helped to reassure patients and their families that everything possible was being done. They also served as protection for the medical practitioners involved, should the patient fail to improve or die.

In addition, patients sometimes chose to consult several healers, particularly when suffering from an acute or chronic disorder. As we have seen, Hooke consulted four healers when Tom Gyles had smallpox. Ralph Josselin sought help from two physicians and two surgeons regarding his diseased leg during the last ten years of his life.[17] And Pepys consulted both a physician and a surgeon when he feared a recurrence of bladder stones.[18]

Regardless of whether or not a medical practitioner was consulted, family members and friends continued to help, give advice and sometimes even undermine the healer's authority. We have seen that the medical writers were suspicious of the activities of the well-meaning but 'ignorant' women who surrounded their patients.[19] Disagreements between healers and such women sometimes led to the healer being dismissed or leaving the case.[20] Male friends might also challenge a medical practitioner's decisions. Two examples of this sort of interference have already been cited from Pepys's diaries. In one instance, Pepys took a remedy for itching recommended by Sir J. Mennes in preference to any prescribed by a surgeon.[21] And, when his brother Tom was dying, Pepys himself challenged the diagnosis of syphilis made by Tom's physician.

Whether minor or serious, acute or chronic, most disorders entitled the sufferer to visits from friends, relatives and acquaintances. Even when physic-taking confined an individual to his or her chamber, and no illness existed, visitors were welcomed. Modern conventions which protect the privacy of people excreting excrement or giving birth simply did not exist in seventeenth-century England. Apparently no one ever wanted to be left alone. Thus, visiting the sick or confined was a social duty.

Such visits served a number of purposes. As we have seen, both clerical and lay visitors prayed with the sick. Ralph Josselin was summoned in his dual role as vicar and friend to pray with ailing parishioners on a number of occasions. Roger Lowe prayed with fellow-Presbyterians. A good deal of moral support found its way into these visits. The fact that Josselin stayed the night with his friend Mr R. H. during a spiritual crisis surely did R. H. as much good as the prayers they said and the physician Josselin summoned to let R. H.'s blood.[22]

Sometimes practical secular services were performed during visits. Roger Lowe was asked to draw up wills for dying acquaintances on more than one occasion. Any educated person might be asked to write a will. Lowe was a mercer. Perhaps more frequently approached were ministers, physicians and lawyers.[23]

In addition, visitors undertook nursing care and household tasks. Mothers routinely travelled to be with married daughters when the daughters gave birth.[24] They also frequently visited adult children in times of illness. In return, adult children hurried to the bedsides of ailing parents. The Josselin daughters returned to Earls Colne to visit and nurse their parents during serious illnesses.[25] John Evelyn spent nearly four weeks at his mother's death-bed.[26] And he spent the period June to October 1640 travelling between Oxford and his father's house when the elder Evelyn was suffering from the illness which finally killed him.[27] More distant relatives also helped each other. Lady Margaret Hoby offered her help during the confinements of her cousins.[28]

Friends sometimes performed nursing services for one another during illnesses. Jane Josselin applied leeches to Mary Church's leg when Mary, a close friend, was unwell. And Dorothy Osborne attended Lady Diana Rich when Lady Diana was staying with a nearby gentlewoman who was treating her for sore eyes. Dorothy said that she would not leave the area until Lady Diana did.[29]

In addition, as indicated above, it was customary for married women to be present at childbirth. They sometimes helped deliver the babies. More often they provided moral support, took care of the housework and other children, and acted as witnesses of the birth.

Helping out during times of illness was a service people offered their patrons. The best examples of this kind of behaviour come from Samuel Pepys's diary. Not only did Pepys visit Lord Sandwich himself when the great man was ill, but also he supervised the care taken of at least one of the Montague children during medical treatment. In 1660 Lady Jemima Montague was living at the house of Mr Scott, a surgeon, for treatment of 'malformation of the neck'.[30] Pepys and his wife visited her frequently, even consulting with Scott about the collar he wished to fit to the lady's neck to correct her condition.[31]

Visiting persons confined to bed sometimes took on a kind of ritual character. The Pepyses went to several christening parties held in the new mother's bedroom.[32] Even when there was no party, it was certainly traditional to visit a recently delivered woman before her month of lying-in was over.[33]

It was also traditional to visit the dying. Evelyn described the scene in his dying mother's chamber as follows:

> Therefore, summoning all her Children then living . . . she expressed herself in a manner so heavenly, with instructions so pious, and Christian, as made us strangely sensible of the extraordinary loss then imminent; after which, embracing every one of us in particular, she gave to each a Ring with her blessing, and dismissed us. Then taking my Father by the hand, she recommended us to his care . . . and so having importuned him that what he designed to bestow on her Funeral, he would rather dispose among the poor. . . . She laboured to compose herself for the blessed change which she now expected.[34]

And Pepys, who had spent two days at his brother's death-bed, left when he thought he heard the death rattle beginning, because 'I had no mind to see him die'.[35]

Most visits made to sufferers were simply courtesy visits. All of the diarists made this sort of visit. Pepys and Hooke reported the greatest number of sick visits. However, this is not surprising since they lived in London, had large numbers of acquaintances, and depended on the goodwill of others for their social opportunities, promotions and increases in income. None the less, the identity of those they visited makes obvious that personal interest did not consciously affect their visiting habits. For instance, Hooke visited the Bishop of Chester three times in five days, when the bishop was dying of the stone.[36]

He also visited his ex-servant and -mistress, Nell, after she miscarried of a baby girl.[37] By the same token, Pepys made numerous visits to ailing members of Lord Sandwich's family.[38] He also visited Mrs Betty Michell, a poor woman of his acquaintance, after her babies were born.[39]

On only one occasion recorded in a diary were visitors turned away from a sick-room. This was when Samuel and Elizabeth Pepys attempted to visit Samuel's cousin Scott who lay dying after a miscarriage. Samuel wrote, 'My wife could not be admitted to see her, nor anybody'.[40]

Even diseases known to be contagious did not prevent sufferers from receiving visitors. Pepys visited Lady Jemima Montague when it was feared she had smallpox.[41] As it happened, she only had chickenpox. He also visited Sir R. Slingsby, 'our Comptroller, when Slingsby lay ill of the "new disease" – an ague and fever'. Slingsby died the following week.[42]

The above discussion has concentrated upon conventional behaviour and the benefits the sufferer derived from sick-room visits. It should not be forgotten that the visitor also benefited. In an age when illness and death took place at home, suffering cemented relationships between people. Supplying services and comfort to the sufferer allowed visitors to feel that they were helping. Proximity prevented the mystification of illness and death and the alienation of sufferers and the dying which are so apparent today. Visitors, confronted with the truth of their own mortality, were both comforted by the assurance that they also would have social support during their own crises and taught behaviour which they might themselves employ. Pious responses to suffering and the spiritual satisfaction of a 'good' death fulfilled the needs of both sufferers and visitors.

The evidence indicates that seventeenth-century sufferers expected to be visited and seventeenth-century men, women and children expected to visit. However, social responses to diseases varied.[43] There were respectable illnesses, such as gout and ague; frightening, but nearly inevitable diseases, such as smallpox; disreputable diseases, such as syphilis; and terrifying diseases, such as the plague.

Non-infectious chronic disorders, although unpleasant, could bring the sufferer years of sympathy and attention from those surrounding him or her. Pepys visited Lord Brouncker during attacks of gout in the 1660s.[44] Hooke visited him when he suffered from the same disorder in the 1670s.[45]

Infectious diseases, because they were more feared, were

also avoided. Although no coherent 'theory of infection' was articulated in the diaries and autobiographies consulted, people certainly distinguished between infectious and non-infectious ailments, feeling much safer in the presence of the latter. Ralph Josselin, for instance, found comfort, after his daughter Mary's death from worms, in the fact that her 'disease was not infectious'.[46] Infection was believed to pass directly from person to person. It also could lurk in contaminated clothing or bed-linen.[47] John Evelyn was certain he had contracted smallpox by sleeping in a bed previously occupied by a girl whose mother had reported as recently recovered from an ague. Evelyn concluded 'by the smell of franc incense . . . [that] she had been newly recovered of the Small Pox'.[48] Although sufferers from contagious diseases were visited, they were approached with caution.

The response to disfiguring diseases was not always sympathetic. Lady Anne Clifford reported in February 1619,

> My Lady of Suffolk at Northampton House about this time had the smallpox which spoiled that good face of hers, which had brought to others much misery, and to herself greatness which ended with much unhappiness.[49]

And individuals were distressed by even transitory alterations of their own appearances due to minor ailments. When Pepys was troubled with itching and swelling in February 1663, he wrote that he was 'not only sick but ashamed of myself to see myself so changed in my countenance'.[50] And when he developed cold sores in September 1664, he reported 'my mouth very scabby, my cold being going away – so that I was forced to wear a great black patch'.[51]

The shame attached to such temporary problems or even the scarring produced by smallpox was minor. So many people survived smallpox that its effects were almost to be expected and, except in severe cases, unworthy of remark. Patches and make-up disguised pits in the face. Wigs and gloves concealed hair loss and disfigurement of the hands.

The same cannot be said about syphilis. It was indeed the foul disease. Its symptoms, which have been described above, were disgusting to both the sufferer and those caring for him or her.[52] And its foul reputation caused social responses ranging from snide gossip to ostracism. It is no wonder that attempts were made to deny the presence of syphilis in the living and to conceal it as a cause of death.[53] Rather than pity, the stereotyped reaction to the pox was humour.

Indeed, syphilis provided subject matter for a large number of seventeenth-century dramatists. Sufferers were figures of fun. Shadwell's character Crazy was typical of the genre.

Crazy.	Good morrow Mrs. Errant.
Errant.	How does the pain in your head?
Crazy.	Oh I am on the rack: no primitive Christian under Diocletian ever sufferd so much as I do under this rascal: this villain that like a hangman destroys mankind, and has the law for 't. Oh abominable quacks! that devour more than all the diseases would do, were they let alone, which they pretend to cure.
Errant.	Ay, but sir, yours is a French surgeon, and who so fit to cure the French Disease as a French-surgeon?
Crazy.	Yes, as one poison expels another; but if this rogue should cure me, he can cure me of nothing but what he has given me himself; 'twas nothing when I put myself into his hands; he brought it to what it is, and I think I must deal with him as they do that are bitten with a viper, crush the rogue's head and apply it to the part, for if I do not kill him, he'll be the death of me.[54]

Dramatists ridiculed the symptoms of the pox, the practitioners who treated it, the people who suffered from it, the remedies taken for it, and even its name.

Syphilis was no respecter of social class. It tarnished the reputation of Court ladies. Thus a character in a Restoration drama commented:

> Your proud women are a company of proud, vain, fops and jilts, abominably daubed and painted; and I had rather kiss a blackamoor, with a natural complexion, than any such: and, besides, many of them are so unsound, that making love is as dangerous as making war; and the wounds and scars are dishonourable to boot.[55]

And as early as 1619 Beaumont and Fletcher wrote:

Leontius.	Here's one has served now under Captain Cupid, And crack't a pike in' youth: you see what's come on't.
Lieutenant.	No, my disease will never prove so honourable.
Leontius.	Why, sure, thou hast the best pox.
Lieutenant.	If I have 'em, I am sure I got 'em in the best company.[56]

However, the pox afflicted those of lower status as well. Whores were well known to give and receive syphilis when they sold their services.

Regarding syphilis, drama mirrored the attitudes found in general society. Pepys's shock at the news that his brother Tom had the pox has already been described.[57] However, despite his fear of malicious gossip causing shame to his own family, he was more than willing to participate in gossip about other people. For instance, in 1667 he noted that

> Mr. Lowder is come to use the Tubb, that is, to bathe and sweat himself, and that his Lady is come to use the Tubb too; which he [Pepys's informant] takes to be that he hath and hath given the pox.[58]

Later in the year, Mr Lowther was known to have a sore mouth. Still later, Pepys reported that he could no longer look at Lady Lowther with any pleasure because she had developed a sore nose.[59]

John Aubrey, whose appetite for gossip was even larger than that of Pepys, wrote that Eleanor Ratcliffe, Countess of Sussex was

> a great and sad example of the power of lust and slavery to it. She was as great a beauty as any in England and had a good wit. After her lord's death (he was jealous) she sends for —— (formerly) her footman, and makes him groom of the chamber. He had the pox and she knew it; a damnable sot. He was not very handsome but his body of an exquisite shape. . . . His nostrils were stuffed and borne out with corks in which were quills to breathe through. About 1666 this countess died of the pox.[60]

Apparently the shame of syphilis was not sufficient to deter either Mr Lowther or Lady Eleanor Ratcliffe in their pursuit of pleasure. None the less, this shame was very real, motivating numerous attempts to disguise its presence. John Graunt's remarks about the routine concealment of syphilis as a cause of death have been quoted above. And Joseph Binns's syphilis patients who attempted to obtain treatment while remaining unwilling to name their illness have also been referred to.

While syphilis was the only killing disease which was generally ridiculed, it was certainly not the only one people wished to avoid. More fearful than the pox, and never a subject for humour, was the plague. The plague was a disaster set apart from other diseases by both societal and individual reactions to it.

As indicated above, the plague was so dreaded that even people dwelling out of its range, such as Ralph Josselin, lived in fear of it.[61] It was the only illness concerning which embryonic public health legislation was passed. From 1564, plague regulations required that when a person contracted the plague, he or she and all other persons living in the same dwelling (which might house as many as six families in poor neighbourhoods) were ordered to be confined within the building. Houses thus closed were marked with a cross on the door.[62] Needless to say, these regulations were unpopular. In 1603, 'The spread of plague to Westminster discovered a "very unruly" body of citizens "near St. Clements Church and the fields" who had to be forcibly imprisoned in their infected houses'.[63] And early in the 1665 outbreak, Noorthouck reported that

> At the beginning of the disorder there were great knavery and collusion in the reports of deaths, for while it was possible to conceal the infection, they were attributed to fevers of all kinds, which began to swell the bills [of Mortality]; this was done to prevent their houses being shut up, and families shunned by their neighbours.[64]

Thus, not only did plague sufferers have to cope with the discomfort of their symptoms and the fear of death, but also they were faced with the frantic terror of those immured with them. They also had to endure isolation from friends, neighbours and family members. Considering what has been said above about conventions regarding visiting the sick, such isolation must surely have been nearly as painful as the disease itself.

Beginning in the 1590s pest-houses were set up in plague-stricken localities to deal with epidemics. In 1665 there were five pest-houses in London.[65] For the pest-house established for the sixteen parishes outside the walls of the City of London, mortality has been estimated at 98.1 per cent during 1665.[66] Plague sufferers must surely have viewed being sent to a pest-house as a death sentence.

Prevailing theory held that plague was passed directly from person to person. Thus, the Royal College of Physicians approved of the plague legislation, although few of its members stayed around to help deal with the resulting terror and mortality. In their dread of the disease, people became afraid of each other, avoiding one another on the streets and particularly shunning those who had recently come from a plague-stricken area.[67] Masters deserted servants, ministers abandoned congregations, adults were cruel to children, and healers abandoned patients.

Fear of the plague thus caused a breakdown in normal social relations and conventions. It even separated families. When Sir Dudley North and his younger sister Mary contracted the plague as children, they 'were confined to their father's house in London'. Their father moved out 'because of his promiscuous converse'.[68]

According to Pepys, when Mr Wright's serving-maid came down with the plague in early August 1665, Wright put her in an outhouse, presumably to avoid having his house shut up. The maid escaped, so when her master caught her he had her taken to the pest-house. On the way, two young men, presumably in search of flirtation, looked into the coach which was carrying her, 'and there saw somebody look very ill, and in a sick dress and stunk mightily'. One of the young men was nearly frightened to death when he realised the girl had the plague.[69]

Pepys himself had his maid Susan removed from his house in 1666 when he thought she might have the plague. Although he offered to pay the nurse hired to care for her, he was mightily relieved at her departure. However, he was quite pleased to take her back a week later when it was discovered that she merely had ague.[70]

And he told the story, with more distaste than surprise, of a man who in September 1665 had taken

> a child from London from an infected house . . . it was the child of a very able citizen in Gracious Street, a saddler, who had buried all the rest of his children of the plague; and himself and his wife now being shut up, and in despair of escaping, did desire only to save the life of this little child; and so prevailed to have it received stark-naked into the arms of a friend, who brought it (having put it into fresh clothes) to Greenwich.

A complaint was lodged against this Good Samaritan for his pains.[71]

Those who were even suspected of having had contact with a plague sufferer were avoided. Pepys told of Captain Cocke whose man-servant was reputed to have died of the plague.

> By and by Captain Cocke came to the office, and Sir W. Batten and I did send to him that he would either forbear the office or forbear going to his own office. However, meeting with the

> Searchers with their rods in their hands coming from his house, I did overhear them say that the fellow did not die of the plague.[72]

It is no wonder that those who had to stay within reach of the plague grew reckless. In some cases the sick openly flouted the plague regulations.

> They abused constables who tried to enforce household segregation and broke out of their houses in Westminster and Southwark in 1630. One widow got out and marched deliberately into Westminster Abbey, to the horror of the people there. In Holborn a watchman went round tearing padlocks off the doors of infected houses.[73]

Mr Caesar, the lutemaster Pepys hired to teach his boy, reported that at the height of the 1665 plague in Westminster,

> bold people there were to go in sport to one another's burials. And in spite to well people, would breathe in the faces (out of their windows) of well people going by.[74]

Such folk had indeed become abandoned – abandoned by God, by medicine, by their government, by their neighbours. They, in turn, abandoned courtesy, common sense and, finally, fear.[75]

The plague was no more typical of seventeenth-century diseases than a hurricane is of rainstorms. In cases of almost all other illnesses, medical practitioners were more than eager to attend patients – provided, of course, that the patients could afford their services. Even in plague time, when physicians and many surgeons left London, the city was not totally deprived of medical care. People dosed themselves with prophylactics in enormous quantities.[76] In addition, many apothecaries remained in London, both selling medications and giving medical advice. The fact that they stayed, 'providing that general medical care which the mass of the population needed', was not forgotten by the general public.[77] The apothecaries' star was rising, despite the physicians' attempt to subordinate them.

The seventeenth-century experience of illness included the activities of medical practitioners. These practitioners served, sometimes as learned authorities, sometimes as skilled craftsmen, sometimes as suppliers of necessary commodities, sometimes as experts in the occult. Despite the physicians' efforts to ignore the financial relationship existing between themselves and their patients, all healers sold their services. To a great extent these services were determined and defined by the clients purchasing them. White witches diagnosed witchcraft as the cause of illnesses partly because the patients seeking their help already suspected that they were tormented by witches. Surgeons let blood, made issues and applied blisters on demand. Apothecaries gave medical advice because visitors to their shops requested it. Physicians continued to examine urine long after the Royal College of Physicians denounced the practice as useless, because patients believed in uroscopy. The medical marketplace, then, operated on a supply and demand basis.

At this point in our discussion, it must be reiterated that there was no seventeenth-century medical profession. Although occupational organisations existed and aspired to the kind of control over the provision of medical services their descendants would actually attain, in the seventeenth century they supervised the activities of relatively few healers and affected the behaviour of the lay public almost not at all. Even within licensed groups of practitioners, there was little unity. Learned surgeons despised unlearned ones. Fellows of the Royal College of Physicians distrusted licentiates and physicians authorised to practise by universities and bishops. Female midwives were suspicious of man-midwives: man-midwives, in turn, were contemptuous of their female rivals.

Between groups of authorised practitioners there was even greater dissension. Physicians accused surgeons and apothecaries of usurping their own rights by prescribing internal medicines. Surgeons and apothecaries, in their turn, rejected the subservient roles the physicians recommended for them. Surgeons claimed the right to prescribe internal medication to their patients without first asking the permission of a physician. Apothecaries demanded official recognition of their already habitual practice of giving advice to the clients patronising their shops. And, of course, between licensed healers and unlicensed ones there was only competition and enmity.

The authorities, although basically sympathetic with the aims of those who wished to raise the standards of medical and surgical care, were unreliable supporters. As the 1543 'Quacks' Charter' demonstrates, unlearned and unlicensed practice had its protectors.[78] In addition, seventeenth-century courts and parliaments were fickle, switching support from the physicians to the apothecaries and back again in the controversy over who should be allowed to participate in the practice of general internal medicine.[79] This is not surprising, because courtiers and MPs, like other members of the lay population, reserved the personal right to consult any healer they wished to consult. They patronised medical renegades, such as Simon Forman and Gideon Harvey, along with orthodox physicians and surgeons. Even on them, the medical propaganda promulgated by such writers as the anti-quack authors had a less than successful effect.[80] Thus, although learned and licensed physicians sound very 'modern' in their defence of high standards in medical education and practice, theirs were indeed lonely voices crying in the wilderness. The classical learning they defended was doomed to obsolescence. The privileges they coveted would descend to bastard heirs emerging from surgery and apothecary as well as physic.

All healers claimed expertise in their own areas of practice. However, the question of what constituted such expertise was an open one in seventeenth-century England. Indeed, many lay-people claimed to be expert in the treatment of certain ailments. Sometimes their recipes were even adopted by licensed physicians and surgeons.[81]

Of all licensed healers, the surgeons were best able to sell their services by claiming expertise. Despite the prevalence of self-treatment, rare indeed was the man who would let himself blood, set his own fractured bones, 'cut' himself for the stone or amputate his own limbs. Surgeons routinely performed these and other procedures with success. It is therefore ironic that the diaries and correspondence consulted give so little information about surgery, and so much about internal medicine. With the exception of the Pepyses, the people mentioned in these sources depended mainly on self-treatment and on physicians. Joseph Binns's casebook, therefore, is helpful in giving insight into the career of at least one practising surgeon. Without this insight, this study might have passed over in silence the too-often neglected work of seventeenth-century surgeons. Unlike those of the physicians, the surgeons' services were rarely suspected of being unnecessary. If they were criticised, it was for lack of skill.

Yet even surgery was undertaken by lay-people. The Barbersurgeons' Company of London issued special licences to experts in a number of surgical procedures, regardless of a lack of proper apprenticeship.[82] Lady Margaret Hoby's surgical activities have already been cited, as have those of the two female bone-setters mentioned in Ralph Josselin's diary. Thus, not even surgeons could claim a monopoly over expertise in their area of practice.

In physic and apothecary, of course, such claims were even less secure. Almost everyone diagnosed his or her own ailments. Most people either bought remedies from apothecaries' shops, made their own medicines, or both. Laywomen considered healing a 'natural' duty. Indeed, considering the evidence, one wonders why licensed healers were ever consulted and paid.

The answer lies outside the realm of reason and expertise. At no time are human beings more emotionally vulnerable than during illness. The more acute the symptoms and the longer they last, the more desperate the sufferer and his or her loved ones become to find relief. The promise or hope of a cure supplied by a respectable licensed healer provides at least temporary ease. Perhaps more important, the medical practitioner assumes responsibility for decisions and therapy for a period of time.

Thackeray's explanation, published in 1850, although perhaps more appropriate in the twentieth century, none the less applied in the seventeenth:

> It is not only for the sick man, it is for the sick man's friends that the Doctor comes. His presence is often as good for them as for the patient, and they long for him yet more eagerly. How we have all watched after him! What an emotion the thrill of his carriage-wheels in the street, and at length at the door, has made us feel! How we hang upon his words, and what a comfort we get from a smile or two, if he can vouchsafe that sunshine to lighten our darkness! . . . Over the patient in fever, the wife expectant, the children unconscious, the doctor stands as if he were Fate, the dispenser of life and death.[83]

The doctor is, to a great extent, what patients have made him – not only what his teachers and organisations expected him to be. The Latin phrases, velvet gowns, luxurious coaches and huge fees of the seventeenth-century society physician increased his value in the eyes of prospective patients, even while he was ridiculed for them.

To the aid of both healers and sufferers of the seventeenth century came natural death. This boon to humanity covered a multitude of sins. It excused the healers' failure to cure, while reassuring survivors that they had done everything possible for the deceased. Along with the promise of heavenly health, it comforted the grief-stricken. And if a sufferer, whose survival had been given up by friends and medical practitioners alike, should happen to recover, such an event could be hailed as the providential intervention of a beneficent God.

Natural death came in many guises. It was considered natural for infants and the very old to die of almost any illness. Indeed, these age groups were so at risk that mention of the age group itself was sufficient explanation of the cause of death.[84] It was also natural for people to die of epidemic diseases, childbirth and certain chronic disorders, such as cancer. Even death from minor ailments could be regarded as natural if the symptoms were unusually severe and the sufferer's needs had not been neglected.

Certain deaths were not natural. Murder and suicide were unnatural causes of death. So were deaths caused by witchcraft. However, such calamities were outside the realm of medicine, either in the hands of healers or in the hands of lay-people.

Thus, death was usually not considered to be anyone's fault. Only in rare cases was a healer blamed for causing death. For instance, when the Duke of Gloucester died of smallpox in 1660, Pepys reported that he had perished through 'the great negligence of the Doctors' who 'had forecast recovery and had prescribed nothing'.[85] Of course, healers insulted each other by accusing one another of murder. Sometimes such accusations resulted in trials for malpractice.[86] More often these accusations were merely a part of the general attack made on one sort of healer by another.[87] Although lay-people amused themselves with cynical jokes about the harm the foul-tasting remedies they took might do, they almost never blamed any individual for the death of a loved one. Indeed, approaching death virtually removed the dying person from the realm of medical responsibility.

The process of dying, although often surrounded by healers and medical treatment, was both conventionally and actually a situation where therapeutics gave way to economic, family and spiritual concerns. In his seminal study *The Hour of our Death*, Philippe Aries describes the 'good' death in traditional Europe as one in which the dying person was able to put his or her spiritual and temporal house in order before taking leave of earthly life.[88] Worldly goods were distributed, funerals described and provided for. In addition, the dying sufferer made peace with God and set an example for the living by his or her pious behaviour.

As we have seen, death in seventeenth-century England was often a leisurely affair. Loved ones often spent weeks in or near death-chambers. While the suffering of the dying relative or friend was pitied and occasionally abhorred, time was necessary to produce the desirable end. Sudden death, death alone, death under disreputable circumstances were bad deaths, feared and avoided. Like illness, death was encompassed by general personal and social responsibilities. It was not relegated to professionals.

This book has concentrated, not upon death, but upon illness, an important part of life in any era. It has returned repeatedly to the joint issues of responsibility and power. Sufferers and healers shared the responsibility of dealing with illness, injury, handicap, childbirth and ageing. They also shared the power of decision-making, although ultimately that power rested in the hands of sufferers and their 'friends'.

Neither sufferers nor healers had a great deal of power over illness itself. That power, when it arrived as the gift of medical science and public health initiatives, transformed the relationship between sufferers and healers so dramatically that it is difficult for present-day scholars to avoid seeing in the sufferers and healers of earlier ages their modern counterparts. This book attempts, however imperfectly, to improve the clarity of our vision regarding the medical world of seventeenth-century England. Its exploration is woefully incomplete, but it may perhaps suggest directions for further investigation.

ABBREVIATIONS

Aveling, *English Midwives*: J. H. Aveling, *English Midwives: their History and Prospects*, London (1872).
Barker: British Library Sloane MS 78 or 663.
A Brief Account: *A Brief Account of Mr. Valentine Greatraks*, London (1666 and 1668).
Clark, *Royal College*: G. N. Clark, *A History of the Royal College of Physicians of London*, vols I and II, Oxford (1964).
Clifford, *Diary*: *The Diary of the Lady Anne Clifford with an introductory Note by V. Sackville-West*, London (1923).
Cotta, *A Short Discovery*: J. Cotta, *A Short Discovery of the Unobserved Dangers of Several Sorts of Ignorant and Unconsiderate Practisers of Physic in England*, London (1612).
Evelyn, *Diary*: *The Diary of John Evelyn*, E. S. de Beer, ed., London (1959).
Halkett: *The Autobiography of Anne Lady Halkett*, J. G. Nichols, ed., Camden Society, new series, 13 (1875).
Hoby, *Diary*: *Diary of Lady Margaret Hoby, 1599–1605*, D. M. Meads, ed., London (1930).
Hooke, *Diary*: *The Diary of Robert Hooke, 1672–1680*, H. W. Robinson and W. Adams, eds, London (1968 and 1935).
Josselin, *Diary*: *The Diary of Ralph Josselin, 1616–1683*, A. Macfarlane, ed., Oxford (1976).
Lowe, *Diary*: *Diary of Roger Lowe of Ashton-in-Makerfield, Lancashire, 1663–74*, W. L. Sachse, ed., London (1938).
MacDonald, *Mystical Bedlam*: M. MacDonald, *Mystical Bedlam: Madness, Anxiety and Healing in Seventeenth-Century England*, Cambridge (1981).
Macfarlane, *Family Life*: A. Macfarlane, *The Family Life of Ralph Josselin. A Seventeenth-Century Clergyman: An Essay in Historical Anthropology*, Cambridge (1970).
Macfarlane, *Witchcraft*: A. Macfarlane, *Witchcraft in Tudor and Stuart England: A Regional and Comparative Study*, London (1970).
Osborne, *Letters*: *The Letters of Dorothy Osborne to William Temple*, G. C. Moore Smith, ed., Oxford (1928).
Pelling, 'Appearance and Reality': M. Pelling, 'Appearance and Reality: Barbersurgeons, the Body and Venereal Disease in Early Modern London', in A. L. Beier and R. Finlay, eds, *The Making of the Metropolis: London 1500–1700*, London (1986), pp. 82–112.

Pelling, 'Occupational Diversity': M. Pelling, 'Occupational Diversity: Barbersurgeons and the Trades of Norwich, 1550–1640', *Bulletin of the History of Medicine*, LVI (1982), 484–511.

Pepys, *Diary*: *The Diary of Samuel Pepys*, R. Latham and W. Matthews, eds, vols I–IX, London (1970–82).

Roberts, thesis: R. S. Roberts, 'The London Apothecaries and Medical Practice in Tudor and Stuart England', unpublished London University Ph.D thesis (1964).

Roberts, 'The Personnel and Practice': R. S. Roberts, 'The Personnel and Practice of Medicine in Tudor and Stuart England', *Medical History*, VI (1962), 363–82, and VII (1964), 217–34.

Sl. 1112:: 'The casebook of a provincial physician, 1619–1622', British Library Sloane MS 1112.

Slack, 'Metropolitan Government': P. Slack, 'Metropolitan Government in Crisis: London's Response to Plague, 1563–1665', in A. L. Beier and R. Finlay, eds, *The Making of the Metropolis: London 1500–1700*, London (1986), pp. 60–81.

Stone, *The Family, Sex and Marriage*: L. Stone, *The Family, Sex and Marriage in England, 1500–1800*, London (1977).

Symcotts: *A Seventeenth-Century Doctor and his Patients: John Symcotts, 1592?–1662*, F. N. L. Poynter and W. J. Bishop, eds, Bedfordshire Historical Record Society, vol. 31, Streatley, Beds (1950).

Thomas, *Religion and Magic*: K. Thomas, *Religion and the Decline of Magic*, Harmondsworth (1973).

Thornton: *The Autobiography of Mrs. Alice Thornton of East Newton, Co. York*, C. Jackson, ed., Surtees Society, vol. 62 (1875).

Young, *Barber-Surgeons*: S. Young, ed., *The Annals of the Barber-Surgeons*, London (1890).

NOTES

1. INTRODUCTION

1. C. Singer, *A Short History of Anatomy and Physiology from the Greeks to Harvey*, New York (1957, first published 1925); E. H. Ackerknecht, *A Short History of Medicine*, New York (1955); L. S. King, *The Growth of Medical Thought*, Chicago, Ill. (1963).
2. K. Dewhurst, *Thomas Willis as a Physician*, Los Angeles (1964); G. Keynes, *The Life of William Harvey*, Oxford (1966).
3. E.g. P. Slack, *The Impact of Plague in Tudor and Stuart England*, London (1985); E. Shorter, *A History of Women's Bodies*, Harmondsworth (1984); J. Donnison, *Midwives and Medical Men: A History of Inter-Professional Rivalries and Women's Rights*, London (1977).
4. K. Thomas, *Religion and the Decline of Magic*, Harmondsworth (1973); L. Stone, *The Family, Sex and Marriage in England, 1500–1800*, London (1977).
5. A. Macfarlane, *Witchcraft in Tudor and Stuart England: A Regional and Comparative Study*, London (1970).
6. C. Webster, ed., *Health, Medicine and Mortality in the Sixteenth Century*, Cambridge (1979).
7. M. MacDonald, *Mystical Bedlam: Madness, Anxiety and Healing in Seventeenth-Century England*, Cambridge (1981).
8. P. Slack, op. cit.
9. H. Cook, *The Decline of the Old Medical Regime in Stuart London*, London and Ithaca (1986).
10. See e.g. R. Porter, ed., *Patients and Practitioners: Lay Perceptions of Medicine in Pre-Industrial Society*, Cambridge (1985); M. Pelling, 'Appearance and Reality: Barbersurgeons, the Body and Venereal Disease in Early Modern London', in A. L. Beier and R. Finlay, eds, *The Making of the Metropolis: London 1500–1700*, London (1986).

2. THE MEDICAL MARKETPLACE

1. G. S. Holmes, *Augustan England: Professions, State and Society 1680–1730*, London (1982), p. 3.
2. Ibid., p. 170; J. H. Raach, *A Directory of English Country Physicians, 1603–1643*, London (1962).

3. See Chapter 5.
4. 'Medical Practice in the Early Modern Period. Trade or Profession?', *The Society for the Social History of Medicine Bulletin*, XXXII (1983), 27–8.
5. M. Pelling, 'Occupational Diversity: Barbersurgeons and the Trades of Norwich, 1550–1640', *Bulletin of the History of Medicine*, LVI (1982), 490–1.
6. The best information about the licensing of English physicians, surgeons and midwives is to be found in M. Pelling and C. Webster, 'Medical Practitioners', in C. Webster, ed., *Health, Medicine and Mortality in the Sixteenth Century*, Cambridge (1979), pp. 165–235.
7. See R. S. Roberts, 'The London Apothecaries and Medical Practice in Tudor and Stuart England', unpublished London University Ph.D thesis (1964).
8. J. Oberndoerffer, *The Anatomies of the True Physician and Counterfeit Mountebank . . .* , F. H[erring], trans., London (1602), pp. 29–30.
9. For information on the education of physicians, see P. Allen, 'Medical Education in Seventeenth-Century England', *Journal of the History of Medicine*, I (1946), 115–43; G. N. Clark, *A History of the Royal College of Physicians of London*, vols I and II, Oxford (1965); V. L. Bullough, *The Development of Medicine as a Profession*, Basel and New York (1966); Pelling and Webster, op. cit.; A. H. T. Robb-Smith, 'Cambridge Medicine', in A. G. Debus, ed., *Medicine in Seventeenth-Century England*, Los Angeles (1974), pp. 327–70.
10. Robb-Smith, op. cit., p. 329.
11. 3 Henry VIII *cap*. 11, An Act for the appointing of physicians and surgeons, 1512: *Statutes of the Realm*, London (1810–28, repr. 1963), III, pp. 31–2.
12. Pelling and Webster, op. cit., p. 185.
13. *Statutes*, loc. cit.
14. M. MacDonald, *Mystical Bedlam: Madness, Anxiety and Healing in Seventeenth-Century England*, Cambridge (1981). See also *Diary of the Rev. John Ward, A.M., Vicar of Stratford-upon-Avon*, C. Severn, ed., London (1839).
15. Pelling and Webster, op. cit., p. 185.
16. Ibid.
17. G. Keynes, *Dr. Timothy Bright, 1550–1615: A Survey of his Life with a Bibliography of his Writings*, London (1962).
18. R. S. Roberts, 'The Personnel and Practice of Medicine in Tudor and Stuart England', *Medical History*, VI (1962), p. 366.
19. The best description of these efforts is to be found in Roberts, thesis.
20. Clark, *Royal College*, I, pp. 208–10; Pelling and Webster, op. cit., p. 185.
21. M. Pelling, 'Appearance and Reality: Barbersurgeons, the Body and Venereal Disease in Early Modern London', in A. L.

Beier and R. Finlay, eds, *The Making of the Metropolis: London 1500–1700*, London (1986), p. 83.
22. *Statutes of the Realm*, III, p. 31.
23. Pelling, 'Appearance and Reality', p. 83, and Pelling, 'Occupational Diversity', 489.
24. Pelling, 'Appearance and Reality', p. 84.
25. *Certain Works of Chirurgerie*, London (1564), p. 1.
26. E.g. T. Brugis, *Vade Mecum: or, A Companion for a Surgeon*, London (1652); G. Fabrice, *His Experiments in Chyrurgerie*, London (1642); J. Cooke, *Mellificum Chirurgerie. Or the Marrow . . .* , London (1648); J. Woodall, *The Surgeon's Mate . . .* , London (1655, numerous earlier eds, first published 1617).
27. S. Young, ed., *The Annals of the Barber-Surgeons*, London (1890), pp. 77, 119, 182, 316, 336, 341, 342.
28. Ibid., pp. 335–6, 340.
29. See Chapter 3.
30. See Roberts, thesis. See also C. Wall, H. C. Cannon and E. Ashworth Underwood, *A History of the Worshipful Society of Apothecaries of London*, vol. I, 1617–1815, Oxford (1963).
31. See Roberts, thesis; also the small body of polemical literature on the subject, e.g. Dr Cox, *A Discourse Wherein the Interest of the Patient in Reference to Physick and Physicians is Soberly Debated . . .* , London (1699); *An Essay for the Regulation of the Practice of Physick . . .*, London (1673); *A Letter Concerning the Present State of Physick . . .* , London (1665).
32. For an important provincial case of an apothecary winning the right to prescribe, see Roberts, 'The Personnel and Practice', VI (1962), 371–4.
33. See Roberts, thesis.
34. See J. H. Aveling, *English Midwives: their History and Prospects*, London (1872). He indicates that in 1577 baptism by midwives became illegal for Protestants. None the less, baptismal records show that even among Protestants the practice continued for some time. See also W. D., 'Midwives Formerly Baptized Infants', *Gentleman's Magazine*, LV, 2 (1785), 939.
35. J. Hitchcock, 'A Sixteenth-Century Midwife's License', *Bulletin of the History of Medicine*, XLI (1967), 75–6.
36. M. Stocks, in her *A Hundred Years of District Nursing*, London (1960), p. 123, indicates that nurse-midwives of the late nineteenth century sometimes performed like services. Florence Nightingale disapproved of nurses and nurse-midwives doing housework because of her desire to raise the status of nursing.
37. P. Willughby, *Observations in Midwifery*, H. Blenkinsop, ed., Yorkshire (1972).
38. Ibid., p. 305.
39. E.g. E. Roesslin, *The Byrth of Mankynde*, R. Jonas, trans., London (1540); J. Rueff, *The Expert Midwife*, London (1637). For a review of the sixteenth- and seventeenth-century

literature on midwifery, see A. Eccles, *Obstetrics and Gynaecology in Tudor and Stuart England*, London (1982). See also E. Shorter, *A History of Women's Bodies*, Harmondsworth (1984), pp. 35–47.

40. J. H. Aveling, *The Chamberlens and the Midwifery Forceps*, London (1882).
41. Ibid., pp. 20–1.
42. Ibid.
43. Ibid. See also Clark, *Royal College*, I, pp. 253–4.
44. *Harleian Miscellany*, IV, London (1744); J. Donnison, *Midwives and Medical Men: A History of Inter-Professional Rivalries and Women's Rights*, London (1977), p. 19; A. Fraser, *The Weaker Vessel: Woman's Lot in Seventeenth-Century England*, London (1985), pp. 513–22.
45. Aveling, *English Midwives*, p. 2.
46. Quoted in Donnison, op. cit., p. 34, from M. Stephen's *The Domestic Midwife*, London (1795), p. 105.
47. Examples of works attacking man-midwives on moral grounds are J. Blunt, *Man-midwifery Dissected: or the Obstetric Family-Instructor*, London (1793), and [P. Thickness], *Man-Midwifery Analysed: And the Tendency of the Practice Detected and Exposed*, London (1765). Sairey Gamp is a character in Dickens's *Martin Chuzzlewit*, London (1843–4).
48. C. Goodall, *The Royal College of Physicians of London . . .* , London (1684), pp. 1–2.
49. No good general study of unlicensed practitioners exists, although there are some popular works on 'quacks'. R. S. Roberts's thesis contains a discussion of the Royal College of Physicians' attacks on many such healers. Pelling and Webster's article in *Health, Medicine and Mortality* has good information about the activities and numerical strength of unlicensed healers in sixteenth-century England. K. Thomas's *Religion and the Decline of Magic*, Harmondsworth (1973), pp. 209–300, and A. Macfarlane's *Witchcraft in Tudor and Stuart England: A Regional and Comparative Study*, London (1970), pp. 115–34, 178–85, pay particular attention to magical healers. And Pelling's article, 'Appearance and Reality', contains information about seventeenth-century unlicensed healers operating in London and its environs. For a discussion of vagrancy, I depend upon A. L. Beier's *Masterless Men: The Vagrancy Problem in England, 1560–1640*, London (1985).
50. See Chapter 2.
51. Pelling and Webster, op. cit., p. 183.
52. Fioravanti, *A Short Discourse of the Excellent Doctor . . .* , J. Hester, trans., London (1580), The Proheme.
53. Quoted in K. Dewhurst, *Dr. Thomas Sydenham (1642–1689). His Life and Original Writings*, London (1966), p. 124.
54. I have identified at least forty books published in the period 1500–1700 which fall into this category.

55. J. Goeurot, *The Regiment of Life . . .* , T. Phayer, trans., London (1544), Translator's Preface.
56. The large number of do-it-yourself medical handbooks published in the period might, in this context, be considered works by empirical writers.
57. Roberts, thesis, p. 100, and Young, *Barber-Surgeons*, pp. 330 and 340.
58. Ralph Josselin's family employed two local bone-setters. See Chapter 6. The best account of itinerant practitioners is J. Halle's 'An Historical Expostulation . . . ', in Lanfranc of Milan, *A Most Excellent and Learned Work of Chirurgery . . .* , London (1565).
59. Halle, op. cit., no pagination.
60. See Chapter 3.
61. Brain, London (1637), Preface.
62. See Chapter 6.
63. For a discussion of some popular applications of astrology, see B. Capp, *Astrology and the Popular Press: English Almanacs 1500–1800*, London (1979).
64. *The Infallible True and Assured Witch*, 2nd ed., London (1624).
65. See Thomas, *Religion and Magic*; Pelling and Webster, op. cit., p. 183; A. L. Rowse, *Simon Forman: Sex and Society in Shakespeare's Age*, London (1974); 'The Diary of John Dee', J. O. Halliwell, ed., *Camden Society*, XIX (1847).
66. MacDonald, *Mystical Bedlam*; J. Aubrey, *Aubrey's Brief Lives*, O. L. Dick, ed., Harmondsworth (1972), p. 78.
67. J. O. Halliwell, ed., *The Autobiography and Personal Diary of Simon Forman the Celebrated Astronomer from A.D. 1552 to A.D. 1602*, London (for private circulation only) (1849), e.g. pp. 15–19.
68. Clark, *Royal College*, I, p. 259; *A Brief Description of the Notorious Life of J. Lambe*, Amsterdam and London (1628); M. Parker, *The Tragedy of Doctor Lambe*, London (1628).
69. See Thomas, *Religion and Magic*; Macfarlane, *Witchcraft*; also E. Poeton, 'The Winnowing of White Witchcraft', British Library Sloane MS 1954; Cotta, *The Infallible, True and Assured Witch*, London (1624, second edition).
70. Thomas, *Religion and Magic*, pp. 244–5 and 296–8.
71. Ibid., p. 216.
72. Ibid., pp. 217–22.
73. MacDonald, *Mystical Bedlam*, pp. 17–19. See D. P. Walker, *Unclean Spirits: Possession and Exorcism in France and England in the Late Sixteenth and Early Seventeenth Centuries*, London (1981), pp. 57–9, for a case of a cunning-man, hired to heal children thought to be bewitched, who was executed for conjuring.
74. Thomas, *Religion and Magic*, pp. 237 and 240–2.
75. *A Brief Account of Mr. Valentine Greatraks*, London (1666 and

1668) and *The Great Cures and Strange Miracles of Mr. Valentine Gertrux* [sic] (1666). Thomas, *Religion and Magic*, p. 241, lists several other pamphlets which I have not seen.
76. *A Brief Account*, p. 30.
77. In one case he did lance a wen: ibid., p. 65.
78. Ibid., p. 40.
79. Ibid., p. 37.
80. Ibid., p. 1.
81. Thomas, *Religion and Magic*, p. 240.
82. M. Bloch, *The Royal Touch: Sacred Monarchy and Scrofula in England and France*, J. E. Anderson, trans., London (1973), and Thomas, *Religion and Magic*, pp. 192–201.
83. Thomas, *Religion and Magic*, p. 228, based on entries in the King's Register of Healing.
84. Ibid., p. 227.
85. British Library Sloane MS 153, 259/506. (See Notes for Chapter 3 for explanation of case notation.)
86. Thomas, *Religion and Magic*, p. 228.
87. Ibid., pp. 235–6.
88. Ibid., p. 235.
89. 34 and 35 H VIII *cap.* 8, *Statutes of the Realm*, III, p. 906. For information on the use of this act as a defence against prosecution by the RCP, see Roberts, thesis.
90. Macfarlane, *Witchcraft*, p. 120.
91. Pelling and Webster, op. cit., p. 183.
92. J. H. Raach, *A Directory of English Country Physicians, 1603–1643*, London (1962), p. 14.
93. Ibid.
94. Ibid., pp. 13–14.
95. Roberts, 'The Personnel and Practice', VI (1962), 364.
96. Pelling, 'Occupational Diversity', 495.
97. Roberts, 'The Personnel and Practice', VI (1962), 376.
98. Ibid.
99. *Diary of Lady Margaret Hoby, 1599–1605*, D. M. Meads, ed., London (1930), p. 184.
100. See Roberts, thesis, and 'The Personnel and Practice' for information on the blurring of these distinctions. Also see Clark, *Royal College*, I, and Young, *Barber-Surgeons*, for discussions of occupational organisations – particularly the RCP – attempting to enforce monopolies over certain types of practice.
101. See Z. Cope, *The Royal College of Surgeons of England*, London (1959), and C. Wall, *The History of the Surgeon's Company, 1745–1800*, London (1937).
102. Pelling, 'Occupational Diversity', 504–5.
103. Aveling, *English Midwives*, p. 2.
104. Act III, scene 1.
105. *A Most Excellent and Learned Work of Chirurgery*, Epistle.
106. D. Landy, ed., *Culture, Disease and Healing: Studies in Medical*

Anthropology, New York and London (1977), pp. 468–81 and 495–503.

107. F. N. L. Poynter, ed., *Medicine and Culture*, London (1969), p. 2.
108. *Devils, Drugs and Doctors: The Story of the Science of Healing from Medicine Man to Doctor*, London (1929), p. 384.
109. E.g. C. Singer, *From Magic to Science: Essays on the Scientific Twilight*, New York (1958), ch. IV, 'Early English Magic and Medicine'.
110. See U. Maclean, 'Some Aspects of Sickness Behaviour among the Yoruba', in J. B. Loudon, ed., *Social Anthropology and Medicine*, London and New York (1976), pp. 294–5.
111. Thomas, *Religion and Magic*, pp. 223–5.
112. A good example of a compilation of this lore, combined with the basic principles of natural magic, is contained in A. Magnus, *Secrets of the Vertues of Herbes*, London (1549).
113. Robert Hooke, for instance, took chemical remedies and 'Galenicals' in order to purge his system. See Chapter 5.
114. Thomas, *Religion and Magic*, p. 224.
115. Sloane MS 153 op. cit., 105/171, 318/666.
116. Thomas, *Religion and Magic*, p. 225.
117. One edition is Sir Kenelm Digby, *Of the Sympathetic Powder*, London (1669).
118. See P. Slack, 'Mirrors of Health and Treasures of Poor Men: The Uses of the Vernacular Medical Literature of Tudor England', in C. Webster, ed., *Health, Medicine and Mortality in the Sixteenth Century*, Cambridge (1979), pp. 237–73.
119. See Roberts, thesis; Clark, *Royal College*, I. The surgeons' efforts to control surgical practice in London have received less attention than the physicians' activities, but many examples of the Barbersurgeons' Company's efforts in this direction appear in Young, *Barber-Surgeons*.
120. *The Anatomie of the Bodie of Man*, F. J. Furnivall and P. Furnivall, eds, Early English Text Society, extra series, LIII (1888, repr. 1975), p. 6.
121. J. Guillemeau, *Childbirth* . . . , London (1635), Introduction. The eighteenth-century *accoucheur*, William Smellie, called Hippocrates the Father of midwifery: *A Treatise on the Theory and Practice of Midwifery*, 3 vols, London (1779), I, xxx.
122. Cotta, *A Short Discovery of the Unobserved Dangers of Several Sorts of Ignorant and Unconsiderate Practisers of Physic in England*, London (1612), p. 119.
123. Arcaeus, *A Most Excellent and Compendious Method of Curing Wounds in the Head, and in Other Parts of the Body* . . . , J. Read, trans., London (1588).
124. *A Short Discourse of Discovery of Certain Stratagems, Whereby our London Empericks have been Observed Strongly to Oppugne, and oft times to Expugne their Poore Patient's Purses*, London (1602), p. 24.

125. Boorde, *The Breviary of Health*, London (1587), Prologue. This book was published in many editions; I have also seen the 1552 edition.
126. *The Copy of a Letter Written by E. D., Doctor of Physick, to a Gentleman* . . . , London (1606), p. 335.
127. *A Detection and Querimonie of the Daily Enormities and Abuses Committed in Physick* . . . , London (1566), Preface.
128. *A Right Profitable Book of all Diseases, called the Pathway to Health* . . . , London (1632), 'To the Reader'.
129. *The Marrow of Physick* . . . , London (1640), Preface.
130. P. P. Valentinus, *Enchiridion Medicum: Containing an Epitome of the Whole Course of Physic* . . . , London (1608), fo. 3.
131. J. Hart, *KλINIKH, or the Diet of the Diseased* . . . , London (1633).
132. Boorde, op. cit. (1552), p. 2.
133. W. Folkingham, *Panala Medica* . . . , London (1628), 'To the Reader'.
134. *The Character of a Quack Doctor*, London (1676); Cotta, *A Short Discovery*; Cotta, *Cotta contra Antonium* . . . , Oxford (1625); E. D., *The Copy of a Letter*, op. cit.; P. Forestus, *The Arraignment of Urines* . . . , J. Hart, trans., London (1623); J. Halle, 'An Historicall Expostulation', op. cit.; J. Hart, *The Anatomy of Urines* . . . , London (1624); J. Oberndoerffer, *The Anatomies of the True Physician and Counterfeit Mountebank*, London (1602); E. Poeton, 'Medical Treatises', British Library Sloane MS 1954; J. Securis, *A Detection and Querimonie*, op. cit.; F. Herring, *A Short Discourse* of *Discovery of Certain Stratagems*, London (1602); [C. Merret], *A Short View of the Frauds* . . . , London (1669).
135. Oberndoerffer, op. cit., Preface.
136. Cotta, *A Short Discovery*, pp. 11, 17.
137. E. D., op. cit., p. 16.
138. Halle, op. cit. [no pagination].
139. Ibid.
140. Cotta, *A Short Discovery*, p. 4.
141. Cotta, *Cotta contra Antonium* . . . , Oxford (1625), Preface.
142. Gale, *Certain Works of Chirurgerie*, London (1564), Preface.
143. Securis, op. cit. [no pagination].
144. Cotta, *A Short Discovery*, p. 42.
145. Hart, op. cit., Preface.
146. E. D., op. cit., p. 17.
147. E.g. *Here Beginneth the Seeing of Urines* . . . , London (1525), 2nd edn, London (1526); *Hereafter Followeth the Judgement of all Urines* . . . , London (? early sixteenth century).
148. Forestus, op. cit., p. 16.
149. See p. 23.
150. Principally Forestus, Hart, Poeton and Cotta, *A Short Discovery*.
151. Forestus, op. cit., pp. 45–6.

152. Cotta was also worried about the problem of itinerants: *A Short Discovery*, pp. 113–14.
153. Halle, op. cit. [no pagination].
154. Cotta, *A Short Discovery*, p. 34.
155. Ibid., p. 112.
156. Ibid., pp. 113–14.
157. Ibid., p. 25.
158. See Young, *Barber-Surgeons*, p. 260.
159. Some general works reflecting seventeenth-century mysogynism are F. Beaumont, *The Woman Hater*, London (1648); W. Blake, *The Trial of the Ladies*, Hyde Park (1656); *A Brief Anatomy of Women: Being An Invective*, London (1653); *A Description of Wanton Women*, [1690?]; *An Invective Against the Pride of Women*, [London (1657)]; [J. Swetnam], *The Arraignment of Lewd, Idle . . . Women*, London (1645).
160. J. Rueff, *The Expert Midwife*, London (1637), Preface.
161. Ibid.
162. Willughby, *Observations in Midwifery*, op. cit., p. 9.
163. Ibid., p. 57.
164. Ibid., p. 135.
165. Smellie, op. cit., Preface.
166. See Donnison, *Midwives and Medical Men*, op. cit., pp. 21–41. For objections to men-midwives, see [Thickness], *Man-Midwifery Analysed*, op. cit.; Blunt, *Man-Midwifery Dissected*, op. cit.; S. Stone, *A Complete Practice of Midwifery*, London (1737); and J. Sharp, *The Midwives Book*, London (1671).
167. Poeton, 'The Winnowing of White Witchcraft', op. cit.
168. Oberndoerffer, op. cit., p. 15.
169. Forestus, op. cit., p. 53.
170. G. Gifford, *A Discourse of the Subtle Practices of Devils by Witches and Sorcerers*, London (1587) [no page numbers]; see also Hart, *The Anatomy of Urines*, op. cit., Conclusion.
171. Cotta, *A Short Discovery*, p. 86. See also Forestus, op. cit., 'To the Reader'.
172. Cotta, *A Short Discovery*, p. 87.
173. Ibid., p. 88.
174. Securis, op. cit. [no pagination].
175. See Oberndoerffer, op. cit., p. 21.
176. N. Culpeper, *A Directory for Midwives*, London (1651), p. 4.
177. Sharp, op. cit., Introduction.
178. P. Barrough, *The Method of Physick . . .* , London (1583), Introduction.
179. E. D., op. cit., p. 17.
180. See E. Freidson, *Profession of Medicine: A Study of the Sociology of Applied Knowledge*, New York (1972); J. L. Berlant, *Profession and Monopoly: A Study of Medicine in the United States and Great Britain*, Los Angeles (1975); N. Parry and J. Parry, *The Rise of the Medical Profession*, London (1976).
181. Freidson, op. cit., pp. 19–20.

3. A LONDON SURGEON'S CAREER: JOSEPH BINNS

General note: Most of the notes for this chapter refer to a numbering system devised to locate individual cases in a transcription made of Joseph Binns's surgical casebook, British Library Sloane MS 153. The numbers given are double, referring to page numbers of the transcription and individual case numbers.

1. Napier's treatment of patients with emotional disorders has been explored in M. MacDonald's *Mystical Bedlam: Madness, Anxiety and Healing in Seventeenth-Century England*, Cambridge (1981).
2. See e.g. British Library Sloane MS 663, Dr Barker of Shrewsbury's 'Observations on cases in physick, 1595–1605'; British Library Sloane MS 1112, 'The casebook of a provincial physician, 1619–1622'.
3. Sloane MS 153.
4. Mayerne's casebook for the years 1607–51 is housed in the Library of the Royal College of Physicians, MS 444. King's casebook for 1676–96 is British Library Sloane MS 1589.
5. Guildhall Library, MS 5625/1 fo. 89; V. C. Medvei and J. L. Thornton, eds, *The Royal Hospital of St. Bartholomew 1123–1973*, London (1974), p. 388.
6. Public Record Office, PCC 1664, 47, 52.
7. Ibid., PCC 1664, 47. See C. Gittings, *Death, Burial and the Individual in Early Modern England*, London (1984), pp. 117–25, for a discussion of such bequests.
8. 214/429, 311/621, 313/633.
9. PCC 1664, 47.
10. Young, *Barber-Surgeons*, p. 345.
11. 229/450.
12. 39/78.
13. 199/393.
14. 191/372.
15. Young, *Barber-Surgeons*, pp. 77, 119, 182.
16. Pelling, 'Appearance and Reality', pp. 3–4.
17. 185/358.
18. E.g. 168/325, 252/497, 289/561.
19. E.g. 53/86, 100/146, 140/250.
20. E.g. 57/89, 191/372, 259/506, 265/519.
21. 191/372.
22. 12/31.
23. 168/327.
24. 192/379.
25. 217/437–8.
26. 152/288–91.
27. 241/473.
28. 217/437–8.
29. 8/22.
30. 12/31.

31. 6/17, 10/25.
32. 192/379.
33. 123/217, 19/45.
34. 96/142.
35. 24/55.
36. 205/411.
37. 111/190.
38. 123/215.
39. 105/171.
40. 197/388.
41. *The Diary of John Evelyn*, E. S. de Beer, ed., London (1959), p. 264.
42. L. Stone, *The Crisis of the Aristocracy, 1558–1641*, Oxford (1965), pp. 223–4.
43. 213/427.
44. 190/370.
45. E.g. 23/53, 198/391.
46. 176/343, 190/371, 34/67.
47. 125/219.
48. 139/249.
49. 190/371.
50. 213/427.
51. 96/142.
52. 190/370. See also A. L. Beier, *Masterless Men: The Vagrancy Problem in England, 1560–1640*, London (1985).
53. See K. Thomas, *Religion and the Decline of Magic*, Harmondsworth (1973), pp. 628–37; and A. Macfarlane, *Witchcraft in Tudor and Stuart England: A Regional and Comparative Study*, London (1970), pp. 173–6.
54. 191/372.
55. 156/300.
56. 155/297.
57. 155/297.
58. 155/299.
59. 200/394.
60. 12/31.
61. 72/102.
62. 201/396.
63. 86/129.
64. 134/231.
65. 188/365.
66. 163/317.
67. 66/93.
68. 78/115.
69. 140/251.
70. 85/128.
71. 105/171.
72. 29/61.
73. 159/309.

74. 202/402.
75. 67/96.
76. 8/21.
77. 213/425.
78. 141/253.
79. Explanation of this and other medical terms supplied by Dr R. M. McCray, MD.
80. 89/134.
81. 157/301.
82. 100/145.
83. 214/429, 311/621, 313/633.
84. J. Woodall, *The Surgeon's Mate . . .* , London (first published 1617). See also W. J. Bishop, *The Early History of Surgery*, London (1961), pp. 92–3 and 95–6.
85. 96/142, 85/128.
86. 214/429.
87. 207/416.
88. Head wounds are discussed at greater length below.
89. 163/317.
90. 147/269.
91. E.g. 86/129, 147/269.
92. 147/269.
93. 66/93.
94. 239/465.
95. E.g. 116/202.
96. E.g. 72/102, 122/213.
97. 140/251.
98. 8/21, 8/22, 9/24, 167/323.
99. 8/21, 9/24, 167/323.
100. 8/21, 9/24.
101. 198/391.
102. 8/22.
103. 167/323.
104. 32/13.
105. 219/441.
106. E.g. 236/459, 208/417.
107. 200/394.
108. E.g. 29/61, 105/281, 202/401.
109. 202/401.
110. 105/171. The practice of treating certain ailments by touching the hand of a recently hanged criminal is discussed in C. Gittings, *Death, Burial and the Individual in Early Modern England*, London (1984), pp. 67–8.
111. 29/61.
112. This might have been a case where a seriously injured patient was presented to the Court of the Barbersurgeons' Company, and a senior surgeon was called in to consult.
113. 150/281.
114. 112/191.

115. 16/42.
116. 203/404.
117. See Pelling, 'Appearance and Reality', pp. 89–95.
118. 369/526.
119. 169/330.
120. 27/60.
121. For a similar case, see 43/81. In both cases autopsies were performed.
122. 140/250.
123. E.g. 168/325, 229/450, 257/505.
124. 214/429, 294/567.
125. E.g. 25/55, 197/389, 210/421, 278/542, 300/579, 301/583.
126. E.g. 46/83, 81/122, 105/166, 139/248.
127. E.g. 80/121, 82/123, 94/140, 137/244.
128. E.g. 80/121, 89/135.
129. E.g. 81/122, 137/244.
130. 159/310.
131. 95/141.
132. 220/442.
133. E.g. 236/460.
134. E.g. 89/135.
135. 181/352.
136. 46/83.
137. Binns mentioned assistants very infrequently. While it is likely that he trained apprentices, his casebook says so little about them that no comment is possible.
138. 195/386. One cannot help thinking that Binns and his surgical colleagues neglected a golden opportunity for research on the stomach's function similar to that pursued by William Beaumont between 1824 and 1833.
139. 104/164.
140. 271/530.
141. 259/507.
142. 241/471.
143. 311/623.
144. E.g. 227/449, 229/450, 198/390, 199/393.
145. E.g. 71/101, 297/573.
146. 111/190.
147. Pelling, 'Appearance and Reality', p. 83.
148. 197/387. See also 310/618.
149. 265/520.
150. 267/525.
151. 16/42.
152. 288/556.
153. 259/506.
154. 277/541.
155. 43/81, 27/60.
156. 53/85.
157. 307/605. See also 23/52.

158. 212/424.
159. 213/428.
160. E.g. 314/638, 127/223, 241/473, 312/625.
161. The distinction is unclear. See discussion of gonorrhoea as symptom above.
162. E.g. 102/151, 192/377, 191/373, 275/536. See also I. Veith, *Hysteria: The History of a Disease*, Chicago, Ill. (1965).
163. E.g. 41/80, 141/255.
164. T. Sydenham, *Works*, Dr Greenhill, trans., London (1848), vol. II, pp. 35–6.
165. Beaumont and Fletcher, *Knight of the Burning Pestle*, Act III, scene 1, reprinted in *The Dramatic Works in the Beaumont and Fletcher Canon*, F. Bowers, ed., Cambridge (1966), vol. I, p. 57. See also H. Silvette, *The Doctor on Stage: Medicine and Medical Men in Seventeenth-Century England*, Knoxville, Tenn. (1967), pp. 182–234.
166. E.g. 12/30, 20/47, 36/69.
167. E.g. 30/60, 162/316.
168. 129/226.
169. E.g. 65/90.
170. 209/420–2.
171. 209/415-16.
172. 114/200.
173. 54/87.
174. E.g. 18/44, 131/228.
175. 131/228.
176. 97/143.
177. E.g. 274/534, 57/39.
178. 14/36, 33/65–6, 36/69, 158/304, 183/354, 317/657.
179. 56/88.
180. 131/228.
181. 238/464.
182. 92/138.
183. 122/214.
184. 154/295.
185. 165/320.
186. See Chapter 9.
187. 121/210.
188. 102/154–5.
189. 136/242.
190. 192/379 (316/653).
191. E.g. 216/435, 191/373, 275/536.
192. 191/374. For an in-depth discussion of this disorder, see E. Jorden, *A Brief Discourse of a Disease called the Suffocation of the Mother*, London (1603).
193. 292/565.
194. M. MacDonald, *Mystical Bedlam*, p. 20.
195. Ibid., p. 26.

4. THE PHYSICIAN'S TALE

1. Cambridge (1981).
2. Ibid., p. 16.
3. See Chapter 3.
4. Some of his notes for the years 1607–51 are housed in the Library of the Royal College of Physicians, MS 444.
5. F. N. L. Poynter and W. J. Bishop, eds, *A Seventeenth-Century Doctor and his Patients: John Symcotts, 1592?–1662*, Bedfordshire Historical Record Society, vol. 31, Streatley, Beds (1950), hereafter referred to as *Symcotts*.
6. *Symcotts*, p. x.
7. Ibid., pp. xxi–xxiii.
8. Ibid., p. xi.
9. Ibid.
10. Ibid., p. xii.
11. Ibid., pp. 105–8.
12. Ibid., p. xxvi.
13. Ibid., pp. 57, 70, 72, 76, 77, 81, 82.
14. Ibid., pp. 17, 55, 56, 58, 70, 75.
15. Ibid., pp. 75–6.
16. See G. J. Witkowski, *Accoucheurs et Sages-Femmes Célèbres*, Paris (1891), for some diagrams of midwifery instruments used by surgeons.
17. *Symcotts*, p. 81.
18. Ibid., p. 80.
19. Ibid., p. 81.
20. Ibid., p. 62.
21. Ibid., p. 59.
22. Ibid., p. 68.
23. Ibid., p. 76.
24. Ibid., p. 58.
25. Ibid., p. 52.
26. Ibid., p. xxx.
27. Ibid., p. 73.
28. Ibid., pp. 87–8.
29. Ibid., p. 81.
30. Ibid., p. 82.
31. Ibid., pp. 79–80.
32. Ibid., pp. 38, 51.
33. Ibid., p. 77.
34. Ibid., pp. xix-xx.
35. Ibid., pp. 6–7.
36. Ibid., p. 71.
37. Ibid., pp. 71–2.
38. Ibid., pp. 96–7.
39. Ibid., p. 103.
40. Ibid., p. 70.
41. Ibid., pp. 11–12.

42. Ibid., p. 89.
43. Ibid., pp. 87–8.
44. The Royal College of Physicians codified its disapproval of physicians diagnosing from a carried urine sample in 1601. G. N. Clark, *A History of the Royal College of Physicians of London*, p. 178. See Chapter 2.
45. *Symcotts*, p. 25.
46. Ibid., pp. 15, 41.
47. Ibid., p. 39.
48. Ibid., p. 17.
49. Ibid., p. xiii.
50. E.g. ibid., pp. 30, 37, 39.
51. Ibid., pp. 43, 59.
52. Ibid., p. 19.
53. Ibid., p. 43.
54. Ibid., p. 72.
55. Ibid., p. 81.
56. Ibid., p. 7.
57. Ibid., pp. 9–11.
58. Ibid., p. 38.
59. Ibid., p. 28.
60. Ibid., pp. 28–9.
61. See Chapter 2.
62. *Symcotts*, pp. 55–6, 80–1.
63. Ibid., p. 56.
64. See Chapter 3.
65. See Chapter 3.
66. See L. Stone, *The Crisis of the Aristocracy 1558–1641*, Oxford (1965), p. 41, for a brief discussion of the social position of physicians. 'John Ferne thought it not a very honourable profession, and as late as the middle of the seventeenth century a gentleman was refusing the offer of marriage with the daughter of a rich doctor since "the very thought of the Blister-pipes [*recte* clyster pipe] did Nauseate his Stomach"!'
67. See Chapter 6.
68. *Symcotts*, p. 29.
69. K. Thomas quotes Gregory King in calculating that 'in 1688 over half the population were "decreasing the wealth of the kingdom", that is to say earning less than they consumed. There can be no doubt that between a third and a half of the population lived at subsistence level and were chronically under-employed', *Religion and Magic*, p. 3.
70. *Symcotts*, p. 76.
71. Ibid., pp. 12–13.
72. See Chapter 6.
73. *Symcotts*, pp. 11–12.
74. Ibid., pp. 15–17.
75. Ibid., p. 88.
76. Ibid., p. 20.

77. Ibid., p. 23.
78. Ibid.
79. Ibid., p. 33.
80. Ibid., pp. 40–1.
81. Ibid., pp. 25–6.
82. Ibid., p. 45.
83. Ibid., p. 37.
84. Ibid., p. 35. See also p. 47.
85. Ibid., p. 46.
86. Ibid., p. 47.
87. Ibid., p. xxvi.
88. Barker's casebook, hereafter referred to as *Barker*, is the British Library Sloane MS 78 or 663. Another early healer whose work is mentioned above is the magical practitioner Simon Forman. See Chapter 2.
89. *Barker*, 7/4.
90. Ibid., 22/13, 132/78.
91. Ibid., 27/17.
92. Ibid., 56/40.
93. Ibid., 49/34, 124/73.
94. E.g. ibid., 102/66, 105/68, 110/69, 124/73, 137/82.
95. E.g. ibid., 19/11, 24/14, 27/17, 44/28.
96. See Clark, *Royal College*, p. 178.
97. *Barker*, 120–22b/72.
98. Ibid., 112/69.
99. Ibid., 99/65.
100. *Symcotts*, p. 86.
101. *Barker*, 21/13.
102. E.g. ibid., 14/8, 18/9, 23/14, 33/22, 48/34.
103. The *Oxford English Dictionary* states that betony is a 'plant of the Labiate order, having spiked purple flowers and ovate crenate leaves'. It quotes Burton's *Anatomy of Melancholy* to the effect that the Emperor Augustus used this herb to drive out demons.
104. *Barker*, 33/22.
105. Ibid., 61/45.
106. Ibid., 3/2, 4/3, 49/34, 72/49.
107. Ibid., 134/79.
108. Ibid., 90/59.
109. Ibid., 49/34.
110. British Library Sloane MS 1112, hereafter referred to as *Sl. 1112*.
111. *Sl. 1112*, 14/5, 15/5, 21/7, 22/7, 29/7, 48/12, 51/13.
112. Ibid., 1/1, 6/2, 13/5, 23/7, 47/12, 79/16.
113. Ibid., 3/1.
114. Ibid., 8/2.
115. Ibid., 5/15.
116. Ibid., 19/6.
117. Ibid., 5–6.

118. T. R. Forbes, *The Midwife and the Witch*, London (1966), pp. 64–79.
119. *Sl. 1112*, 29/7, 50/12.
120. I. Veith, *Hysteria: The History of a Disease*, Chicago, Ill. (1965).
121. *Sl. 1112*, 78/16.
122. Ibid., 1/1, 2/1, 3/1, 4/1, 33/9, 61/14.
123. *Symcotts.*, pp. 13, 41.
124. *Sl. 1112*, 1/1, 79/16.
125. Although Binns employed a 'man', there was nothing this apprentice or assistant did which Binns did not also do himself.
126. Sloane MS 153, 267/525.
127. *Symcotts*, pp. 13, 41.
128. See Chapter 6.
129. Ibid.
130. Ibid.
131. *Symcotts*, p. 102.
132. Ibid., p. 34.
133. Ibid., pp. 12–13.
134. Ibid., p. 33.

5. SUFFERERS AND PATIENTS: THE DISEASES OF THE PEOPLE

1. *Leviathan*, pt I, ch. 13, London (1973 edn), p. 65.
2. Thomas, *Religion and Magic*, p. 7.
3. Stone, *The Family, Sex and Marriage*, p. 69; and R. Schofield and E. A. Wrigley, 'Infant and Child Mortality in England in the late Tudor and early Stuart Period', in C. Webster, ed., *Health, Medicine and Mortality in the Sixteenth Century*, Cambridge (1979), pp. 61–96.
4. L. Stone, *The Crisis of the Aristocracy, 1558–1641*, Oxford (1965), pp. 223–4.
5. See C. Creighton, *A History of Epidemics in Britain*, Cambridge (1894 and 1965); J. F. D. Shrewsbury, *A History of Bubonic Plague in the British Isles*, Cambridge (1971); H. Zinsser, *Rats, Lice and History*, London (1935 and 1943); *The Plague Reconsidered: A New Look at its Origins and Effects in Sixteenth- and Seventeenth-Century England*, Matlock, Derbyshire (1977).
6. P. Slack, 'The Local Incidence of Epidemic Disease: The Case of Bristol, 1540–1650', in *The Plague Reconsidered*, op. cit., p. 51.
7. Thomas, *Religion and Magic*, p. 3.
8. J. Graunt, *Natural and Political Observations Made Upon the Bills of Mortality*, P. Laslett, ed., *The Earliest Classics*, Gregg International (1973, first edn 1662), p. 70.
9. Interesting commentary on these sources is made in T. R. Forbes's *Chronicle from Aldgate: Life and Death in Shakespeare's London*, London (1971), pp. 25–51.
10. Graunt, 'The Table of Casualties', op. cit., pp. 76–7.

11. Ibid.
12. Ibid.
13. Ibid., p. 32.
14. W. A. Littledale, *The Registers of St. Vedast, Foster Lane*, London: Harleian Society, Vol. XXX (1903), pp. 199–227.
15. Graunt, op. cit., pp. 25–6.
16. Ibid., pp. 26–8.
17. Ibid., p. 29.
18. Ibid., p. 11.
19. Ibid., p. 13.
20. Ibid., p. 14.
21. Ibid., pp. 23–4.
22. Ibid.
23. Ibid., p. 29.
24. *The Diary of Samuel Pepys*, R. Latham and W. Matthews, eds, London (1970–82), e.g. II, p. 17, IV, p. 59, VIII, p. 198, I, p. 283.
25. *The Diary of Ralph Josselin, 1616–1683*, A. Macfarlane, ed., Oxford (1976), e.g. 5/1/51, 16/3/51, 4/2/55, 3/59. See Chapter 6.
26. *The Diary of Robert Hooke, 1672–1680*, H. W. Robinson and W. Adams, eds, London (1968 and 1935).
27. Ibid., 14/2/78.
28. *The Diary of Lady Margaret Hoby, 1599–1605*, D. M. Meads, ed., London (1930), 13/5/1605, p. 220.
29. Pepys, *Diary*, 13/2/61, II, p. 36.
30. Josselin, *Diary*, 26/4/49 and 30/4/49.
31. *The Diary of John Evelyn*, E. S. de Beer, ed., London (1959), p. 240.
32. Pepys, *Diary*, 1/12/68, IX, p. 381.
33. See Chapter 2.
34. Pepys, *Diary*, IX, pp. 564–5.
35. Ibid., p. 248.
36. Ibid., pp. 507, 537.
37. Evelyn, *Diary*, p. 271.
38. E.g. Hooke, *Diary*, 30/1/74, p. 84; Josselin, *Diary*, 15/6/45; *The Letters of Dorothy Osborne to William Temple*, G. C. Moore Smith, ed., Oxford (1928), letter 4, p. 10.
39. See Chapter 6.
40. Osborne, *Letters*, p. 96.
41. Ibid., p. 40.
42. Ibid., p. 41.
43. *The Diary of the Lady Anne Clifford with an Introductory Note by V. Sackville-West*, London (1923), pp. 51–62.
44. Ibid., pp. 51–2.
45. Evelyn, *Diary*, pp. 380–5.
46. Pepys, *Diary*, IV, p. 21.
47. Ibid., p. 28.
48. Ibid., p. 58.

49. Ibid., 11/3/61, II, p. 53.
50. Ibid., 8/5/61, p. 96.
51. Josselin, *Diary*, 17/7/46.
52. Ibid., 28/2/47.
53. Pepys, *Diary*, 19/8/63–11/12/63, IV.
54. Hooke, *Diary*, p. 98; Josselin, *Diary*, p. 149.
55. Lady Anne Clifford believed a nosebleed had ended her daughter's attack of ague in 1617: Clifford, *Diary*, p. 54.
56. Ibid., pp. 108–10. See Chapter 8.
57. See Chapter 7.
58. See Chapter 7.
59. Evelyn, *Diary*, 5/1/64, p. 458.
60. Ibid., pp. 300, 412, 487.
61. Ibid., p. 300.
62. Ibid., p. 412.
63. Ibid., p. 487.
64. D. McLaren, 'Fertility, Infant Mortality and Breast Feeding in the Seventeenth Century', *Medical History*, XXII (1978), 378–96.
65. Evelyn, *Diary*, p. 4.
66. Ibid., p. 459.
67. See Chapter 7.
68. Ibid.
69. Josselin, *Diary*, 31/1/46, p. 54, and 19/7/46, p. 64.
70. Evelyn, *Diary*, p. 7.
71. Pepys, *Diary*, I, p. 1.
72. Ibid., V, p. 277.
73. Ibid., VIII, p., 177, Lady Margaret Hoby, also childless, attended one cousin's confinement in November 1601, and another's in February 1602: Hoby, op. cit., pp. 191–2 and 195.
74. Pepys, *Diary*, IX, p. 102.
75. Notably Stone, *The Family, Sex and Marriage*, p. 552.
76. Pepys, *Diary*, I, p. 213.
77. Ibid., p. 276.
78. Ibid., II, p. 98.
79. Ibid., IV, p. 384.
80. Ibid., p. 386.
81. Ibid., p. 384.
82. Ibid., p. 386.
83. Ibid.
84. Ibid., V, p. 87.
85. Ibid., IX, p. 211.
86. Ibid., p. 265.
87. Josselin, *Diary*, 6–14/2/47, p. 86.
88. Hooke, *Diary*, 14/2/78.
89. Pepys, *Diary*, IV, p. 118.
90. Ibid., I, pp. 283–310.
91. Ibid., VII, p. 36.

92. Evelyn, *Diary*, p. 529.
93. Ibid., p. 537.
94. Ibid., p. 722.
95. Ibid., p. 952.
96. Ibid., p. 1119.
97. Ibid., p. 1123.
98. Hooke, *Diary*, p. 156.
99. Pepys, *Diary*, VIII, p. 218.
100. Ibid., IX, p. 136.
101. Hooke, *Diary*, p. 14.
102. Pepys, *Diary*, IV, p. 59.
103. Evelyn, *Diary*, p. 529.
104. Pepys, *Diary*, VI, p. 51.
105. E.g. ibid., II, 10/10/61, p. 194, 3/12/61, p. 226; III, 1/8/62, p. 152.
106. Ibid., VI, p. 51.
107. Ibid., p. 52.
108. Ibid., V, p. 167.
109. Ibid., p. 194.
110. Ibid., p. 241.
111. Ibid., IV, p. 329.
112. Ibid., p. 328.
113. Ibid., p. 333.
114. Ibid., pp. 38–9.
115. Ibid., VI, p. 4.
116. *Diary of Roger Lowe of Ashton-in-Makerfield, Lancashire, 1663–74*, W. L. Sachse, ed., London (1938).
117. Hooke, *Diary*, xiv.
118. Ibid., xv.
119. Ibid., xxvi.
120. See Chapter 6.
121. Evelyn, *Diary*, p. 334; Hooke, *Diary*, pp. 60, 92.
122. Evelyn, *Diary*, p. 388.
123. Ibid., p. 387.
124. Osborne, *Letters*, pp. 70–1.
125. Clifford, *Diary*, p. 73; Osborne, *Letters*, p. 7.
126. Josselin, *Diary*, 6–27/6/52.
127. Evelyn, *Diary*, p. 264.
128. Ibid.
129. See Chapter 7.
130. Hooke, *Diary*, p. 312.
131. Ibid.
132. Ibid., pp. 418–27.

6. SUFFERERS AND PATIENTS: APPROACHES TO ILLNESS

1. See Chapter 2.
2. M. W. Bullen and A. H. Bullen, eds, Early English Text

Society, extra series, LII (1888 and 1875). Also published in 1564 and 1573.
3. Ibid., p. 119.
4. Ibid., p. 120.
5. R. Burton, *The Anatomy of Melancholy*, F. Dell and P. Jordan-Smith, eds, New York (1948), p. 156.
6. Ibid., p. 384.
7. Ibid., p. 385.
8. Pepys, *Diary*, III, p. 10.
9. A. Anderson, London (1593).
10. Ibid.
11. Pepys, *Diary*, VI, p. 120.
12. Ibid., p. 186.
13. Ibid., p. 201.
14. Ibid., p. 233.
15. Ibid., p. 268.
16. Evelyn, *Diary*, p. 481.
17. Ibid., p. 480.
18. Pepys, *Diary*, VI, pp. 155, 163.
19. Ibid., p. 174.
20. Ibid., VII, p. 35.
21. Ibid., VI, pp. 125, 205.
22. Ibid., VII, p. 21.
23. See Chapter 7.
24. Josselin, *Diary*, pp. 180–1.
25. Ibid., p. 201.
26. Ibid., p. 447.
27. Ibid., p. 430.
28. Ibid., p. 407.
29. Lowe, *Diary*, p. 83.
30. *Diary of the Rev. John Ward, A.M., Vicar of Stratford-upon-Avon*, C. Severn, ed., London (1839).
31. Pepys, *Diary*, VI, p. 67.
32. Ibid., IV, p. 339; IX, p. 32.
33. Hooke, *Diary*, p. 307.
34. Sloane MS 153, 105/171.
35. Pepys, *Diary*, IX, p. 197.
36. P. Willughby, *Observations in Midwifery*, H. Blenkinsop, ed., Yorkshire (1972), p. 205.
37. See Chapter 2.
38. Cotta, *A Short Discovery*, Preface.
39. E. Poeton, 'The Winnowing of White Witchcraft', British Library Sloane MS 1954, Introduction.
40. Burton, *Anatomy of Melancholy*, op. cit., p. 383.
41. Ibid.
42. Ibid.
43. Poeton, op. cit., pp. 5, 7.
44. A publication issued at intervals after 1618 with the endorsement of the Royal College of Physicians. It was

designed to keep physicians and apothecaries up to date concerning approved medicines.

45. Thomas, *Religion and Magic*, p. 226.
46. There exists a large body of work on the intellectual history of medicine. Examples of works which shed light on the diversity of educated medical opinion in seventeenth-century England are T. M. Brown, 'The College of Physicians and the Acceptance of Iatromechanism in England, 1665–1695', *Bulletin of the History of Medicine*, XIIV (1970), 12–30; N. G. Coley, 'Cures without Care: "Chemical Physicians" and Mineral Waters in Seventeenth-Century English Medicine', *Medical History*, XXIII, 2 (1979), 191–214; H. L. Coulter, *Divided Legacy: A History of the Schism in Medical Thought*, Washington (1973–7); W. Pagel, *Paracelsus: An Introduction to Philosophical Medicine in the Era of the Renaissance*, Basel and New York (1958); P. Rattansi, 'The Helmontian–Galenist Controversy in Restoration England', *Ambix*, XII (1964), 1–23; O. Temkin, *Galenism: Rise and Decline of a Medical Philosophy*, Ithaca, NY and London (1973); C. Webster, 'Alchemical and Paracelsian Medicine', in C. Webster, ed., *Health, Medicine and Mortality in the Sixteenth Century*, Cambridge (1979), pp. 301–34; C. Webster, *The Great Instauration: Science, Medicine and Reform, 1626–60*, London (1975).
47. Evelyn, *Diary*, p. 1.
48. Ibid., p. 264.
49. Ibid., p. 1.
50. See B. Capp, *Astrology and the Popular Press, English Almanacs, 1500–1800*, London (1979).
51. The diaries of Hoby, Josselin, Pepys, Evelyn and Hooke all give evidence of this practice.
52. Pepys, *Diary*, III, p. 247.
53. Ibid., VI, p. 244.
54. Ibid., IV, p. 333.
55. Hooke, *Diary*, p. 246.
56. Ibid., p. 16.
57. E.g. S. Bradwell, *Helps for Sudden Accidents Endangering Life. By which those that live far from Physicians or Chirurgeons may happily preserve the life of a poor Friend or Neighbour, till such a Man may be had to perfect the cure*, London (1633); *The Englishman's Doctor. Or the School of Salerne*, London (1607); P. Levins, *A Right Profitable Book of all Diseases, called the Path-way to Health . . .* , London (1632); *The Countryman's Physician . . .* , London (1680).
58. See J. O'Hara-May, *Elizabethan Dyetary of Health*, Lawrence, Kan. (1977), for a list of such publications.
59. Slack, 'Mirrors of Health and Treasures of Poor Men: The Uses of the Vernacular Literature of Tudor England', in C. Webster, ed., *Health, Medicine and Mortality*, op. cit., p. 237.
60. Hooke, *Diary*, pp. 15, 28, 173, 317, 331.

61. Hoby, *Diary*, p. 52.
62. Ibid.
63. Josselin, *Diary*, pp. 154, 181.
64. F. Beaumont and J. Fletcher, *Monsieur Thomas*, Act II, scene 3, *The Works of Francis Beaumont and John Fletcher*, A. R. Waller, ed., vol. IV, pp. 116–17, Cambridge (1906).
65. E.g. Josselin, *Diary*, p. 117; Pepys, *Diary*, V, p. 241; Hooke, *Diary*, p. 65.
66. Osborne, *Letters*, p. 8.
67. Pepys, *Diary*, VII, p. 208.
68. Hooke, *Diary*, p. 7.
69. Ibid., p. 280.
70. Ibid., p. 58.
71. Ibid., p. 203.
72. Ibid., p. 52.
73. Ibid., p. 99.
74. Ibid., p. 28.
75. Ibid., p. 172.
76. Hooke, *Diary*, p. 172.
77. Pepys, *Diary*, III, p. 57.
78. Osborne, *Letters*, p. 23.
79. Josselin, *Diary*, p. 207.
80. Pepys, *Diary*, e.g. IV, p. 246; IX, p. 233.
81. Ibid., IV, p. 246.
82. Evelyn, *Diary*, p. 321; Osborne, *Letters*, p. 7; Josselin, *Diary*, p. 586.
83. Evelyn, *Diary*, pp. 300, 304, 319.
84. Pepys, *Diary*, IX, p. 261.
85. British Library Sloane MS 153, 214/424, 278/542.
86. Ibid., 294/567.
87. Evelyn, *Diary*, p. 333.
88. Pepys, *Diary*, III, p. 77.
89. Evelyn, *Diary*, pp. 355–6.
90. Hoby, *Diary*, p. 102.
91. Clifford, *Diary*, xxiii.
92. E.g. Josselin, *Diary*, pp. 186, 566.
93. Ibid., p. 131.
94. See Chapter 7.
95. Pepys, *Diary*, IV, p. 39.
96. Ibid., p. 329.
97. Osborne, *Letters*, p. 40.
98. Hooke, *Diary*, p. 368.
99. Ibid., p. 67.
100. Ibid., p. 17.
101. Ibid., p. 25.
102. See Chapter 7.
103. Josselin, *Diary*, p. 112.
104. E.g. Evelyn, *Diary*, pp. 241, 264–8, 271, 277–8, 301, 319, 333, 335.

105. Ibid., pp. 31, 163, 241.
106. Ibid., pp. 284–5.
107. Ibid., p. 570.
108. Ibid., p. 387.
109. See e.g. Hooke, *Diary*, pp. 4, 163, 240; Pepys, *Diary*, II, p. 17; V, pp. 1–2; IX, p. 522.
110. Pepys, *Diary*, VI, p. 226.
111. Ibid., V, p. 194.
112. Pepys, *Diary*, V, p. 165.
113. Ibid., V, p. 241.
114. Ibid., p. 86.
115. Ibid., p. 84.
116. E.g. ibid., I, pp. 215, 276.
117. Hooke, *Diary*, p. 105.
118. Ibid., pp. 106 and 115.
119. E.g. Hoby, *Diary*, pp. 114, 120, 123, 146.
120. Lowe, *Diary*.
121. E.g. T. Brown, *Physick Lies a Bleeding or the Apothecary Turned Doctor . . .* , London (1697); G. Harvey, *The Conclave of Physicians, Detecting their Intrigues, Frauds and Plots Against their Patients . . .* , London (1683); P. Mexia, *A Delectable Dialogue wherein is contained a Pleasant Disputation between two Spanish Gentlemen, concerning Physick and Physicians with Sentence of a learned master given upon their argument*, T. N., trans., London (1580); *The Skillful Mountebank . . .* , London (1638).
122. See Chapter 2.
123. An extreme example of this tendency is L. R. C. Agnew's 'Quackery', in A. G. Debus, ed., *Medicine in Seventeenth Century England*, Los Angeles (1974), pp. 313–26.
124. Harvey, op. cit., p. 5.
125. Mexia, op. cit. (no pagination).
126. Mexia, op. cit.
127. Harvey, op. cit., pp. 8–9.
128. *All's Well that Ends Well*, Act I, scene 1.
129. *Volpone*, Act I, scene 4: *Ben Jonson*, C. H. Herford and P. Simpson, eds, Oxford (1937), pp. 35–6.
130. Beaumont and Fletcher, *Thierry and Theodoret*, Act I, scene 5, *The Works*, op. cit., vol. X, p. 64.
131. Lacy, *Dumb Lady*, V, quoted in H. Silvette, *The Doctor on Stage: Medicine and Medical Men in Seventeenth-Century England*, Knoxville, Tenn. (1967), p. 128.
132. Chapman, *All Fooles*, Act III, scene 1: *The Plays of George Chapman*, T. M. Parrott, ed., New York (1961), vol. I, pp. 139–40.
133. See Chapter 2.
134. *Macbeth*, Act IV, scene 1.
135. *The Comedy of Errors*, Act V, scene 1.
136. Mexia, op. cit.

7. IN SICKNESS AND IN HEALTH: THE JOSSELINS' EXPERIENCE

1. *The Diary of Ralph Josselin, 1616–1683*, A. Macfarlane, ed., London (1976), hereafter cited as Josselin, *Diary* with dates (unless cited in text) and page references.
2. A. Macfarlane, *The Family Life of Ralph Josselin. A Seventeenth-Century Clergyman: An Essay in Historical Anthropology*, Cambridge (1970).
3. L. Lessius' *Hygiasticon, or the Right Course of Preserving Life and Health unto Extreme Old Age*, London (1634), and D. Sennertus' *Institutionum Medicinae* (many Latin and English eds). See Josselin, *Diary*, 22/1/49 and 9/10/49, pp. 154, 181.
4. See e.g. Stone, *The Family, Sex and Marriage*, pp. 66–7, and R. Schofield and E. A. Wrigley, 'Infant and Child Mortality in England in the late Tudor and early Stuart Period', in C. Webster, ed., *Health, Medicine and Mortality in the Sixteenth Century*, Cambridge (1979), pp. 61–96.
5. See Chapter 5.
6. Macfarlane, *Family Life*, p. 87.
7. E.g. Josselin, *Diary*, 28/12/44, p. 30; 7/10/44, p. 24; 18/7/50, p. 210.
8. Definite mention is made of Jane feeding her first, second, third and sixth babies. The weaning of all the children is noted. Since Josselin would probably have remarked upon the employment of wet-nurses (which he did not), and since conception of the next child usually followed the weaning of the preceding one by a few months, I think it can safely be assumed that Jane fed all of her children herself.
9. Josselin, *Diary*, 18/6/56, p. 371.
10. E.g. Josselin, *Diary*, 3/4/45, p. 37; 24/11/45, p. 50; 5/9/47, p. 102; 5/12/47, p. 108; 30/10/53, p. 313.
11. Ibid., pp. 313 and 315.
12. Ibid., 23/10/53, p. 313.
13. Ibid., 20/3/47, p. 89.
14. See Chapter 2. I deliberately avoid mentioning the notorious forceps of the Chamberlen family, since very few women had the benefit of this family monopoly, and no other surgeons knew about it. See also A. Fraser, *The Weaker Vessel: Woman's Lot in Seventeenth-Century England*, London (1985), pp. 65–88.
15. E. Jocelin, *The Mother's Legacy to her Unborn Child*, New York and London (1894, repr. of 1632 edn) from 'The Approbation'.
16. Josselin, *Diary*, 23/6/57, pp. 402–3.
17. Ibid., 24/11/45, p. 50. See also 29/3/49, p. 162.
18. Ibid., 5/12/47, p. 108.
19. Ibid., 31/1/46, p. 54, and 19/7/46, p. 64.
20. Ibid., 25/8/61, p. 482.
21. See e.g. J. Hitchcock, 'A Sixteenth-Century Midwife's Licence', *Bulletin of the History of Medicine*, XLI (1967), 75–6. These women witnessed the mother's conversation during

labour and could report on statements made concerning the paternity of the child. They could also protect the mother and the midwife from accusations of infanticide in cases of stillbirth. See A. Wilson, 'Participant or Patient? Seventeenth-Century Childbirth from the Mother's Point of View', pp. 129–44, in R. Porter, ed., *Patients and Practitioners: Lay Perceptions of Medicine in Pre-Industrial Society*, Cambridge (1985), for a discussion of the social ritual surrounding birth.
22. Josselin, *Diary*, p. 50.
23. Ibid., 11/2/48, p. 110.
24. E.g. ibid., 7/9/50, p. 215; 21/10/73, p. 570; 4/11/77, p. 604; 27/10/78, p. 615.
25. Ibid., 7/9/50, p. 215.
26. Ibid., 25/11/45, p. 50; 14/1/58, p. 415; 20/6/60, p. 465; 26/11/63, p. 502.
27. Ibid., 11/2/48, p. 110; 5/5/49, p. 165.
28. Ibid., 14/1/58, p. 415.
29. Ibid., 12/4/42, p. 12.
30. Ibid., 24/2/48, p. 115.
31. E.g. ibid., 27/1/50, p. 189; 17/7/46, p. 64; 9/8/58, p. 429; 30/9/55, p. 354.
32. Ibid., 8/7/56, p. 374; 10/8/56, p. 376.
33. Ibid., 18/6/56, p. 371.
34. Ibid., 27/11/72, p. 566.
35. Ibid., 14/11/80, p. 630.
36. Ibid., 7/11/48, p. 145; 27/12/48, p. 150.
37. See Chapter 5.
38. Ibid., 17/2/48, p. 145; 27/12/48, p. 150.
39. Ibid., 20/2/48, p. 113.
40. Ibid., 17/2/48, p. 112.
41. Ibid., 21/2/48, p. 114.
42. Ibid., 25/11/49, p. 184.
43. Ibid., p. 185.
44. Ibid., p. 186.
45. Ibid., p. 190.
46. Ibid.
47. Ibid., p. 192.
48. Ibid., p. 194.
49. Ibid., p. 197.
50. Ibid., p. 200. See also Chapter 5.
51. Ibid., p. 205.
52. Ibid., p. 198.
53. Ibid., p. 200.
54. Ibid., p. 201.
55. Ibid., p. 202.
56. Ibid.
57. Ibid., p. 203.
58. Ibid., p. 212.
59. Ibid. Similar feelings were expressed by John Evelyn when his

5-year-old son, Richard, died in January 1658. See Evelyn, *Diary*, pp. 385–7.
60. Josselin, *Diary*, p. 203.
61. E.g. ibid., 27/10/44, p. 26; 20/12/46, p. 80; 25/11/49, p. 184; 18/2/52, p. 272.
62. Ibid., 23/10/45, p. 48; 14/1/49, p. 152; 28/3/52, p. 275; 23/5/54, p. 508.
63. Ibid., 1/12/44, p. 29; 23/3/45, p. 37; 21/1/55, p. 338.
64. E.g. ibid., 8/12/44, p. 29; 17/7/47, p. 64; 13/1/50, p. 187; 18/2/50, p. 190.
65. Ibid., 21/12/49, p. 186; 20/6/47, p. 97.
66. Ibid., 8/7/49, p. 172.
67. Ibid., 23/3/56, p. 364.
68. Ibid., p. 428.
69. Ibid., 1/8/52, p. 283.
70. Ibid., 11/6/59, p. 447; 18/4/69, p. 546; 10/11/68, p. 545; 3/11/78, p. 615.
71. E.g. ibid., 24/11/44, p. 28; 14/1/55, p. 337.
72. Ibid., 25–8/5/45, pp. 40–1.
73. Ibid., 13/11/44, p. 27.
74. Ibid., 3/2–14/4/61, pp. 475–8.
75. Ibid., 7–19/2/48, pp. 111–13.
76. Ibid., p. 24.
77. Ibid., pp. 113, 156.
78. Ibid., 9/12/60, p. 473.
79. Ibid., p. 433.
80. Ibid., 13/1/69, p. 545.
81. Ibid., p. 565.
82. Ibid., p. 210.
83. Ibid., p. 314.
84. Ibid., p. 330.
85. Ibid., 22/8/60, p. 468.
86. Ibid., p. 113.
87. Ibid., 1/9/54, p. 330.
88. Ibid., 28/12/44, p. 30.
89. Ibid., 27/1/72, p. 566.
90. Other marginal notes refer to such topics as the weather, Josselin's income, religious events, and so on.
91. E.g. ibid., 16/11/45, p. 49; 12/9/47, p. 103; 7/9/48, p. 134; 9/5/50, p. 200.
92. Ibid., p. 63.
93. Ibid., p. 79.
94. Ibid., 21/10/77, p. 603.
95. He took hyssop syrup made by his wife for a cold: 13/10/50, p. 218.
96. See above, this chapter.
97. Ibid., 5/9/47, p. 102.
98. E.g. ibid., 8/12/44, p. 29; 15/6/45, p. 42; 19/3/46, p. 56; 23/5/47, p. 94.

99. E.g. ibid., 2–3/12/46, p. 77; 16/10/46, p. 72; 18/9/47, p. 103.
100. Ibid., 4/2/47, p. 86.
101. Ibid., p. 152.
102. E.g. ibid., 23/9/46, p. 70; 24/12/46, p. 81.
103. Ibid., 6/12/52, p. 290.
104. Ibid., 20/4/46, p. 58.
105. Ibid., 17/12/48, p. 149.
106. Ibid., 10/8/59, p. 450.
107. Ibid., pp. 319, 566.
108. Ibid., 21/3–8/5/55, pp. 342–5.
109. Ibid., 10/5/55, pp. 345–6.
110. Ibid., p. 348.
111. E.g. ibid., 10–11/5/50, p. 200.
112. Ibid., p. 64.
113. Ibid., 7–20/2/48, pp. 111–13.
114. Ibid., pp. 544–6.
115. Ibid., 15/10/48, p. 141, to 18/4/52, p. 277.
116. Ibid., p. 159.
117. Ibid., p. 253.
118. Ibid., 27/11/72, p. 566.
119. Ibid., 26/12/72, p. 566.
120. Ibid.
121. Ibid., 18/2/83, p. 642; 25/2/83, p. 642; 17/3/83, p. 642.
122. Ibid., 15/4/83, p. 643.
123. Ibid., p. 644.
124. Macfarlane, *Family Life*, p. 119.
125. Josselin, *Diary*, p. 567.
126. Ibid.
127. Ibid.
128. Ibid., p. 568.
129. By the end of his life he was also employing a man-servant: ibid., 8/8/80, p. 629.
130. Ibid., 28/4/45, p. 39.
131. Ibid., 6/3/48, p. 118.
132. Ibid., 10/3/50, p. 192.
133. Ibid., 23/1/49, p. 154.
134. Ibid., 4/8/58, p. 429.
135. Ibid., 3/9/44, p. 19.
136. Ibid., p. 62.
137. E.g. ibid., 16/4/47, p. 91; 19/8/48, p. 131; 7/9/50, p. 215; 9/5/52, p. 278.
138. Ibid., p. 18.
139. Ibid., p. 68.
140. Ibid., p. 402.
141. Ibid., 17/3/57, p. 394.
142. Ibid., 19/2/60, p. 460.
143. E.g. ibid., 9/5/52, p. 278; 6/6/52, p. 280; 27/6/52, p. 281; 18/7/52, p. 282.
144. Ibid., 25/2/61, p. 476.

145. Ibid., 18/3/75, p. 583.
146. Ibid., 26/2/53, p. 297.
147. Ibid., 4/8/50, p. 212.
148. Ibid., 27/10/49, p. 183.
149. Ibid., 19/5/51, p. 246.
150. Ibid., 9/8/58, p. 429; 27/9/74, p. 579.
151. Ibid., 28/1/45, p. 33.
152. Ibid., 22/5/65, p. 518.
153. Ibid., 4/3/48, p. 117.
154. Ibid., 28/4/45, p. 39.
155. Ibid., 14/2/48, p. 112.
156. Ibid., p. 76.
157. Ibid., 23/5/47, p. 94; 7/5/50, p. 200; 20–7/6/52, p. 281.
158. Ibid., 27/10/50, p. 219.
159. Ibid., 20–1/12/49, p. 186.
160. Ibid., 31/5/46, p. 61, and 13/10/50, p. 218.
161. E.g. ibid., 13/10/50, p. 218; 9/12/57, p. 412; 25/4/75, p. 584; 4/11/77, p. 604; 21/10/73, p. 570.
162. E.g. ibid., 27/1/50, p. 189; 23/5/64, p. 508.
163. Ibid., p. 595.
164. Ibid., p. 91.
165. Ibid., p. 131.
166. Ibid., p. 64.
167. Ibid., 5/9/44, p. 19.
168. Ibid., 17–18/3/45, p. 36; 14/2/48, p. 112; 26/11/48, pp. 147–8.
169. Ibid., 1/3/50, p. 191; 15/6/59, p. 447.
170. Stibium is black antimony, used as an emetic or poison: *Oxford English Dictionary*.
171. Josselin, *Diary*, 18/5/75, p. 584; 16/3/83, p. 642; 4/5/83, p. 643.
172. Ibid., 7/6/75, p. 585.
173. Ibid., 17/5/75, p. 584; 18/6/76, p. 591; 27/6/80, p. 628; 25/7/80, p. 629; 19/9/80, p. 630.
174. Ibid., 13/10/78, p. 615; 14/5/83, p. 644; 20/5/83, p. 644.
175. See Chapter 6.
176. Josselin, *Diary*, 22/5/50, p. 202.
177. Ibid., 23/6/50, p. 207.
178. Ibid., 4/5/83, p. 643.
179. Ibid., 8/5/83, p. 643.
180. Ibid., p. 64.
181. Ibid., 24/12/46, p. 81.
182. Ibid., 28/5/45, p. 41; 21/12/49, p. 186; 27/1/73, p. 566.
183. Ibid., p. 566.
184. Ibid., 22/5/50, p. 212.
185. Ibid., p. 111.
186. Ibid., 4/8/50, p. 212.
187. Ibid., 27–9/11/53, p. 314.
188. Ibid., 22/8/60, p. 460.
189. See above, this chapter.

190. Josselin, *Diary*, 5/5/49, p. 165.
191. Ibid., 21/12/45, p. 51; 28/2/48, p. 116.
192. Ibid., 1/2/58, p. 418.
193. Ibid., 17/2/48, p. 112.
194. Ibid., 2/8/43, p. 14.
195. Ibid., 7/6/75, p. 585; 15/4–4/5/83, p. 643.
196. Ibid., 29/10/76, p. 594; 20/11/76, p. 595; 17/9/78, p. 614.
197. Ibid., 4/5/83, p. 643.
198. Ibid., 1–19/8/64, pp. 510–11.
199. Macfarlane, *Family Life*, pp. 174–6.
200. Josselin, *Diary*, 23/2/48, p. 114.
201. Macfarlane, *Family Life*, pp. 174–6.
202. Josselin, *Diary*, 23/2/48, p. 114.
203. Ibid., p. 121.
204. Ibid., 8/7/56, p. 374.
205. E.g. ibid., 21/11/54, p. 333; 30/9/57, p. 407; 27/3/65, p. 516.
206. Ibid., 15/8/47, p. 101.
207. Ibid., p. 15.
208. Macfarlane, *Family Life*, pp. 28–9.
209. Josselin, *Diary*, 19 and 26/6/59, p. 447.
210. E.g. ibid., 27/5/49, pp. 168–9.
211. Ibid., p. 198.
212. Ibid., p. 71.
213. Ibid., p. 204.
214. E.g. ibid., 5/1/51, p. 230; 16/3/51, p. 238; 4/2/55, p. 339.
215. Ibid., p. 520–1.
216. See K. Dewhurst, *Dr. Thomas Sydenham (1624–1689), His Life and Original Writings*, London (1966), pp. 105–14.
217. Josselin, *Diary*, 15/8/47, p. 101.
218. Ibid., 3/11/67, p. 538.
219. E.g. ibid., 2/9/49, p. 178; 16/3/51, p. 238; 26/6/53, p. 307.
220. Ibid., 4/12/45, p. 51.
221. Ibid., 14/11/51, p. 262.
222. Ibid., 31/7/73, p. 568; 27–8/5/50, pp. 203–4.
223. Stone, *The Family, Sex and Marriage*, p. 70. See L. Pollock, *Forgotten Children*, Cambridge (1983) for further development of this argument.
224. Ibid., pp. 67, 69, 71.

8. THE CHARACTER OF A GOOD WOMAN: WOMEN AND ILLNESS

1. J. Hoch-Smith and A. Spring, 'Introduction' in J. Hoch-Smith and A. Spring, eds, *Women in Ritual and Symbolic Roles*, London (1978), p. 20.
2. Morningside Heights, NY (1943).
3. Ibid., p. 62.

4. K. C. Hurd-Mead, *A History of Women in Medicine*, Haddam, Conn. (1938).
5. A. Clark, *Working Life of Women in the Seventeenth Century*, London (1919), p. 285. For critiques of Clark's seminal theory, see J. Thirsk, 'Foreword', in M. Prior, ed., *Women in English Society 1500–1800*, London (1985), pp. 8–12, and L. Charles, 'Introduction', in L. Charles and L. Duffin, eds, *Women and Work in Pre-Industrial England*, London (1985), pp. 1–23.
6. S. Young, *The Annals of the Barber-Surgeons of London*, London (1890), p. 260.
7. A. Clark, op. cit., p. 260.
8. V. L. Bullough, 'Medieval Medical and Scientific Views of Women', *Viator*, 4, (1973), 499.
9. I. Maclean, *The Renaissance Notion of Woman: A Study in the Fortunes of Scholasticism and Medical Science in European Intellectual Life*, Cambridge (1980), p. 30.
10. P. Crawford, 'Attitudes to Menstruation in Seventeenth-Century England', *Past and Present*, 91 (1981), 59.
11. Ibid., 61.
12. *The Woman's Doctor or an Exact and Distinct Explanation of all such Diseases as are Peculiar to that Sex*, London (1652), p. 4.
13. V. L. Bullough, op. cit., 495.
14. M. Summers, ed., London (1928 and 1971).
15. Ibid., Question VI, 'Contents'.
16. Ibid., Question IX, 'Contents'.
17. B. Ehrenreich and D. English, *Witches, Midwives and Nurses: A History of Women Healers*, Oyster Bay, NY (n.d.).
18. I. Maclean, op. cit., p. 46.
19. *Character of a Good Woman*, London (1697), pp. 42–3. Italics in original.
20. See Chapters 2 and 4.
21. Quoted from R. Thompson, *Women in Stuart England and America*, London (1974), p. 208.
22. Quoted in the *Diary of Lady Margaret Hoby*, D. M. Meads, ed., London (1930), p. 50, hereafter referred to as Hoby, *Diary*.
23. Ibid., p. 53.
24. See Chapter 2.
25. See Chapter 4.
26. A. Clark, op. cit., pp. 243–52.
27. See Chapter 2.
28. See Chapter 7.
29. Hoby, *Diary*, p. 5. See also A. Fraser, *The Weaker Vessel: Woman's Lot in Seventeenth-Century England*, London (1985), pp. 502–3.
30. Hoby, *Diary*, pp. 8–11.
31. Ibid., pp. 12–28.
32. Ibid., p. 29.
33. Ibid., pp. 30–1.

34. Ibid., pp. 39, 43.
35. Ibid., pp. 168, 170, 180.
36. Ibid., p. 100.
37. Ibid., p. 96.
38. Ibid., p. 72.
39. E.g., ibid., pp. 102–5, 108–12.
40. Ibid., p. 193.
41. Ibid., p. 220.
42. E.g. ibid., pp. 167, 169, 189.
43. Ibid., p. 160.
44. Ibid., pp. 67, 106, 146, 161, 171, 174, 186.
45. Ibid., pp. 165, 179.
46. Ibid., pp. 103, 107, 159, 201, 220.
47. Ibid., p. 68.
48. Ibid., pp. 72, 220.
49. Ibid., p. 106.
50. Ibid., pp. 113–15.
51. Ibid., p. 73.
52. Ibid., p. 68.
53. E.g. ibid., pp. 147, 153, 155.
54. Ibid., p. 147.
55. Ibid., p. 157.
56. Ibid., p. 159.
57. Ibid. Mrs Thornborowe was the wife of the Dean of York.
58. Ibid., p. 147.
59. E.g. ibid., pp. 162, 181, 191–2.
60. Ibid., p. 100.
61. Ibid., pp. 101–3.
62. Ibid., pp. 168–70.
63. Ibid., pp. 145, 168.
64. See Chapter 2.
65. Hoby, *Diary*, pp. 131, 134.
66. Ibid., pp. 63, 191–2, 195.
67. *The Autobiography of Mrs. Alice Thornton of East Newton, Co. York*, C. Jackson, ed., Surtees Society, vol. 62 (1875), p. vii, hereafter referred to as *Thornton*. See also A. Fraser, op. cit., pp. 83–4, 86, 88, 108, 143, 150, 154, 169, 504.
68. *Thornton*, p. 43.
69. Ibid., p. viii.
70. Ibid., pp. 78–9.
71. Ibid., p. 75.
72. Ibid., pp. 78–9.
73. Ibid., p. 83.
74. Ibid., pp. xi–xii.
75. It has already served as an important source of information on breast-feeding and child mortality. See D. McLaren, 'Fertility, Infant Mortality and Breast Feeding in the Seventeenth Century', *Medical History*, XXII (1978), 378–96.
76. *Thornton*, p. 3.

77. Ibid., p. 129.
78. Ibid.
79. Ibid., p. 91.
80. Ibid., pp. 139–42.
81. Ibid., pp. 5–6.
82. John Evelyn's physician told him that, had he not been bled in the early stages of smallpox, his disease might have turned to plague or spotted fever.
83. *Thornton*, p. 91.
84. Ibid., pp. 128–9.
85. Ibid., p. 6.
86. Ibid., pp. 33–4.
87. Ibid., pp. 34–5.
88. See P. Aries, *The Hour of our Death*, H. Weaver, trans., London (1981) for lengthy discussion of the good death and changes in conventions over time.
89. *Thornton*, p. 124.
90. Ibid., p. 166.
91. Ibid., pp. 157–9.
92. Ibid.,p. 4.
93. Ibid.,p. 11.
94. Ibid., p. 133.
95. Ibid., pp. 129–30.
96. See Chapter 6.
97. *Thornton*, p. 164.
98. Ibid., p. 65.
99. Ibid., p. 273.
100. Ibid., p. 95.
101. Ibid., p. 139.
102. Stone, *The Family, Sex and Marriage*, pp. 74–5, 114; D. McLaren, op. cit.
103. *Thornton*, p. 87.
104. Ibid., p. 94.
105. Ibid., pp. 96, 123–4.
106. Ibid., pp. 139–42, 145, 148, 150–1, 166.
107. Ibid., p. 98.
108. Ibid., pp. 84–8.
109. Ibid., p. 140.
110. Ibid., p. 126.
111. Ibid., p. 95.
112. Ibid., pp. 92, 141.
113. Ibid., pp. 96–7.
114. Ibid., pp. 51–3.
115. Ibid., pp. 144–8.
116. Ibid., pp. 164–5.
117. See Chapter 7.
118. *Thornton*, pp. 13, 39–42, 54, 98, 149, 165, 172–5.
119. Ibid., pp. 5–6, 54, 151.
120. Ibid., pp. 81, 52, 157, 149, 173.

121. Ibid., p. 235.
122. Ibid., pp. 39, 81, 87, 157, 172–5, 223.
123. Ibid., pp. 93, 158, 164.
124. Ibid., p. 23.
125. Ibid., pp. 4, 10–11, 33–5.
126. Ibid., pp. 124, 133.
127. Ibid., p. 130.
128. Macfarlane, *Family Life*, pp. 172–7.
129. *Thornton*, pp. 9, 28–32, 48–9, 133, 144, 151, 157.
130. Ibid., p. 159.
131. P. White sees the main difference as being Puritans' 'rigid predestinarian doctrines' – an issue which does not arise in medical matters. See 'The Rise of Arminianism Reconsidered', *Past and Present*, 101 (1983), 34–54. For a discussion of 'Puritan Perceptions of Illness in Seventeenth Century England', see A. Wear, in R. Porter, ed., *Patients and Practitioners: Lay Perceptions of Medicine in Pre-Industrial Society*, Cambridge (1985), pp. 55–100.
132. Hoby, *Diary*, p. 54.
133. *The Autobiography of Anne Lady Halkett*, J. G. Nichols, ed., Camden Society, new series, 13 (1875), hereafter referred to as *Halkett*. See also A. Fraser, op. cit., pp. 68–9, 162–3, 211–13.
134. *Halkett*, pp. 62–3.
135. Ibid., pp. 82, 32–3.
136. Ibid., pp. 32–3, 36, 65, 87.
137. Ibid., pp. 104–5.

9. CONCLUSION: THE EXPERIENCE OF ILLNESS

1. See Chapter 3.
2. See Chapter 7.
3. Pepys, *Diary*, VI, p. 67.
4. Ibid., V, p. 78.
5. See Chapter 5.
6. See D. Mechanic, *Medical Sociology: A Selective View*, London and New York (1968), p. 116.
7. See Chapter 7.
8. Lowe, *Diary*, pp. 19, 100, 109.
9. Hooke, *Diary*, pp. 311–12.
10. Pepys, *Diary*, VI, p. 174.
11. Ibid., III, p. 65.
12. E.g. P. Laslett, *The World We have Lost*, London (1971).
13. See Chapter 7.
14. Pepys, *Diary*, I, p. 187.
15. See e.g. Chapter 3.
16. See Chapter 3.
17. See Chapter 7.
18. See Chapter 6.
19. See Chapter 2.

20. See e.g. Sloane MS 153, 37/76.
21. See Chapter 6.
22. See Chapter 7.
23. See M. Spufford, *Contrasting Communities: English Villages in the Sixteenth and Seventeenth Centuries*, Cambridge (1974 and 1979), p. 322.
24. E.g. Chapter 7; also Evelyn, *Diary*, p. 1023.
25. See Chapter 7.
26. Evelyn, *Diary*, pp. 8–9.
27. Ibid., pp. 14–16.
28. See Chapter 6.
29. Osborne, *Letters*, p. 10.
30. Pepys, *Diary*, I, p. 5.
31. Ibid., p. 36.
32. E.g. ibid., VII, pp. 49, 329–30.
33. Ibid., VI, p. 55; IX, p. 265.
34. Evelyn, *Diary*, p. 8.
35. Pepys, *Diary*, V, pp. 78–86.
36. Hooke, *Diary*, p. 13.
37. Ibid., p. 160.
38. E.g. Pepys, *Diary*, I, p. 5; IV, p. 24; V, p. 136.
39. E.g. ibid., IX, p. 264.
40. Ibid., V, p. 40.
41. Ibid., I, p. 15.
42. Ibid., II, p. 200.
43. See Chapters 5 and 6.
44. Pepys, *Diary*, IX, p. 546.
45. Hooke, *Diary*, p. 44.
46. Josselin, *Diary*, p. 204.
47. See below, this chapter.
48. Evelyn, *Diary*, p. 263.
49. Clifford, *Diary*, p. 87.
50. Pepys, *Diary*, IV, pp. 38–9.
51. Ibid., V, p. 280. See also Pelling, 'Appearance and Reality'
52. See Chapter 3.
53. See Chapters 3, 5 and 6.
54. T. Shadwell, *The Humorists*, Act I, scene 1, *The Complete Works of Thomas Shadwell*, M. Summers, ed., vol. I, p. 193, London (1968 and 1927).
55. Shadwell, *Bury Fair*, Act III: *The Complete Works*, op. cit., IV, p. 337.
56. F. Beaumont and J. Fletcher, *Humourous Lieutenant*, Act I, scene 1, *The Works of Francis Beaumont and John Fletcher*, A. R. Waller, ed., vol. II, pp. 291–2, Cambridge (1906).
57. See Chapter 6.
58. Pepys, *Diary*, VIII, p. 219.
59. Ibid., VIII, p. 435.
60. *Aubrey's Brief Lives*, O. L. Dick, ed., Harmondsworth (1972), pp. 414–15.

61. See Chapter 7.
62. See P. Slack, 'Metropolitan Government in Crisis: London's Response to Plague, 1563–1665', in A. L. Beier and R. Finlay, eds, *The Making of the Metropolis: London 1500–1700*, London (1986), pp. 65–7.
63. J. F. D. Shrewsbury, *A History of Bubonic Plague in the British Isles*, Cambridge (1971), p. 269.
64. Quoted in ibid., p. 446.
65. Slack, 'Metropolitan Government', p. 67.
66. Shrewsbury, op. cit., p. 476.
67. Ibid., p. 450.
68. Ibid., p. 479.
69. Pepys, *Diary*, VI, p. 181.
70. Ibid., VII, p. 116.
71. Ibid., VI, p. 212.
72. Ibid., p. 283.
73. Slack, 'Metropolitan Government', p. 73.
74. Pepys, *Diary*, VII, p. 41.
75. For a description of social unrest in a plague-stricken Italian village, see C. M. Cipolla, *Faith, Reason and the Plague: A Tuscan Story of the Seventeenth Century*, Brighton (1979).
76. Shrewsbury, op. cit., pp. 464, 480.
77. Roberts, thesis, p. 358.
78. See Chapter 2.
79. See Roberts, thesis.
80. See Chapter 2.
81. See e.g. F. N. L. Poynter and W. J. Bishop, eds, 'A Seventeenth-Century Doctor and his Patients: John Symcotts, 1592?–1662', *Bedfordshire Historical Record Society*, vol. 31, Streatley, Beds (1950), xx–xxi; *Diary of the Rev. John Ward, A.M., Vicar of Stratford-upon-Avon*, C. Severn, ed., London (1839).
82. See Chapter 2.
83. Thackeray, *History of Pendennis*, II, New York (1968), pp. 174–5.
84. See Chapter 5.
85. Pepys, *Diary*, I, p. 244.
86. See Clark, *Royal College*; Young, *Barber-Surgeons*; Roberts, thesis.
87. See Chapter 2.
88. P. Aries, *The Hour of our Death*, H. Weaver, trans., London (1981).

BIBLIOGRAPHY

MANUSCRIPT SOURCES

Barker, Dr, 'Observations on cases in physick, 1595–1605', British Library Sloane MS 78 or 663.

Binns, J., 'Surgical Casebook, 1633–1663', British Library Sloane MS 153.

'The casebook of a provincial physician, 1619–1622', British Library Sloane MS 1112.

Guildhall Library, London, MS 5625/1 fo. 89.

King, Sir Edmund, 'Casebook, 1676–1696', British Library Sloane MS 1589.

Mayerne, Sir Theodore Turquet de, Casebook, Library of the Royal College of Physicians, MS 444.

Poeton, E., 'Medical Treatises', including 'The Winnowing of White Witchcraft', British Library Sloane MS 1954.

Public Record Office, PCC 1664, 47, 52: Joseph Binns's wills.

SIXTEENTH- AND SEVENTEENTH-CENTURY WORKS

Anderson, A., *An Approved Medicine Against the Deserved Plague*, London (1593).

Andrewes, L., *A Sermon of the Pestilence*, London (1636).

Arcaeus, F., *A Most Excellent and Compendious Method of Curing Wounds in the Head, and in Other Parts of the Body . . .* , J. Read, trans., London (1588).

Aubrey's Brief Lives, O. L. Dick, ed., Harmondsworth (1972).

The Autobiography and Personal Diary of Simon Forman the Celebrated Astronomer from A.D. 1552 to A.D. 1602, J. O. Halliwell, ed., London: for private circulation only (1849).

The Autobiography of Anne Lady Halkett, J. G. Nichols, ed., Camden Society, new series, 13 (1875).

The Autobiography of Mrs. Alice Thornton of East Newton, Co. York, C. Jackson, ed., Surtees Society, vol. 62 (1875).

Barrough, P., *The Method of Physick . . .* , London (1583).

Beaumont, F., *The Woman Hater*, London (1648).

Beaumont, F. and J. Fletcher, *Humourous Lieutenant*, in *The Works of*

Francis Beaumont and John Fletcher, A. R. Waller, ed., vol. II, Cambridge (1906).
Beaumont, F. and J. Fletcher, *Monsieur Thomas,* in *The Works of Francis Beaumont and John Fletcher*, A. R. Waller, ed., vol. IV, Cambridge (1906).
Beaumont, F. and J. Fletcher, *Thierry and Theodoret,* in *The Works of Francis Beaumont and J. Fletcher*, A. R. Waller, ed., vol. X, Cambridge (1906).
Beaumont, F. and J. Fletcher, *Knight of the Burning Pestle,* in *The Dramatic Works in the Beaumont and Fletcher Canon*, F. Bowers, ed., vol. I, Cambridge (1966).
Blake, W., *The Trial of the Ladies*, Hyde Park (1656).
Blunt, J., *Man-midwifery Dissected: or the Obstetric Family-Instructor*, London (1793).
Boorde, A., *The Breviary of Health*, London (1587).
Bradwell, S., *Helps for Sudden Accidents Endangering Life* . . . , London (1633).
Brain, T., *The Piss-Prophet, or Certain Piss-Pot Lectures* . . . , London (1637).
A Brief Account of Mr. Valentine Greatraks, London (1666 and 1668).
A Brief Anatomy of Women: Being an Invective, London (1653).
A Brief Description of the Notorious Life of J. Lambe, Amsterdam and London (1628).
Brown, T., *Physick Lies a Bleeding or the Apothecary Turned Doctor* . . . , London (1697).
Brugis, T., *The Marrow of Physick* . . . , London (1640).
Brugis, T., *Vade Mecum: or, a Companion for a Surgeon*, London (1652).
Bullein, W., *A Dialogue against the Fever Pestilence*, M. W. Bullen and A. H. Bullen, eds, Early English Text Society, extra series, LII (1888 and 1975). Also published in 1564 and 1573.
Burton, R., *The Anatomy of Melancholy*, F. Dell and P. Jordan-Smith, eds, New York (1948, first published 1621).
Cellier, E., 'Petition . . .', *Harleian Miscellany*, vol. IV, London (1744).
Chapman, G., *All Fooles,* in *The Plays of George Chapman*, T. M. Parrott, ed., vol. I, New York (1961).
Character of a Good Woman, London (1697).
The Character of a Quack-Doctor, London (1676).
Cooke, J., *Mellificium Chirurgerie. Or the Marrow* . . . , London (1648).
Cotta, J., *Cotta Contra Antonium* . . . , Oxford (1625).
Cotta, J., *The Infallible True and Assured Witch*, 2nd edn, London (1624).
Cotta, J., *A Short Discovery of the Unobserved Dangers of Several Sorts of Ignorant and Unconsiderate Practisers of Physic in England*, London (1612).
The Countryman's Physician . . . , London (1680).
Cox, Dr, *A Discourse Wherein the Interest of the Patient in Reference to*

Physick and Physicians is Soberly Debated . . . , London (1699).
Culpeper, N., *A Directory for Midwives*, London (1651).
D. E., *The Copy of a Letter Written by E. D., Doctor of Physick, to a Gentleman . . .* , London (1606).
A Description of Wanton Women, (1690?).
The Diary of John Dee, J. O. Halliwell, ed., *Camden Society*, XIX (1847).
The Diary of John Evelyn, E. S. de Beer, ed., London (1959).
Diary of Lady Margaret Hoby, 1599–1605, D. M. Meads, ed., London (1930).
The Diary of Ralph Josselin, 1616–1683, A. Macfarlane, ed., Oxford (1976).
The Diary of Robert Hooke, 1672–1680, H. W. Robinson and W. Adams, eds, London (1968 and 1935).
Diary of Roger Lowe of Ashton-in-Makerfield, Lancashire, 1663–74, W. L. Sachse, ed., London (1938).
The Diary of Samuel Pepys, R. Latham and W. Matthews, eds, vols I–IX, London (1970–82).
The Diary of the Lady Anne Clifford with an introductory note by V. Sackville-West, London (1923).
Diary of the Rev. John Ward, A.M., Vicar of Stratford-upon-Avon, C. Severn, ed., London (1839).
Digby, Sir Kenelm, *Of the Sympathetic Powder*, London (1669).
The Englishman's Doctor. Or the School of Salerne, London (1607).
An Essay for the Regulation of the Practice of Physick . . . , London (1673).
Fabrice, G., *His Experiments in Chyrurgerie*, London (1642).
Fioravanti, L., *A Short Discourse of the Excellent Doctor . . .* , J. Hester, trans., London (1580).
Folkingham, W., *Panala Medica . . .* , London (1628).
Forestus, P., *The Arraignment of Urines . . .* , J. Hart, trans., London (1623).
Gale, T., *Certain Works of Chirurgerie*, London (1564).
Gifford, G., *A Discourse of the Subtle Practices of Devils by Witches and Sorcerers*, London (1587).
Goeurot, J., *The Regiment of Life . . .* , T. Phayer, trans., London (1544).
Goodall, C., *The Royal College of Physicians of London . . .* , London (1684).
Graunt, J., *Natural and Political Observations Made Upon the Bills of Mortality*, P. Laslett, ed., *The Earliest Classics*, Gregg International (1973, first edn 1662).
The Great Cures and Strange Miracles of Mr. Valentine Gertrux [sic], n.p. (1666).
Guillemeau, J., *Childbirth . . .* , London (1635).
Halle, J., 'An Historical Expostulation . . .', in Lanfranc of Milan, *A Most Excellent and Learned Work of Chirurgery . . .* , J. Halle, trans., London (1565).
Hart, J., *The Anatomy of Urines . . .* , London (1624).

Hart, J., *KλINIKH, or the Diet of the Diseased*, London (1633).
Harvey, G., *The Conclave of Physicians, Detecting their Intrigues, Frauds and Plots Against their Patients . . .* , London (1683).
Hereafter Followeth the Judgement of all Urines . . . , London (? early sixteenth century).
Here Beginneth the Seeing of Urines . . . , London (1525 and 1526).
Herring, F., *A Short Discourse of Discovery of Certain Stratagems, Whereby our London Empericks have been Observed Strongly to Oppugne, and oft times to Expugne their Poore Patient's Purses*, London (1602).
Hobbes, T., *Leviathan*, London (1973).
An Invective Against the Pride of Women, [London (1657)].
Joceline, E., *The Mother's Legacy to her Unborn Child*, New York and London (1894, repr. of 1632 edn).
Jonson, B., *Volpone*, in *Ben Jonson*, C. H. Herford and P. Simpson, eds, Oxford (1937).
Jorden, E., *A Brief Discourse of a Disease called the Suffocation of the Mother*, London (1603).
Lanfranc of Milan, *A Most Excellent and Learned Work of Chirurgerie*, J. Halle, trans., London (1565).
Lessius, L., *Hygiasticon, or the Right Course of Preserving Life and Health unto Extreme Old Age*, London (1634).
A Letter Concerning the Present State of Physick . . . , London (1665).
The Letters of Dorothy Osborne to William Temple, G. C. Moore Smith, ed., Oxford (1928).
Levins, P., *A Right Profitable Book of all Diseases, called the Pathway to Health . . .* , London (1632).
Magnus, A., *Secrets of the Vertues of Herbes*, London (1549).
[Merrett, C.], *A Short View of the Frauds . . .* , London (1669).
Mexia, P., *A Delectable Dialogue . . .* , T. N., trans., London (1580).
Oberndoerffer, J., *The Anatomies of the True Physician and Counterfeit Mountebank . . .* , F. H[erring], trans., London (1602).
Parker, M., *The Tragedy of Doctor Lambe*, London (1628).
Roesslin, E., *The Byrth of Mankynde*, R. Jonas, trans., London (1540).
Rueff, J., *The Expert Midwife*, London (1637).
Securis, J., *A Detection and Querimonie of the Daily Enormities and Abuses Committed in Physick . . .* , London (1566).
Sennertus, D., *Institutionum Medicinae* (many Latin and English editions, mid-seventeenth century).
Shadwell, T., *The Humorists*, in *The Complete Works of Thomas Shadwell*, M. Summers, ed., vol. I, London (1968 and 1927).
Shadwell, T., *Bury Fair*, in *The Complete Works of Thomas Shadwell*, M. Summers, ed., vol. IV, London (1968 and 1927).
Shakespeare, W., *The Comedy of Errors* (1592–3).
Shakespeare, W., *All's Well that Ends Well* (1602–3).
Shakespeare, W., *Macbeth* (1605–6).
Sharp, J., *The Midwives Book*, London (1671).

The Skillful Mountebank . . . , London (1638).
[Swetnam, J.], *The Arraignment of Lewd, Idle . . . Women*, London (1645).
Sydenham, T., *Works*, vol. II, Dr Greenhill, trans., London (1848).
Valentinus, P. P., *Enchiridion Medicum: Containing an Epitome of the Whole Course of Physic . . .* , London (1608).
Vicary, T., *The Anatomie of the Bodie of Man*, F. J. and P. Furnivall, eds, Early English Text Society, extra series, LIII (1888 and 1975).
Willughby, P., *Observations in Midwifery*, H. Blenkinsop, ed., Yorkshire (1972).
The Woman's Doctor or an Exact and Distinct Explanation of all such Diseases as are Peculiar to that Sex, London (1652).
Woodall, J., *The Surgeon's Mate . . .* , London (1655, numerous earlier edns, first published 1617).

SECONDARY SOURCES

Ackerknecht, E. H., *A Short History of Medicine*, New York (1955).
Agnew, L. R. C., 'Quackery', in A. G. Debus, ed., *Medicine in Seventeenth-Century England*, Los Angeles (1974), pp. 313–26.
Allderidge, P., 'Management and Mismanagement at Bedlam, 1547–1633', in C. Webster, ed., *Health, Medicine and Mortality in the Sixteenth Century*, Cambridge (1979), pp. 141–64.
Allen, P., 'Medical Education in Seventeenth-Century England', *Journal of the History of Medicine*, I (1946), 115–43.
Aries, P., *The Hour of our Death*, H. Weaver, trans., London (1981).
Aveling, J. H., *English Midwives: their History and Prospects*, London (1872).
Aveling, J. H., *The Chamberlens and the Midwifery Forceps*, London (1882).
Beier, A. L., *Masterless Men: The Vagrancy Problem in England, 1560–1640*, London (1985).
Beier, A. L. and R. Finlay, *The Making of the Metropolis: London 1500–1700*, London (1986).
Berlant, J. L., *Profession and Monopoly: A Study of Medicine in the United States and Great Britain*, Los Angeles (1975).
Bishop, W. J., *The Early History of Surgery*, London (1961).
Bloch, M., *The Royal Touch: Sacred Monarchy and Scrofula in England and France*, J. E. Anderson, trans., London (1973).
Boss, J., 'The Medical Philosophy of Francis Bacon (1561–1626)', *Med. Hypotheses*, IV (1978), 208–20.
Brown, T. M., 'The College of Physicians and the Acceptance of Iatromechanism in England, 1665–1695', *Bulletin of the History of Medicine*, XLIV (1970), 12–30.
Bruce-Chwatt, L. J. and J. de Zulueta, *The Rise and Fall of Malaria in Europe: A Historico-Epidemiological Study*, Oxford (1980).
Bullough, V. L., *The Development of Medicine as a Profession*, Basel and New York (1966).

Bullough, V. L., 'Medieval Medical and Scientific Views of Women', *Viator*, 4 (1973).

Capp, B., *Astrology and the Popular Press: English Almanacs, 1500–1800*, London (1979).

Charles, L. and L. Duffin, eds, *Women and Work in Pre-Industrial England*, London (1985).

Cipolla, C. M., *Faith, Reason and the Plague: A Tuscan Story of the Seventeenth Century*, Brighton (1979).

Clark, A., *Working Life of Women in the Seventeenth Century*, London (1919).

Clark, G. N., *A History of the Royal College of Physicians of London*, vols I and II, Oxford (1964).

Coley, N. G., 'Cures without Care: "Chemical Physicians" and Mineral Waters in Seventeenth-Century English Medicine', *Medical History*, XXIII, 2 (1979), 191–214.

Cope, Z., *The Royal College of Surgeons of England*, London (1959).

Copeman, W. S. C., *Doctors and Disease in Tudor England*, London (1960).

Coulter, H. L., *Divided Legacy: A History of the Schism in Medical Thought*, Washington (1973–7).

Crawford, P., 'Attitudes to Menstruation in Seventeenth-Century England', *Past and Present*, 91 (1981).

Creighton, C., *A History of Epidemics in Britain*, Cambridge (1894 and 1965).

D., W., 'Midwives Formerly Baptised Infants', *Gentleman's Magazine*, LV, 2 (1785).

Dainton, C., *The Story of England's Hospitals*, London (1961).

Debus, A. G., *The English Paracelsians*, New York (1966).

Debus, A. G., ed., *Medicine in Seventeenth-Century England*, Los Angeles (1974).

Dewhurst, K., *Thomas Willis as a Physician*, Los Angeles (1964).

Dewhurst, K., *Dr. Thomas Sydenham (1624–1689). His Life and Original Writings*, London (1966).

Dickens, C., *Martin Chuzzlewit*, London (1843–4).

Dingwall, R. and P. Lewis, eds, *The Sociology of the Professions: Lawyers, Doctors and Others*, London and Basingstoke (1983).

Donnison, J., *Midwives and Medical Men: A History of Inter-Professional Rivalries and Women's Rights*, London (1977).

Eccles, A., *Obstetrics and Gynaecology in Tudor and Stuart England*, London (1982).

Ehrenreich, B., and D. English, *Witches, Midwives and Nurses: A History of Women Healers*, Oyster Bay, NY (n.d.).

Forbes, T. R., *The Midwife and the Witch*, London (1966).

Forbes, T. R., *Chronicle from Aldgate: Life and Death in Shakespeare's London*, London (1971).

Fraser, A., *The Weaker Vessel: Woman's Lot in Seventeenth-Century England*, London (1985).

Freidson, E., *Profession of Medicine: A Study of the Sociology of Applied Knowledge*, New York (1972).

Freidson, E., 'The Theory of Professions: State of the Art', in R. Dingwall and P. Lewis, eds, *The Sociology of the Professions: Lawyers, Doctors and Others*, London and Basingstoke (1983), pp. 19–37.
Gittings, C., *Death, Burial and the Individual in Early Modern England*, London (1984).
Guthrie, D., *A History of Medicine*, London (1945 and 1946).
Haggard, H. M., *Devils, Drugs and Doctors: The Story of the Science of Healing from Medicine Man to Doctor*, London (1929).
Harleian Miscellany, IV, London (1744).
Hitchcock, J., 'A Sixteenth-Century Midwife's Licence', *Bulletin of the History of Medicine*, XLI (1967), 75–6.
Hoch-Smith, J., and A. Spring, eds, *Women in Ritual and Symbolic Roles*, London (1978).
Holmes, G., *Augustan England: Professions, State and Society, 1680–1730*, London (1982).
Hughes, M. J., *Women Healers in Medieval Life and Literature*, Morningside Heights, NY (1943).
Hurd-Mead, K. C., *A History of Women in Medicine*, Haddam, Conn. (1938).
Keynes, G., *Dr. Timothy Bright, 1550–1615: A Survey of his Life with a Bibliography of his Writings*, London (1962).
Keynes, G., *The Life of William Harvey*, Oxford (1966).
King, L. S., *The Growth of Medical Thought*, Chicago (1963).
King, L. S., ed., *A History of Medicine: Selected Readings*, Harmondsworth (1971).
Landy, D., ed., *Culture, Disease and Healing: Studies in Medical Anthropology*, New York and London (1977).
Laslett, P., *The World We Have Lost*, London (1971).
Littledale, W. A., ed., *The Registers of St. Vedast, Foster Lane*, London: Harleian Society, vol. XXX (1903).
MacDonald, M., *Mystical Bedlam: Madness, Anxiety and Healing in Seventeenth-Century England*, Cambridge (1981).
Macfarlane, A., *The Family Life of Ralph Josselin. A Seventeenth-Century Clergyman: An Essay in Historical Anthropology*, Cambridge (1970).
Macfarlane, A., *Witchcraft in Tudor and Stuart England: A Regional and Comparative Study*, London (1970).
McLaren, D., 'Fertility, Infant Mortality and Breast Feeding in the Seventeenth Century', *Medical History*, XXII (1978), 378–96.
Maclean, I., *The Renaissance Notion of Woman: A Study in the Fortunes of Scholasticism and Medical Science in European Intellectual Life*, Cambridge (1980).
Maclean, U., 'Some Aspects of Sickness Behaviour among the Yoruba', in J. B. Loudon, ed., *Social Anthropology and Medicine*, London and New York (1976).
Mechanic, D., *Medical Sociology: A Selective View*, London and New York (1968).
Medvei, V. C. and J. L. Thornton, eds, *The Royal Hospital of St.*

Bartholomew 1123–1973, London (1974).
O'Hara-May, J., *Elizabethan Dyetary of Health*, Lawrence, Kan. (1977).
Pagel, W., *Paracelsus: An Introduction to Philosophical Medicine in the Era of the Renaissance*, Basel and New York (1958).
Parry, N. and J. Parry, *The Rise of the Medical Profession*, London (1976).
Pelling, M., 'Occupational Diversity: Barbersurgeons and the Trades of Norwich, 1550–1640', *Bulletin of the History of Medicine*, LVI (1982), 484–511.
Pelling, M., 'Medical Practice in the Early Modern Period. Trade or Profession?', *The Society for the Social History of Medicine Bulletin*, XXXII (1983), 27–8.
Pelling, M., 'Appearance and Reality: Barbersurgeons, the Body and Venereal Disease in Early Modern London', in A. L. Beier and R. Finlay, eds, *The Making of the Metropolis: London 1500–1700*, London (1986).
Pelling, M. and C. Webster, 'Medical Practitioners', in C. Webster, ed., *Health, Medicine and Mortality in the Sixteenth Century*, Cambridge (1979), pp. 165–235.
The Plague Reconsidered: A New Look at its Origins and Effects in Sixteenth- and Seventeenth-Century England, Matlock, Derbyshire (1977).
Pollock, L., *Forgotten Children*, Cambridge (1983).
Porter, R., ed., *Patients and Practitioners: Lay Perceptions of Medicine in Pre-Industrial Society*, Cambridge (1985).
Poynter, F. N. L., ed., *Medicine and Culture*, London (1969).
Poynter, F. N. L., and W. J. Bishop, eds, *A Seventeenth-Century Doctor and his Patients: John Symcotts, 1592?–1662*, Bedfordshire Historical Record Society, vol. 31, Streatley, Beds (1950).
Prior, M., ed., *Women in English Society 1500–1800*, London (1985).
Raach, J. H., *A Directory of English Country Physicians, 1603–1643*, London (1962).
Rattansi, P., 'The Helmontian–Galenist Controversy in Restoration England', *Ambix*, XII (1964), 1–23.
Robb-Smith, A. H. T., 'Cambridge Medicine', in A. G. Debus, ed., *Medicine in Seventeenth-Century England*, Los Angeles (1974), pp. 327–70.
Roberts, R. S., 'The London Apothecaries and Medical Practice in Tudor and Stuart England', unpublished London University Ph.D thesis (1964).
Roberts, R. S., 'The Personnel and Practice of Medicine in Tudor and Stuart England', *Medical History*, VI (1962), 363–82, and VII (1964), 217–34.
Rowse, A. L., *Simon Forman: Sex and Society in Shakespeare's Age*, London (1974).
Schofield, R. and E. A. Wrigley, 'Infant and Child Mortality in England in the late Tudor and early Stuart Period', in C. Webster, ed., *Health, Medicine and Mortality in the Sixteenth Century*, Cambridge (1979), pp. 61–96.

Shorter, E., *A History of Women's Bodies*, Harmondsworth (1984).
Shrewsbury, J. F. D., *A History of Bubonic Plague in the British Isles*, Cambridge (1971).
Silvette, H., *The Doctor on Stage: Medicine and Medical Men in Seventeenth-Century England*, Knoxville, Tenn. (1967).
Sinclair, H. M., 'Oxford Medicine', in A. G. Debus, ed., *Medicine in Seventeenth-Century England*, Los Angeles (1974), pp. 371–92.
Singer, C., *A Short History of Anatomy and Physiology from the Greeks to Harvey*, New York (1957, first published 1925).
Singer, C., *From Magic to Science: Essays on the Scientific Twilight*, New York (1958).
Singer, C., and E. Ashworth Underwood, *A Short History of Medicine*, Oxford (1962).
Slack, P., 'The Local Incidence of Epidemic Disease: The Case of Bristol, 1540–1650', in *The Plague Reconsidered: A New Look at its Origins and Effects in Sixteenth- and Seventeenth-Century England*, Matlock, Derbyshire (1977), pp. 49–62.
Slack, P., 'Mirrors of Health and Treasures of Poor Men: The Uses of the Vernacular Medical Literature of Tudor England', in C. Webster, ed., *Health, Medicine and Mortality in the Sixteenth Century*, Cambridge (1979), pp. 237–73.
Slack, P., *The Impact of Plague in Tudor and Stuart England*, London (1985).
Slack, P., 'Metropolitan Government in Crisis: London's Response to Plague, 1563–1665', in A. L. Beier and R. Finlay, eds, *The Making of the Metropolis: London 1500–1700*, London (1986), pp. 60–81.
Smellie, W., *A Treatise on the Theory and Practice of Midwifery*, 3 vols, London (1779).
Spufford, M., *Contrasting Communities: English Villages in the Sixteenth and Seventeenth Centuries*, Cambridge (1974 and 1979).
Statutes of the Realm, London (1810–1828: repr. 1963).
Stephen, M., *The Domestic Midwife*, London (1795).
Stocks, M., *A Hundred Years of District Nursing*, London (1960).
Stone, L., *The Crisis of the Aristocracy, 1558–1641*, Oxford (1965).
Stone, L., *The Family, Sex and Marriage in England, 1500–1800*, London (1977).
Stone, S., *A Complete Practice of Midwifery*, London (1737).
Summers, M., ed., *Malleus Maleficarum*, London (1928 and 1971).
Temkin, O., *Galenism: Rise and Decline of a Medical Philosophy*, Ithaca, NY and London (1973).
Thackeray, W. M., *History of Pendennis*, New York (1968).
[Thickness, P.], *Man-Midwifery Analysed: And the Tendency of the Practice Detected and Exposed*, London (1765).
Thomas, K., *Religion and the Decline of Magic*, Harmondsworth (1973).
Thompson, R., *Women in Stuart England and America*, London (1974).
Veith, I., *Hysteria: The History of a Disease*, Chicago, Ill. (1965).
Walker, D. P., *Unclean Spirits: Possession and Exorcism in France and*

England in the Late Sixteenth and Early Seventeenth Centuries, London (1981).
Wall, C., *The History of the Surgeon's Company, 1745–1800*, London (1937).
Wall, C., H. C. Cannon and E. Ashworth Underwood, *A History of the Worshipful Society of Apothecaries of London*, vol. I, 1617–1815, Oxford (1963).
Webster, C., 'Alchemical and Paracelsian Medicine', in C. Webster, ed., *Health, Medicine and Mortality in the Sixteenth Century*, Cambridge (1979), pp. 301–34.
Webster, C., *The Great Instauration: Science, Medicine and Reform, 1626–60*, London (1975).
White, P., 'The Rise of Arminianism Reconsidered', *Past and Present*, 101 (1983), pp. 34–54.
Wilson, A., 'Participant or Patient? Seventeenth-Century Childbirth from the Mother's Point of View', in R. Porter, ed., *Patients and Practitioners: Lay Perceptions of Medicine in Pre-Industrial Society*, Cambridge (1985), pp. 129–44.
Witkowski, G. J., *Accoucheurs et Sages-Femmes Célèbres*, Paris (1891).
Young, S., ed., *The Annals of the Barber-Surgeons*, London (1890).
Zinsser, H., *Rats, Lice and History*, London (1935 and 1943).

GLOSSARY

ague: an intermittent fever, sometimes identified with malaria. The form of an ague is determined by the interval between fits. A quotidian ague is characterised by daily fits, a tertian ague by fits every second day, and a quartan ague by fits every third day.

apostem: a matter-filled swelling.

clyster or **glister:** an enema.

cachexia: a depraved condition of the body characterised by pervasive malnutrition.

cupping: letting blood by means of suction.

dropsy: a condition characterised by the accumulation of fluid in one or more parts of the body.

fistula: a hollowness, usually long and narrow, which will not heal.

issue: an artificially produced ulcer which is not allowed to heal.

ligature: a thread of silk, flax wire, or other material, used by surgeons to tie arteries or other parts of the body.

livergrown: a condition, primarily affecting children, which involved having an enlarged liver.

pannado: bread boiled to a pulp and flavoured with sugar, nutmeg, etc.

phlebotomy: therapeutic bleeding.

pleagett: a bandage or dressing.

posset: hot milk which has been curdled by means of wine.

rheum: mucous discharge, common in colds.

rotula: patella or knee-cap.

scarification: letting blood by means of shallow cuts.

scrofula or King's Evil: swellings, sometimes ulcerated, on the neck and other parts of the body.

squinsey or quinsy: a severe sore throat.

suffocation of the Mother: fits caused by a wandering womb.

tent: a roll of dressing used to keep an orifice open.

trepan or trephine: instruments used to open the skull.

INDEX

HUNGER AND FAMINE IN THE LONG NINETEENTH CENTURY

HUNGER AND FAMINE IN THE LONG NINETEENTH CENTURY

Edited by Gail Turley Houston

Volume I

'Guttling and Guzzling': The Immiseration of the Poor, or 'Perish[ing] from the Table of Nature' (1795–1839)

Routledge
Taylor & Francis Group
LONDON AND NEW YORK

First published 2022
by Routledge
4 Park Square, Milton Park, Abingdon, Oxon OX14 4RN

and by Routledge
605 Third Avenue, New York, NY 10158

Routledge is an imprint of the Taylor & Francis Group, an informa business

British Library Cataloguing-in-Publication Data
A catalogue record for this book is available from the British Library

Library of Congress Cataloging-in-Publication Data
Names: Houston, Gail Turley, 1950- editor.
Title: Hunger and famine in the long nineteenth century / edited by Gail Turley Houston.
Description: 1st Edition. | New York, NY : Routledge, 2022. | Includes bibliographical references and index. | Contents: v. 1. -- v. 2. -- v. 3. -- v. 4. -- Set | Identifiers: LCCN 2021041236 (print) | LCCN 2021041237 (ebook) | ISBN 9780367187514 (v. 1 ; hardback) | ISBN 9780367187521 (v. 2 ; hardback) | ISBN 9780367187538 (v. 3 ; hardback) | ISBN 9780367187545 (v. 4 ; hardback) | ISBN 9780367187507 (set) | ISBN 9780429198038 (set ; ebook) | ISBN 9780429198052 (v. 1 ; ebook) | ISBN 9780429198069 (v. 2 ; ebook) | ISBN 9780429198076 (v. 3 ; ebook) | ISBN 9780429198083 (v. 4 ; ebook)
Subjects: LCSH: Famines--Great Britain--History--19th century. | Poor--Government policy--Great Britain--History--19th century. | Great Britain--Economic policy--19th century. | Great Britain--Social conditions--19th century.
Classification: LCC HC79.F3 H845 2022 (print) | LCC HC79.F3 (ebook) | DDC 363.80941--dc23/eng/20211208
LC record available at https://lccn.loc.gov/2021041236
LC ebook record available at https://lccn.loc.gov/2021041237

ISBN: 978-0-367-18750-7 (set)
eISBN: 978-0-429-19803-8 (set)
ISBN: 978-0-367-18751-4 (volume I)
eISBN: 978-0-429-19805-2 (volume I)

DOI: 10.4324/9780429198052

Typeset in Times New Roman
by Deanta Global Publishing Services, Chennai, India

FOR GEORGE FLOYD

CONTENTS

ACKNOWLEDGEMENTS

This set of volumes on the topic of hunger, starvation and famine in the long nineteenth century was written during the Covid-19 pandemic and was affected by that catastrophic ongoing event in numerous ways. A research trip to Ireland and England was cancelled on the eve of the lockdown in California, where I reside. Likewise, the Huntington Library and University of California, Los Angeles (UCLA)'s Graduate Library became unavailable sites for research and quiet study. As a result, the bulk of the research was done at home online. Thus, I must express my gratitude to all those invisible staff at various research sites for having done the laborious work of digitising archival materials over the last three decades. This set of volumes simply could not have been done without that massive effort to save archival materials in the virtual sphere. As a result of these efforts, I have been able to use the British Library (periodicals and newspapers), as well as the Nineteenth Century Collections Online, the Wellcome Collection, Hathi Trust, Parliamentary Papers, The National Archives at Kew, and Irish Newpapers Online, and though there may be documents I missed because I could not actually visit the archives in Britain, I am assured that the digital archive is rich and effulgent. Meanwhile, the folks at Proquest and Cengage have been more than patient with my copyright queries. I also must thank Routledge for inviting me to edit these volumes, as well as for the timely, efficient, meticulous publishing practices they exhibited throughout this process.

Other resources have been most helpful and timely; the University of New Mexico (UNM)'s interlibrary loan staff has always provided requested materials in a timely, efficient fashion; the Librarian for the UNM English Department, Glenn Koelling, has extended her help and insights at key points in my research journey. As always, the Victoria list-serve, with its lively and collegial discussions, has lent tremendous advice and suggestions along the way. I extend gratitude, as well, to my department chair for her support, as well as to Sinae Kang, Austin Patenaude-Arroyo, Kate Alexander and Johnbosco Ozuruome.

Writing and editing this collection during Covid-19 has also impacted the arguments and insights achieved regarding the existence of hunger, starvation and famine in Britain and its colonies during the long nineteenth century. Both may be seen as catastrophic events that affect the nation-State and put under interrogation what the purpose of the State is if it does not seek to shield its citizenry from disease, want and disaster. The nineteenth-century British government's response to starvation amongst its poor in the State's centre alongside its reactions to famine in the colonies is cause to remark a familiar refrain during the response to Covid-19 in the United States: why was the most powerful country in the world not prepared for such a disaster? And, why, when disaster came, did this most powerful government in the world not respond more forcefully to protect its citizens? Likewise, why did these governments prioritise the economy over the lives of their people?

Clearly, Covid-19 coloured my investigation of hunger, famine and starvation. I did expect to find shocking instances of poverty, hunger and starvation in Britain, especially across the first half of the nineteenth century, what with the enclosure acts, the new Poor Law, the Corn Laws, the gleaning laws, the enormous debt after the Napoleonic Wars, the potato famine and the combination of capitalist economics and Malthusian philosophy. Not as focused on the history of the British colonies in my previous work, I was all but stupefied by the relentless inaction of the British State when faced with repeated famines across the nineteenth century, in India, in particular. But setting these occurrences of starvation and famine at home and abroad in the British Empire side-by-side, as they were historically, implies a kind of malevolence or determined incompetence that is as impossible to fathom as is the U.S. government's response to Covid-19 under the leadership of the 45th President of the United States. In this interrogation of the State, one has to factor in Lord Cranborne's remarkable statement to the House of Commons (1867): that allowing so many to die in India during the Orissa Bengal Famine of 1866–1867 indicated England's blatant racism against those with brown or black skin. The enfolding of race in the midst of Covid-19 with George Floyd's murder also puts into question not only the State's refusal to protect its citizens but also its willingness to do them harm based on race, class and gender. Thus, the actions of the two most powerful countries in the long nineteenth century and the twenty-first century in response to catastrophic events have merged or combined in my mind to form a kind of virtual metempsychosis. There is no way to overstate the connections or trajectories.

As always, children and their partners, and my beloved grandchild, as well as my six siblings (bless you, Mark) have been cause for a degree of support and kindness I cannot overestimate.

The following articles were all reproduced with the kind permission of ProQuest LLC:

2. Anon., 'The Grumblers', *Town and Country Magazine, or, Universal Repository of Knowledge, Instruction, and Entertainment.*
3. Sir Francis Burdett, 'Speech', Commons sitting.
6. Anon., 'ART. XI. 1. *An Inquiry into the Causes of General Poverty and Dependance of Mankind; Including a Full Investigation of the Corn Laws*', *Quarterly Review.*

9. T. William, 'Address to the Industrious Classes of Britain and Ireland, Particularly to our Neighbours, the Distressed Spitalfields Weavers', *Co-operative Magazine and Monthly Herald.*
10. D. W. Harvey, Speech, 'State of the Country', Commons sitting.
11. Anon., 'Domestic Policy. No. III. *The Condition of the Lower Orders*', *Blackwood's Edinburgh Magazine.*
12. MP Mr. Samuel Whitbread, 'Poor-Laws Bill', Commons sitting.
13. Anon., 'Liber Sine Titulo; or, Copy of a Manuscript-Fragment Found at a Certain Mountain in Derbyshire, which Takes its Name from the Devil', *The Scourge, or, Literary, Theatrical, and Miscellaneous Magazine.*
14. George Ensor, 'An Inquiry Concerning the Population of Nations; Containing a Refutation of Mr Malthus's Essay on Population', *Monthly Magazine, or, British Register.*
15. 'Poor Relief Bill'; MPs James Scarlett, Robert Thomas Wilson, Matthew F. Lewis, John Bennet, Commons sitting.
18. David Robinson, 'The Poor Laws', *Blackwood's Edinburgh Magazine.*
19. Anon., 'The Population Question.—Mr. Sadler and the Political Economists', *The Monthly Magazine, or, British Register.*
30. Anon., 'Corn Laws-Petition of the Starving Weavers of Blackburn', Commons sitting.
32. Anon., '*The following Report seems to us to be drawn up with so much judgment.* Report of the Association, formed in London, on the 23rd Day of May, 1812, for the Relief and Benefit of the Manufacturing and the Labouring Poor', *Universal Magazine.*
39. Anon., 'Alarming State of the People', *The Examiner.*
40. Anon., 'Causes and Cures of the Present Distress', *Manchester Times.*
41. 'J. R.', 'Art. IX. Domestic Arrangements of the Working Classes', *London and Westminster Review*
42. 'M', 'On Making Bread From Wood', *Edinburgh Magazine and Literary Miscellany.*
43. Anon., 'Real Relief for the Sufferings of the Poor', *Moral Reformer, and Protestor Against the Vices, Abuses, and Corruptions of the Age.*
44. Anon., 'The General Fast', *Figaro in London.*
45. 'Dietary Tables Issued by the Poor Law Commissioners for Cirencester Union, December 1836', Hansard.
47. 'Testimony from Mr. Thomas Bourne, *Select Committee on Poor Law Amendment Act: Third Report'*, Hansard.
49. John Eagles, 'New Scheme for Maintaining the Poor', *Blackwood's Edinburgh Magazine.*
50. Testimony from Rev. D. Williams (Curate of Shalbourne), 11 May 1838, and Testimony from John Bowen (Guardian of Bridgwater Union), 5 July 1838, *Select Committee of House of Lords on Operation of Poor Law Amendment Act. Report, Minutes of Evidence, Index*, Hansard.

51. Charles Horace Wall, 'How Do Poor Men Live?', *Tait's Edinburgh Magazine.*
55. William Johnston, 'The Present Crisis', *Blackwood's Edinburgh Magazine.*
56. William Cobbett, 'Feelosofical Quackery', *Cobbett's Weekly Political Register.*
57. Anon., 'The Interpreter: Where May One Starve?', *Figaro in London.*
60. Testimony from Rev. George Stringer Bull, 14 August 1838, *Select Committee of House of Lords on Operation of Poor Law Amendment Act. Report, Minutes of Evidence, Index*, Hansard.
61. Anon., 'Stealing from Starvation', *The Champion and Weekly Herald.*
62. A Commissioner, 'Intercepted Report of a Poor Law Commissioner', *Figaro in London.*

The following primary documents were reproduced with the kind permission of the National Archives, Kew:

4. The weavers and townspeople of Royton 'Handbill issued by the weavers and townspeople of Royton in May 1808, after Partiament rejected a bill to guarantee the weavers a minimum wage', 30 May 1808. Catalogue ref: HO 42/95f.375.
5. 'A Sufferer', 'Letter to Prince Regent', 23 May 1812. *Letters and Papers. 1812, May. May 1812.* MS Home Office Papers and Records: Part Five: HO 42, Box 123.
23. Richard Taylor, 'To the Manfacturers, Mechanics, Artisans, and Others, (Inhabitants of Manchester and its Vicinity) Who Signed and Supported the late Petition to the House of Commons'. *Letters and Papers Supplementary*, September to November 1811, MS Home Office Papers and Records, Part Five, HO 42, Box 117.
24. Anon., 'An Address from the Framework-Knitters to the Gentlemen Hosiers of the Town of Nottingham', *Nottingham Review & General Advertiser for the Midland Counties*, 4, 29 November 1811. *Letters and Papers Supplementary*, September to November 1811. MS Home Office Papers and Records, Part Five, HO 42, Box 117.
25. William Crump, 'Address of the Plain Silk Stocking-Makers to the Gentlemen Hosiers, Who Have Agreed to Give an Advance of Sixpence per Pair for the Making of Black Silk Hose', *The Nottingham Review* 4, November 29, 1811. *Letters and Papers Supplementary*, September to November 1811. MS Home Office Papers and Records, Part Five, HO 42, Box 117.
26. Charles Prescott, local magistrate, 'Letter' regarding the Stockport weavers' petition to Parliament, 21 May 1816.

ABBREVIATIONS

BL	British Library
BLN	British Library Newspapers
BP	British Periodicals
ECCO	Eighteenth Century Collections Online
HC	House of Commons
HL	House of Lords
HT	HathiTrust
NA	National Archives
NCCO	Nineteenth Century Collections Online
TDA	*The Times* Digital Archive

GENERAL INTRODUCTION

Persons are perpetually being brought to the police-offices under the awful imputation of daring to be seen in the public thorough fares unfed.

(Anon., 'The Reform Egg', 1833)

How can I sing, by Poverty depress'd?
Can Genius, in a narrow garret cramp'd,
Expand her eagle-wings? For bread I write:
Be BREAD my theme: let me not want its aid.
O thou, our chief, our best, support below!
Suppliant I thee invoke, to aid my song;
For without thee can I have pow'r to sing?

(S. N., 'Bread.—A Poem', 1809)

Hunger, starvation and famine can never be seen outside the infrastructure of State power manifesting itself in uneven but systemic ways in Britain and its colonies across the long nineteenth century. During this time the State wrestled with developing understandings of what Amartya Sen refers to as 'entitlements', that is, the individual's or group's ability to demand food, a dynamic heavily based on class, race and gender.[1] Stephen Devereux's ideas about the vulnerabilities that 'set up' the poor for annihilation during natural calamities can be seen in how the Indian poor were already burdened with high taxation and debt by the British government during the course of its colonisation so that any juddering of the weather could lead to a tipping point of mass starvation.[2] Indeed, the Third World *became* the Third World during the nineteenth century as European powers scrambled for colonies in Africa, South America and Asia. The 'death by starvation' of members of the lower classes during the Irish Famine and the repeated and devastating famines in India are manifestations of those lacking entitlement. Who was allowed to experience ongoing, debilitating hunger is at issue in each of these instances. This ideological approach suggests that the State was making choices about who had entitlement to food, and, thus, that the famines and death by starvation taking place in the British Empire at this time were choices—in other words, the millions of untimely deaths that occurred due to famine and starvation during the long nineteenth century did not have to happen.

My work has always leaned in the direction of studying class and gender in Victorian literature and culture. I began my career with *Consuming Fictions: Gender, Class, and Hunger in Dickens's Novels* (Southern Illinois University Press, 1994), where I examined Dickens's metaphorical figurations of hunger as a means to express systematic forms of oppression imposed upon the lives of those without power or privilege based on gender and class constructs. My study *From Dickens to Dracula: Economics, Gothic, and Victorian Fiction* (Cambridge University Press, 2005) continued to explore class constructs vis-à-vis capitalism in more theoretical terms. Studying hunger and famine from a more materialist approach by gathering documents across a range of contemporary perspectives on hunger and famine has been astonishingly gratifying, though heartbreaking. But the need for such a study has been supported by the hundreds of periodical, governmental, epistolary, political and other documents gleaned during the two years I have had the privilege to work in the archive on this topic. I only regret I did not have the ability to read any of the languages of those who were colonised by the British in the nineteenth century—it would certainly have made for a richer analysis and historical awareness.

While hunger, starvation and famine in Britain and its colonies during the long nineteenth century cannot possibly be covered or summarised completely, a gathering of archival documents such as this illustrates how important engaging a range of people, voices, issues and events constellated around this topic is to understanding the British Empire. This is certainly a unique project given its goal of bringing together primary documents from the long nineteenth century as representative of issues around hunger and famine; though many historical and theoretical essay-length and book-length studies are in print regarding approaches to hunger and famine, none, to this author's knowledge, gather such a vast array of primary documents. These studies on hunger and famine or related issues and events are foundational for examining the meaning of the primary documents assembled here, both individually and as a group. This study could not have been done without the shoulders we all stand on of those who have done the work previous to our own.

Theoretical foundations for the study of mass hunger have been stunning in their clarity and forthright power: Sen's *Poverty and Famines: An Essay on Entitlement and Deprivation* (1981) and Judith N. Shklar's *The Faces of Injustice* (1990) are of this quality, as is also Devereux's *Theories of Famine* (1993). Victor R. Preedy and Vinood B. Patel's *Handbook of Famine, Starvation, and Nutrient Deprivation* (2019) is indispensable regarding the physical understanding of starvation vis-à-vis nutrition. Likewise, Eric Hobsbawm's 'The Machine Breakers' (1952) along with E. P. Thompson's groundbreaking work in *The Making of the*

English Working Class (1962) have been invaluable, as is Alan Kidd's *State, Society and the Poor in Nineteenth-Century England* (1999).

In terms of the British Isles proper, the following are studies that have been central to presenting the primary documents gathered in these four volumes: John Vernon's *Hunger: A Modern History* (2007); Amy Bentley's 'Reading Food Riots: Scarcity, Abundance and National Identity' (2001); John R. Butterly and Jack Shepherd's *Hunger: The Biology and Politics of Starvation* (2010); David Arnold's *Famine: Social Crisis and Historical Change* (1988); John Burnett's *Plenty and Want: A Social History of Food in England from 1815 to the Present Day* (1979); Tara Moore's 'Starvation in Victorian Christmas Fiction' (2008); Bernard Harris, Roderick Floud, Robert W. Fogel, and Sok Chul Hong's 'Diet, Health and Work Intensity in England and Wales, 1700–1914' (2010); Ian Gazeley and Sara Horrell's 'Nutrition in the English Agricultural Labourer's Household over the Course of the Long Nineteenth Century' (2013); Kim Price's '"Where is the Fault?": The Starvation of Edward Cooper at the Isle of Wight Workhouse in 1877' (2012); and Gordon Shepherd's 'Income, Domestic Economy and the Distribution of Poverty Amongst Labouring Families in the Parish of Cardington, Bedfordshire, in the 1780s and 1850s' (2010) are included in this list of foundational studies.

Scholarship on Thomas Malthus also played a role in this study and the following works were crucial for understanding his meaning in the long nineteenth century: Linda Schlossberg's '"The Low, Vague Hum of Numbers": The Malthusian Economies of *Jane Eyre*' (2001); David Reisman's *Thomas Robert Malthus* (2018); and James. P. Huzel's *The Popularization of Malthus in Early Nineteenth-Century England: Martineau, Cobbett and the Pauper Press* (2006). These have provided tremendously important insights, along with Frances Ferguson's 'Malthus, Godwin, Wordsworth, and the Spirit of Solitude' (1988) and Alison Bashford and Joyce E. Chaplin's *The New Worlds of Thomas Robert Malthus: Rereading the* Principle of Population (2016), which contributed much needed background as well. Work on the Poor Laws has been extensive and rich and includes the following influential studies: Anthony Brundage's *The English Poor Laws, 1700–1930* (2002) as well as his *The Making of the New Poor Law: The Politics of Inquiry, Enactment, and Implementation, 1832–1839* (1978); N. C. Edsall's *The Anti-Poor Law Movement, 1834–44* (1995); Peter Mandler's *The Uses of Charity The Poor on Relief in the Nineteenth-Century Metropolis* (2016); Felix Driver's *Power and Pauperism: The Workhouse System, 1834–1884* (1993); Marilyn D. Button and Jessica A. Sheetz-Nguyen's *Victorians and the Case for Charity: Essays on Responses to English Poverty by the State, the Church and the Literati* (2014); and Lynn Hollen Lees's *The Solidarities of Strangers: The English Poor Laws and the People, 1700–1948* (1998).

The Chartist movement, of course, has also received intensive study. Works essential for this area include Dorothy Thompson's 'The Influence of Chartism', 'Chartism as a Historical Subject' (1969); James Epstein and Dorothy Thompson's *The Chartist Experience: Studies in Working-Class Radicalism and Culture, 1830–60* (1982); as well as Edward Royle and Roger Lockyer's *Chartism*

(1980); Joan Allen and Owen R. Ashton's 'Editorial: New Directions in Chartist Studies' (2009); D. G. Paz's 'Researching and Teaching the Chartist Movement: Historiographical Challenges' (2010); Frank F. Rosenblatt's *The Chartist Movement in Its Social and Economic Aspects* (1916); and John K. Walton's *Chartism* (1999). All are key documents driving ongoing debates about Chartism.

Studies on the Irish Famine are numerous, and I have used the following as guides to this event: Charlotte Boyce's 'Representing the "Hungry Forties" in Image and Verse: The Politics of Hunger in Early-Victorian Illustrated Periodicals' (2012); Christophe Gillissen's 'A United Kingdom? Ireland, the Union, and Government Responses to the Great Famine' (2014); Terry Eagleton's *Heathcliff and the Great Hunger: Studies in Irish Culture* (1995); Christine Kinealy and Gerard Mac Atasney's *The Hidden Famine: Poverty, Hunger, and Sectarianism in Belfast 1840–50* (2000); Stuart McLean's *The Event and Its Terrors: Ireland, Famine, Modernity* (2004); Patrick O'Sullivan and Richard Lucking's 'The Famine World Wide: The Irish Famine and the Development of Famine Policy and Famine Theory' (1997); Cormic Ó Gráda's *Black '47 and Beyond: The Great Irish Famine in History, Economy, and Memory* (1999); Christopher Morash's 'Mitchel's Hunger' in *Writing the Irish Famine* (1995). One of the most important studies on the Cotton Famine has been D. J. Oddy's 'Urban Famine in Nineteenth-Century Britain: The Effect of the Lancashire Cotton Famine on Working-Class Diet and Health' (1983), while Peter Shapely's 'Urban Charity, Class Relations and Social Cohesion: Charitable Responses to the Cotton Famine' (2001) has been invaluable as well.

Indian famines have been studied in a number of texts crucial to this study, including B. M. Bhatia's *Famines in India: A Study in Some Aspects of the Economic History of India with Special Reference to Food Problems,1860–1990* (1991); Ajit Kumar Ghose's 'Food Supply and Starvation: A Study of Famines with Reference to the Indian Sub-Continent' (1982); K S S Seshan's 'Famines and Famine Relief Measures' (2008); Jill Bender's 'The Imperial Politics of Famine: The 1873–74 Bengal Famine and Irish Parliamentary Nationalism' (2007); L. Brennan's 'The Development of the Indian Famine Codes: Personalities, Politics, and Policies' (1984); Arup Maharatna's *The Demography of Famines: An Indian Historical Perspective* (1996); Kathryn Edgerton-Tarpley's 'Tough Choices: Grappling with Famine in Qing China, the British Empire and Beyond' (2013); and Mike Davis's *Late Victorian Holocausts; El Niño Famines and the Making of the Third World* (2001).

Clearly, as these texts show, whether about the home front or the colonies abroad, the dialogues about starvation and famine resonate across the long nineteenth century, so that similar, though uneven, interactions, ideas and trajectories intermix and coalesce over the time period through the documents selected. Hence, the documents gathered here perform both a diachronic and synchronic function, with topics developing and merging across the four time periods laid out as well as deeply investigated within a single period or event. As becomes clear in any research on this topic, a web of voices is invoked in a kind of call and response across the long nineteenth century, resulting, if further metaphor be allowed, in echoes cast forwards and backwards through the anxiety, fear, smugness and anger displayed from various political and personal orientations. Making each individual choice for inclusion was like curating an art exhibition in that it was important to bring together a range of voices that would engage with each other robustly while also being part of an apparatus that would allow for other texts and voices to join that conversation from further investigations outside these volumes. Choices about texts to include, then, were based on: their apparent dialogue with each other across the period; their deep representation of important topics addressed in the introductory matter; their exhibition of key events, like Peterloo, Chartist petitions, the New Poor Laws and various famines; their strong rhetorical features that are representative of topics discussed in the introductory matter.

The four volumes presenting this topic are arranged, primarily, by chronology: the first volume covers 1795–1839; the second volume focuses on the Hungry Forties; the third volume takes 1850–1870 as its terrain, with the final volume centring on documents from the 1870s through around 1914. Since the time periods and sub-topics are so unique, broad and diverse across the four volumes, each volume includes an introduction to specific people, movements, issues and dynamics through which to understand the archival matter that reveals and epitomises occurrences of hunger and famine during the chronological period covered. Responses administered through government policies and statements of ideological premises are included as well as forceful petitions to Parliament, letters, speeches, placards and other documents composed by the radical and worker movements developed to counter the government's increasingly draconian measures.

Within each volume, the material is organised around patterns or motifs that emerge organically from a broad reading of the archival documents themselves as well as from the need to contextualise the general topic. Being attentive to these motifs, each volume is unique unto itself while still illustrating arguments and impulses that intersect and reticulate in meaningful if seemingly disparate arrangements across the century. Thus, for example, Volume I features introductory matter around Thomas Malthus, the Poor Laws, the Corn Laws, and rhetorical tropes common to debates about the State's obligations to the poor. It then includes sections grouping archival materials under such topics as 'War, taxation and the end of the social contract'; 'Responses to Malthus, the Poor Laws and the Corn Laws'; 'Distress of the Nation'; 'Labour petitions and reform meetings'; 'Dietary: real and imagined'; and, finally, 'Violence, revolution, crime'. Volume II revolves around the Hungry Forties and provides background on the Great Hunger in Ireland, also known as the Irish Famine; it also addresses the rise of Chartism and the labour movement that responded to the intensifying and ongoing distress and starvation facing the poor as a result of capitalist economic formations. Volumes III and IV target continuing poverty in the lower classes on the home front, while scrutinising Britain's governance of India and other colonies or sites of influence when it came to repeated and calamitous famines occurring during the second half of the nineteenth century. As well, the use of famine or starvation to consolidate political power in the Scramble for Africa comes to the fore.

As noted in the preface, while it was frustrating not to have access to the actual archives because of the Covid-19 pandemic, the digital archive on this period is broad and deep, and it was gratifying to work in the virtual archive to see just how rich are its treasures. Self-published pamphlets, petitions, handbills, lectures, sermons, parliamentary speeches and investigations, letters, dietaries, famine commission reports, medical opinions, newspaper articles and opinions have been set side-by-side to obtain a sense of the competing voices responding to hunger and famine. In terms of competing voices, one would imagine that there was no pro-famine opinion in the debates around hunger and starvation happening in the nation and empire. But, as will be seen, Malthus's approach to population was viewed by many as suggesting that famine was God's way of winnowing what was referred to as the surplus and undeserving population; in any case, it was common to find economic arguments across the nineteenth century supporting Malthus and resisting any disruption of the market through government interference in famine responses.

The poor and people of colour in the empire, who were the targets of this rhetoric, along with those who sympathised with their circumstances, felt the need to find a moving and powerful language to compete with the emergent market economy and its supporters. Within these debates were a range of often complex and conflicted voices. As Peter Mandler notes, it is more difficult to recuperate the voices of the lower classes and, I add, of those who were colonised by the British in the nineteenth century; the voices of the privileged are far more accessible.[3] To get at the range of reformist and radical voices, I rely upon Parliamentary Papers, the Home Office archives, as well as HathiTrust primary documents; I also use the radical periodical press (*Reynolds*, *The Charter*, *Black Dwarf*, *The Northern Star*, etc.) which had a heyday, if you will, savaging the workings of Parliament in regards to the Corn Laws, the Poor Laws and Malthusian economics. *The Times*, *The Morning Chronicle*, *Illustrated London News* and *Blackwood's* could be counted on for mainstream, though often conflicted, approaches. HathiTrust and the Nineteenth Century Collections Online have been a boon for the project, as well as British Periodicals, the National Archives at Kew, and 19th Century British Library Newspapers.

Editorial matters

I have made silent changes in cases of clearly unintended errors in text; and I also change the late eighteenth-, early nineteenth-century convention of using the *f* as a stand-in for 's'. Some inessential misspellings have been edited out, but I have not modernised the language in other cases so as to retain a sense of the powerful language used by members of radical movements. In many instances it is necessary to excise text that is tangential to the topic and I do so using […]. Should I add material to the text for ease of reading it is indicated with square brackets, as follows [ ]. At times, of course, there may be illegible text in the manuscript itself; this is indicated in the text by the following after the problematic word or words: <?>. The conventions regarding capitalisation were so inconsistent in the nineteenth century that I have decided to use current conventions unless they change the tone of the piece.

I provide short biographical information regarding individuals alluded to in the texts in editorial notes, and this will be handled at the first mention of the individual. Many names reappear across the writings and will only be provided a biographical note at first mention to avoid repetition. At times, it is impossible to recuperate information about other individuals referred to, which is noted in the text. I also summarise important topics and events essential to understanding the original text.

INTRODUCTION TO VOLUME I: THE IMMISERATION OF THE POOR (1795–1839): 'GUTTLING AND GUZZLING', OR 'PERISH[ING] FROM THE TABLE OF NATURE'

> [F]athers must die, as an expedient that their children may learn to live without food!
>
> (Anon., 'Reflections on the Poor Law', 1838)

> I see around me starvation in the midst of plenty, such as was never witnessed before in any civilized land; the extreme of luxury on one hand, and the most abject want and degradation on the other; [...] There's something rotten in the state of England!
>
> (J. B. D., 'An Essay on Food', 1839)

> The [rich] lived in luxury and plenty; the labourer in a state of actual starvation, and a degree of distress that would harrow up your very souls.
>
> (Cobbett, 'A General Fast', 1832)

> [G]ive us bread or the appetites of Nature will oblige us to devour you.
>
> (Richard Carlile, 'Le Tocsin', 15 Dec 1820)

Confronting hunger, starvation and famine in the long nineteenth century demands a focused engagement with the visceral, for the first half of the nineteenth century saw the immiseration of a significant portion of the British working classes. If the twentieth century was the first time Blacks, women and children obtained some of their rights, it is, in part, because for so long their bodies were seen as having less value than that of the white male body. It is the catastrophic attacks on the bodies of individual workers and on the working-class body as a group in the British Isles proper with which the first two volumes of this collection are concerned. Indeed, to study hunger, starvation and famine in Britain in the long nineteenth century is to understand how the working-class body became anathema to the rest of the body politic and viewed, as Schlossberg suggests, as 'conveniently dispensable and endlessly replaceable'.[4] As the last two volumes will show, the bodies of people of colour in the colonies were also viewed as dispensible, particularly in times of famine.

In terms of the poor in the British Isles, the intellectual work that made this immiseration possible occurred in what Anthony Brundage refers to as a 'grand clash of ideas about poverty and poor relief' taking place in the 1790s, as total poor relief doubled between 1785 to the early 1800s. Brundage also sees an 'eros[ion] of the social fabric' in the first decades of the nineteenth century as new economic ideas 'burrowed ever deeper into the culture and social values' of the upper classes.[5] Bentley explains E. P. Thompson's work on these issues by noting that England moved from being a 'looser collection of landed gentry to a stronger state', and from a 'mercantilist, feudal economic system to one of laissez-faire market capitalism'.[6] David Reisman explains that by the 1830s the 'detribalized' Englishman was 'experiencing the rootlessness and powerlessness of the internal migrant' as capitalist dynamics replaced an older system of communal engagement and assistance.[7] Samantha Shave notes, too, that in the late eighteenth and early nineteenth centuries the 'revolutions in industry and agriculture' that occurred in England caused labourers to lose their allotments, deprived them of a minimum wage, and subjected them to a 'universal system of pauperism'.[8]

For a large portion of the working classes the new industrial economy overruled the principle enshrined from Elizabethan times, known as 43rd Elizabeth, that the state bore a duty to provide sustenance for the poor in times of need. As *The Bradford Observer* reported in 1838,

> the prevalent idea among the working classes was, that, independent of and paramount to social expediency, they had a claim of right upon the rest of the community for assistance sufficient to supply comforts of life when wages fell short of that point.[9]

With the rise of capitalism, such cultural constructs were being collapsed in what Kidd calls a '"liberal break" with the past' as arguments supporting a 'paternalistic ethos' and the 'mutuality of the "moral economy"' were replaced by market forces.[10] What this meant was that 'the whole of the first half of the nineteenth century was miserably hungry for many'.[11] The following sections provide background on people, laws and rhetorics essential to understanding the debates, discussions and descriptions of starvation and famine in the first half of the century.

In terms of diet itself, Ian Gazeley and Sara Horrell explain that while 'calorie consumption within each wage level demonstrates' that there was a 'fall in per capita calorie consumption' by the poor between the '1790s and the 1830s, a rise to 1863, a decline to 1893', and even further decline to 1912. This seems to correlate with Simon Szreter's suggestion that the rapidity of urban growth gave rise to the '"four Ds" of disruption, deprivation, disease and death', and that these features continued to blight the lives of Britain's urban citizens for much of the nineteenth century. Thus, while food availability and wages may have risen, hunger did also.[12] Meanwhile, scholar Emma Griffin has consciously added a 'new measure for living standards—hunger' to get at the 'human experience of industrialization'. Griffin writes that 'Recent studies of consumption, nutrition, heights, mortality, working hours and child labour have all concluded that life was getting worse for workers during the industrial revolution'. There are still provisos to this general overview, for these markers were uneven across agricultural and manufacturing labourers as well as across gender and age lines. For example, Griffin finds that during the nineteenth century, 'Together, low incomes and external economic shocks were the primary cause of hunger in the rural sector', coupled with the loss of a breadwinner, as the time period saw 'erosion of age-old social pressures upon men to provide for their families'.[13]

Children were the most vulnerable to hunger, with their mothers also experiencing a lowering of sustenance since the male breadwinner was prioritised as needing to retain strength for his job. Often, men were served meat and protein while the women and children in the family survived on the leftovers of bread and tea.[14] With adult women and children regularly consuming a reduced share of the food, it is no surprise that many working-class children had stunted bodies while mothers also experienced a higher mortality rate.[15] Studies of the research done separately by amateur investigators Frederick Morton Eden and Rev. David Davies in the 1790s conclude that the 187 families studied spent 75% of their income on food, with 62% directed to the purchase of bread. With the loss of the commons and the move to the cities, many workers lost the milk (from cows) and vegetables (from the garden) that they depended on to make ends meet. Just the loss of these two items might have affected generations in terms of body mass, height and general health.[16]

The following chart illustrates the ways the weavers' wages were drastically reduced during the first two decades of the nineteenth century; this, of course, would imply a loss of food as wages progressively worsened. Note the dramatic reduction in 1811 and 1812, thus explaining the rise of Luddism in those years, and 1817, pointing to the eventual peaceful demonstration and brutal governmental response at Peterloo in 1819.[17] The chart references shillings and pence (s.d.).

Years.	*June–Dec.*		*Years.*	*June–Dec*	
	s.d.	s.d.		s.d.	s.d.
1798	21 6	21 6	1812	11 6	11 0
1799	22 6	21 0	1813	12 0	15 0
1800	21 0	21 0	1814	16 0	17 0
1801	21 0	22 0	1815	12 6	11 6
1802	24 0	25 0	1816	11 0	10 0
1803	20 0	16 0	1817	7 0	7 0
1804	16 0	20 0	1818	7 0	7 6
1805	19 0	15 0	1819	6 6	6 6
1806	15 0	11 6	1820	7 0	7 0
1807	14 0	14 0	1821	7 0	7 0
1808	11 0	12 6	1822	7 0	7 0
1809	16 0	16 0	1823	6 6	6 6
1810	15 6	10 0	1824	6 6	
1811	11 0	11 0			

The Reverend Thomas Malthus

> [B]y lowering the wages of labour, [you] must devote to starvation that extra population which you have thus incautiously created.
>
> (Anon., 'Sketch of a Petition to Parliament', 1820)

> [B]efore the poor would submit to be driven to perish from the table of nature, they would make trial whether they could not displace some that were already seated; that before such a diabolical law could be carried into execution, there would be such a struggle for existence as the world had never yet seen, and that this convulsion would involve both rich and poor in one common ruin.
>
> (Anon., 'The Malthusian Doctrine', 1834)

The new market economy could not have been established without the intellectual underpinnings of Thomas Malthus's *An Essay on the Principle of Population* (1798, with new editions coming out every few years), which examined the state of the poor vis-à-vis the duties and roles of the State. As Alison Bashford and Joyce Chaplin explain E. A. Wrigley's important discussion of this time period as 'standing between two worlds', Malthus's famous text stood between two different economic understandings of the world, the 'pre-modern organic and agricultural economy' and the 'modern industrial and manufacturing economy'.[18] Helping Britain transition to the latter, Malthus utterly changed the political atmosphere with a shot across the bow targeting the Enlightenment ideas about the economy formulated by Adam Smith (1723–1790), Benjamin Franklin (1706–1790), David Hume (1711–1776) and Jean-Baptiste Say (1767–1832), among others, who claimed that a robust population was a boon for the State. David Hume typifies this belief in *Political Discourses*, when he writes that 'every wise, just, and moral government, by rendering the condition of its subjects easy and secure, will always abound most in people, as well as in commodities and riches'.[19] Aligned with this view was the Christian belief in God's injunction to propagate children as well as the notion that, as God's creation, the earth was capable of supporting the life engendered there.

In contrast, Malthus ominously argued that the food supply could never keep up with an exponentially increasing population, a dynamic that would end in 'vice, misery, and degradation', as Schlossberg pointedly describes Malthus's mordant vision.[20] Drastically changing the economic landscape, Malthus's work, as W. R. Greg wrote, came to be seen as 'the fixed, axiomatic belief of the educated world' over the good part of the nineteenth century.[21] Arguing that those who could not or would not work should be refused a seat at the table, Malthus used an apt metaphor for the hunger and want experienced by the displaced lower classes. Seeing famine as a 'positive check' on the poor, whom he viewed as 'unhappy persons who, in the great lottery of life, have drawn a blank', Malthus believed that starvation, as Schlossberg explains, 'though horrible, ultimately worked to strengthen the remaining (though still struggling) population'.[22]

Boyce suggests, then, that Malthus's work caused hunger, starvation, disease and even famine to be understood not only as inevitable conditions faced by the poor, but as a 'positive' means to slow the growth of the lower classes.[23] Indeed, Malthus devastatingly remarked that 'Gigantic inevitable famine' is 'the last, the most dreadful resource of nature' following upon 'sickly seasons, epidemics, pestilence, and plague' that 'advance in terrific array' to 'sweep off their thousands and ten thousands' of people.[24] If 'Hungry people haunted the cultural imagination of 19th-century England', Malthus's rhetoric made it seem that nature rather than culture responded to a population boom by 'protect[ing] her impoverished young' through 'killing them'.[25] 'Taken to its logical extreme, Malthus's theory', says Schlossberg, made 'physical suffering seem necessary and inevitable'. Henceforth, his theory made pauperism a norm as its existence as a supposed scientific term came to 'permeat[e] the mental world' of many, particularly amongst the gentry and aristocracy.[26]

Not surprisingly, Malthus was reviled by many. One anonymous writer, for example, denounced Malthusian doctrinal belief in 'infanticide' and 'homicide' as means of keeping down the population on an island that could only support so many; the implied conclusion was that 'mental and moral misery' was to be the lot of the poor.[27] In some ways, Malthus's approach assumed that the stomach was where all politics began, particularly for the poor. If many felt that the British should 'dismiss' Malthus 'now and for ever' as 'the heart of flint that has disgraced the beginning of the nineteenth century', it was the stomach he was flinty about.[28] The rise of classical economics and its ostensibly scientific discourse in the first half of the nineteenth century informed fervid debates about the Poor Laws, and Malthus's theory provided lawmakers with the pseudo-scientific support to change the Poor Laws while providing cover to Utilitarian economists who called for ending Elizabeth 43 and replacing it with a harsher version.[29] In addition, demanding a strong work ethic from the poor, Evangelical discourse combined with Malthus's ideas to make for a powerful upending of traditional relief to the lower classes, and, in turn, of the lives of the poor themselves.

A concatenation of natural and political events, coupled with the rising capitalist economy, presented an almost insurmountable tide of desperation. Nature played its part with bad harvests in 1798, 1799, 1800, 1801, 1817, 1818, 1821, 1825, 1826, 1833 and 1836. By 1815 the French Revolutionary Wars, which had begun in 1793, had created a financial depression in Britain that proved difficult to dig out of as soldiers returning from the war found employment opportunities at home scarce. The return to specie payment in 1819 also disrupted the massively over-extended British economy.[30] The Corn Laws, which the poor referred to as the 'Starvation Laws' and which were enacted in 1815 to support the wealthy landowners against the importation of cheap foreign grain, made bread much more expensive for the working classes. A raft of repressive acts combined to worsen the situation. These included the poaching, gleaning and wood laws, along with the enclosure acts, which wove tight restraints on the workers' ability to subsist in a new age wherein he only had his labour to depend upon. Likewise, the rise of industrialisation swiftly destroyed many trade guilds, including that of hand-loom weaving, which had a long and cherished provenance.

The Six Acts, imposed in 1819 after Peterloo, suppressed workers' voices by outlawing seditious meetings and blasphemous and seditious speech. The preamble to the acts included language that inadvertently spoke to the desperation of many in the lower classes: 'in divers parts of this kingdom', great 'numbers of persons', 'collected from various parishes and districts, under the pretext of deliberating upon public grievances', and have 'of late been held in disturbance of the public peace, to the great terror and danger of his Majesty's loyal and peaceable subjects, and in a manner manifestly tending to produce confusion and calamities in the nation'.[31] Many conservatives saw the rise of lower-class activism like Luddism, Chartism, the Swing Riots, etc., as seditious. Facing the ongoing prospect of low wages, high rents and heavy national debt and taxation, the working classes struggled to survive. Assembling a range of materials from the archive makes clear that from 1795 to 1840 there was almost constant distress felt across a broad group of the lower classes, with press articles about 'the state of the country' and the 'present distressed state of the people' a constant during these years.[32] What this tells us is that hunger was at the root of most radicalised movements occurring during this time, including the anti-Corn Law movement, the rise of Luddism, Chartism (including the demand for universal suffrage), Owenite ideas and the strong radical political action of many in the lower classes to unionise and obtain suffrage.

The Corn Laws: 'starved into the bargain'

> [T]he farmers *were compelled* [...] to starve the people who produced the wheat, because the said people had been previously robbed of the means of purchasing it by those said farmers and their accomplices the landlords and capitalists! [...] If I be robbed of my hire—of the due remuneration for my labour, and thereby rendered unable to purchase wheat [...] is that a reason why I am to be starved into the bargain? Is it reason why the food I produce is to be thrown to sheep and hogs, whilst my family is starving?'
>
> (Anon., 'Giving the Food of the People to Sheep and Hogs', *The Operative*, 1839)

> [The working man] spin[s] out the miserable remnant of existence upon black bread and hard cheese doled out in starvation morsels three times a day.
>
> (Anon., 'Great Radical Meeting at Leeds', 1838)

In earlier times the poor in England had come to expect bread at prices based on the communal 'moral economy' of the feudal compact.[33] The Corn Laws, in place between 1815 and 1846, changed that compact. Noting Britain's peculiarity vis-à-vis the Corn Laws, Member of Parliament (MP) Charles Fitzwilliam remarked, 'I know of no other country where a tax has ever been directly upon the bread of the people'.[34] Focused on propping up the price of grain at 80 shillings (s.) a quarter so as to protect the wealthy landowners from cheaper grains that might be imported from outside Britain, it was believed that these laws would reduce the country's reliance on foreign foodstuffs in times of war. Depending on the Corn Laws to maintain their economic and political supremacy, the landed aristocracy fought off the nouveau riche manufacturers, many of whom reviled the Acts, seeing them as a means of voiding free trade. Debates about the Acts were volatile. Indeed, the Corn Laws could be seen as an example of how Parliament was willing to interfere in the markets for the landed aristocracy but not for the hungry poor. As well, Anti-Corn League member Lord Kinnaird argued that the Corn Laws were lowering the actual consumption of bread, which was deleterious to both the lower classes and the landowners; he provided an anecdote to prove his point: 'One of the principal bakers [in Dundee] stated that he now only bakes a batch of bread three times a week instead of one five days in the week, and two on Saturdays'.[35]

On the other side of the debate, *Blackwood's Edinburgh Magazine* also used extreme language, propounding the view that if the Corn Laws were abrogated, thus causing the 'prostration of agricultural property', the 'strife will be a fearful and a mortal one, a *guerra a cuchillo*, of which, indeed, the result may be calculated, but the moral consequences will be felt for generations yet unborn'. The threat is palpable, literally and figuratively going for the gut: it warns that 'half a million of rural population' would be 'thrown upon the high-roads with a corresponding reduction of the prices of labour'.[36] Similarly, no less than Thomas de Quincey remonstrated that the lower classes were being 'agitate[d]' to 'frenzy' and violence by the periodical press and Anti-Corn League activists. Nevertheless, he admitted that the lower classes were they for 'whom "Give us this day our daily bread" is the litany ascending for ever to heaven'.[37]

Apart from these debates, it was clear that high grain prices could not help but affect the price of bread, and thus it is no surprise that, as D. G. Barnes, argues, the labourers 'universally looked on the Corn Laws as the first and greatest source of their distress'. In fact, J. R. Wordie opines that prices for wheat would have been 33% lower if the Corn Laws had not been in place. Free trade in wheat would have made a crucial difference to those in the lower classes, for many of whom the 'largest single item in the expenditure' was bread; as well, it should be remembered that it was the desperately poor who had to pay a higher proportion of their income for this staple.[38]

The Poor Laws: the cancellation of the 'great contract'

> [T]he passing of the Poor Law Amendment Bill [...] virtually cancelled the great contract by which men are bound to society, and enlisted in a

> civilized community. If civilization provides not for the subsistence of the inhabitants of a country, it is worse than barbarism.
>
> ('Anti-Poor Law Amendment Meeting in Blackburn',1837)

> [T]he aristocracy [...] think it must be their interest to preserve the present cannibal society.
>
> (Bronterre O'Brien, 'The Shopocracy', 1836)

Bernard Harris suggests that the Poor Law of 1834 was probably the 'most important single document (or set of documents) in the history of British social policy, certainly in the nineteenth century'. In keeping with this viewpoint, Marilyn D. Button and Jessica Sheetz-Nguyen argue that the New Poor Laws 'proved disastrous in every respect for the people it aimed to help'.[39] Hence, if the literati were experiencing ennui of a spiritual kind, the poor were 'arising eternally to the eternal gruel—the eternal soup and suet-puddings—the eternal cheese and water—the same ever-lasting monotony of solitude and misery!'[40] The journal *Figaro* struck a severe note, as well, saying that the Poor Law 'prefers deliberate murder to the paying of rates' and 'places the saving of human life as a secondary consideration to the saving of sixpence!'[41] Also upbraiding the Poor Laws, *The Eclectic* remarked that they had 'screw[ed] down wages to the "starving place"'. In equally colourful language, *The Morning Post* reported on the 'Guttling and Guzzling system', whereby the Whigs were angry because critics demanded that they cancel their enormous end-of-year banquet in order to give to the poor the funds that would be saved.[42]

With the dramatic rise in population from six million in 1750 to nine million in 1801, and the added burden of higher taxation to pay for the French Revolutionary Wars (1793–1815), landowners were increasingly unwilling to shoulder the burden of relieving the poor. The middling and upper classes saw the poor rates rise from 5.3 million pounds in 1802–1803 to the high of 9.3 million in 1817–1818. Known to its opponents as the 'Starvation Law', the 1834 New Poor Laws rejected the main assumption of the old Poor Laws, the solemn duty, set in place during Elizabethan times (in 1597 and 1601), that the poor deserved aid when in legitimate need. Indeed, that assumption rankled more when the poor violently reminded their so-called betters of this duty. Says Kidd, the main 'catalyst' for reform of the Poor Laws occurred with the 'Captain Swing' disturbance of 1830–1831, following the hard winter of 1829–1830, in which workers protested wages and reduced poor relief in 1,400 parishes. The importunate claims for relief made by the workers frightened and angered the upper classes who, fearing their own French Revolution, felt that social stability had to be restored.[43]

The new Poor Law of 1834 was key to effecting a 'national free market in labour' by obviating relief to the able-bodied male with a family.[44] In other words, no longer would poor relief payments be provided to men who were physically able to work; instead, the poor had to be willing to enter the hated workhouses, known as 'bastiles', where harsh, humiliating regulations (such as separating children from parents and husbands from wives) and often inedible subsistence dietaries were imposed. James P. Huzel explains that the new Poor Laws put in place an important element of the 'revolutionary capitalist market economy: a national labour market where individuals, no longer entitled to monetary relief, would be compelled to earn wages unsupplemented by Poor Law payments'. This argument should be coupled with Karl Polanyi's statement that 'Not until 1834' (the same date the new Poor Law was enacted) was 'a competitive labor market established in England' and thus 'industrial capitalism as a system cannot be said to have existed before that date'.[45]

Between 1800 and 1834 members of Parliament such as Samuel Whitbread II (1764–1815) and James Scarlett (1769–1844) attempted in vain to pass bills that would drastically revise poor law regulations, in 1806–1807 and 1821–1822, respectively. Stating that 43d of Elizabeth was 'considered as the *bible'* on the subject of poor relief, Whitbread remarked that 'the rapid increase of the burthens imposed by that statute' had to be addressed. He pointed to statistics showing that 'in the year 1803, it will appear, that upon a population in England and Wales, (exclusive of your army and navy) of 8,870,000 souls; not less than 1,234,000 are partakers of parochial relief'. Thus, 'nearly one seventh part of your population is indebted to the rest wholly, or in part, for their support'.[46] Brundage points out that people like Malthus, Scarlett, and James Mill (Utilitarian and father of John Stuart Mill; 1773–1836) clearly opposed any form of poor laws; they were combatting a coalition of radicals like William Cobbett (1763–1835) and Henry Hunt (1773–1835) along with paternalist MPs like Thomas Attwood (1783–1856), and many others. Saying that his bill was 'not so much to lower the rates, as to improve the moral condition of the poor', Scarlett essentially argued that only the aged, sick and infirm deserved help from poor laws. Even some conservative voices found his bill too draconian and he eventually withdrew it. In a poignant reminder to Scarlett, MP R. Wilson (1777–1849) asserted that legislators would do well to remember that 43 Elizabeth was 'the Magna Carta of the poor' and was described by the famous jurist William Blackstone (1723–1780) 'as founded upon the first principles of civilized society'.[47]

To understand the human and historical forces that made working-class immiseration possible on such a scale is to recognise that in the wake of the French Revolution, which had called for Liberté, Égalité, and Fraternité, in England, as Thomas Carlyle lamented, the worker had become free to starve.

The 'disguised canibal, and the emaciated helot': rhetorical features of the debates on starvation

> The power of wholesale robbery and murder in the hands of the capitalist is called freedom, and the labourer is said to be free as well as the capitalist, because he may escape the robbery if he pleases, by only

> submitting to starve! Admirable logic!—blissful liberty!—happy, thrice happy country!
>
> (Anon., 'Labour More and More Degraded Every Day', 1835)

If, as Boyce argues, hunger is both a 'material condition and cultural construct', the collection of documents in these volumes is more oriented towards the rhetorical arguments made as the culture struggled to understand the starvation in its midst. Nevertheless, before turning to the archival body of evidence about hunger and famine it is well to begin with a brief description of the material reality of starvation. Starvation occurs when, over a period of time, the body receives fewer calories (energy) than are necessary to fulfill its basic functions. 'Starvation is a state of threat', says Dr. Nancy Zucker, and more threatening the smaller the body, since, for example, there is a smaller supply of body fat in children. As a result, children are much more vulnerable to severe hunger and their bodily organs fail more rapidly when faced with ongoing starvation. Maureen Gallagher, of Action Against Hunger, notes that in the process of starvation the body must turn to 'feeding on itself' as it fights against ongoing food deprivation; no longer receiving nutrients and energy from fats, proteins and carbohydrates, but, rather, being fed upon for those nutrients, bodily organs (including the reproductive organs, the heart and the lungs) begin to shrivel up and shut down as dramatic weight loss occurs. Not surprisingly, bodily movements themselves slow down. Ironically, digestion itself is one of the first corporal functions to be disrupted. Derangement of the digestive tract also may cause diarrhea, another sign that the body's energy supplies have been drastically diminished. A person who is starving might experience a reduced temperature and become more vulnerable to illnesses like anemia, rickets, stunting and beriberi; likewise, the person experiencing starvation can undergo phases of irritability, apathy, hallucinations, convulsions, arrhythmia and pain. In the later stages of starvation, kidney functions begin to fail and by the end stage muscle is eaten up, including the muscles of the heart. Soon thereafter the heart itself ceases to function.[48]

This epidemiology should be brought to mind in any consideration of the materials gathered in these volumes as it underwrites the often convulsive anger and suffering displayed in so many of the texts amassed here. Indeed, in order to understand the harsh reality of hunger and starvation occurring in the British Empire during the long nineteenth century, we must turn to the archive, even though, as Mandler explains it is all but impossible to find many voices of the poor in the historical chronicles.[49] The State's official accounts are always more fulsome, written as they are from the perspective of those privileged enough to view starvation and famine from a safe distance. Certainly it is the very voices of the poor that are needed to gain a clear picture of hunger in the long nineteenth century. But though it is difficult to capture first-hand the bodily experience of the millions who starved, one cannot help but be moved by the trace and trail of devastation exhibited in so many of these documents. And, brought together here for the first time, these extracts go some way towards discerning the hefty material reality of mass hunger and starvation.

It is also important to pay attention to the body of intellectual arguments that attempted to explain the preternatural scenario of mass death from hunger as well as the rationalisations for political and moral retreat from responsibility for the disasters which, to a large degree, could have been avoided. But understanding the debates along the lines of conservative or radical philosophy is too simplistic whenever we look at the nineteenth century. Indeed, it is apparent in the colloquy between the rich and poor that middle-and upper-class apologia at times tips almost sideways into apology, while lower-class protest can sometimes couple astonishing éclat with almost unrepresentable distress.

An article in *The Literary Panorama* in 1807 illustrates Mandler's point about finding the voices of the poor; it also indicates the tin ear so many members of the upper classes had towards the poor. At the same time, the condescending attitude is coupled with the understanding that society could not work without dialogue between the classes:

> The rich cannot enter, *ex animo,* into the sentiments of the poor; the instructed, who never knew ignorance, cannot place themselves exactly in the situation of those who are totally void of information; neither will the untutored individual unbosom himself, without reserve, to a man his superior to a man his superior, how much soever such an one may assure him of his friendship. The cunning which usually attends the uninstructed character forbids it. Yet a thorough knowledge of the natural bias of the human mind, in its unsophisticated state, is indispensably necessary, in order to acquire just ideas of what is practicable, in measures of amelioration and reform: for, to lay down such regulations *as will not* be followed, is little better than to propose such as *cannot* be adopted [....]
>
> [L]owering ourselves down to the level of absolute rusticity, seem to be indispensable pre-requisites for stating and estimating those proposals which the poor will comprehend.[50]

If the new Poor Laws were meant to restore social stability and firmly establish a market economy, they met with powerful protests and political activism by many of the working poor and their allies. The selections in these volumes illustrate that 'Dissent was fueled by a diligent press campaign of Poor Law "horror stories"'. Always at issue in this complex range of voices was the rhetorical jockeying to make the 'pain of other people's hunger' a 'real' thing for those in the middle and upper classes. While John Vernon argues that 'the hungry became figures of humanitarian concern only when novel forms of reporting connected people emotionally with [their] suffering', Boyce reminds us that these rhetorical depictions could also help create powerful demands for reform among the labouring classes. Nevertheless, gritty descriptions of the lives of the poor could also result in the 'distancing or naturalising' of hunger by 'positioning it as the unfortunate but inevitable fate of the indigent "other"'.[51]

It is important, then, to lay out some of the rhetorical features that appear in works addressing this topic across the long nineteenth century, which, using the documents chosen as a yardstick, ends up being roughly between 1795 and 1914, the range of the selected readings. One common approach was to link what the State was experiencing to war, with some comparing the labourers' activism and violence with the radical insurrections of the French Revolution; and, of course, many of those who opposed the government's approach to ongoing hunger did sympathise with the Jacobins. The imagery of class warfare leaks into historian Eric Hobsbawm's suggestion that nineteenth-century British labourers intuitively understood that strikes and violence invoked a kind of 'collective bargaining by riot'.[52] Such actions became the words spoken to the government. The view of the rich as vampires or beasts of prey who gobbled up the starving poor may be found in this same constellation of metaphors. In 'The Relative Condition of Rich and Poor Considered', for instance, the anonymous writer asserts that the rich believed property was 'the right *to expropriate the fruits of other men's services, through an exclusive and usurped power of making those laws and institutions by which all wealth is distributed*' but such a system 'dissolves society into two elements—the disguised canibal, and the emaciated helot—the men of prey, and the men preyed upon'.[53] Similarly, labourers argued that while they produced the country's wealth, the middle and upper classes were 'consuming the capital of the Bee-Hive'.[54]

Though some operatives exclaimed their commitment to peaceful protest, asserting that the 'people's press must be the chief weapon of our warfare', others were more sanguinary.[55] In fiery rhetoric, reformer and MP John Fielden (1784–1849) and Richard Oastler, known as the 'Tory radical' (1789–1861), warned that 'The rights of the poor should be protected, or by the God that made them there should be no protection for the property of the rich'. Hence, as radical Richard Carlile's (1790–1843) epigraph to this section illustrates, a war was going on between the classes about the value of property vis-à-vis the personhood of the labourer. The radical journal *The Northern Star* in an article titled 'The Victimized Cotton Spinners' pictures the capitalists as 'greedy, grinding, all absorbing', while, in another article in the same issue entitled 'The Damnable Act' decries 'devouring self-constituted capitalists'. The 'Consolidation of the Productive Classes' in *The Poor Man's Guardian* (30 August 1834) is even harsher, commenting that capitalists were 'continually turning some of their labourers out to starve'. Thus it harangues against 'Capitalists' who 'derive their subsistence from the sinews of the working classes, and, like beasts of prey or robbers, are continually struggling and quarrelling among themselves for a larger share of the common plunder'. Further, these capitalists work by the 'old starving system' because they have

> sole command of the food, without which the labourers cannot live. Under the present system the capitalists may 'legally' inflict the penalty of death upon every labourer, by refusing him food upon any condition.

> With the power of life and death, they can, of course, compel him to work upon their own terms.[56]

The Black Dwarf features similar radical language. In 'A Comparative View of the Vices and Virtues of the TWO Orders of Society, viz. the RICH and the POOR', (28 May 1817), the latter are described as 'but a short remove from the jaws of starvation'. The writer avers that such discontent 'goad[s]' the poor to that 'acme of phrenzy which though it may proceed through rivers of blood, will ultimately ensue'.[57] This viewpoint mirrors Rev. Stephens, who at a meeting of radical labourers proclaimed that war is 'at your own doors—war in our father land. Have you not a civil war already begun in our own country?' This suggestion that the rich and poor lived utterly separate lives preceded Disraeli's famous comment about the rich and poor in his novel *Sybil*. Stephens added astutely that part of the battle included the rich being 'unionized' in their efforts to 'inflict torture by hunger and nakedness, on working men, their wives and children'.[58] This image of class warfare also appears in Mr. Beaumont, a beloved Scottish radical speaker, vociferating at a huge meeting of the working classes about the 'present state of war of capital against labour', of 'steam against the existence of working men', so that every new mechanical invention brought 'affluence for the few, and misery for the many, whose labour being no more required, they are turned out to starve'.[59]

At the same time that the rhetoric depicts war and violence, there is also a kind of delicacy one would not expect, suggesting the rise of a surprising prudery in the face of starvation, a difficulty in even saying the word, as though it completely broke societal norms to discuss alimentary distress. Thus, the terms 'hunger' and 'starvation' are invisible or only hinted at throughout many of these texts. Dickens was on to something when he had his famed orphan declare 'I want some more', a pronunciation whose aggressive demand cannot be undone by the smarmy 'Please, sir', that precedes it. Hence, the term 'distress' often becomes a placeholder and equivalent to the more visceral term 'starvation'. One journalist succinctly explained this connection: 'it is the scarcity of food, be it known to all men, that causes the distress of England'.[60] Thomas Sokoll's recuperation of letters from the poor to workhouse guardians illustrates this awareness of the need to use formulaic words, though at times the letter writers do name 'starvation'. The words 'distress', 'misery' and 'calamity' often work to avoid using the more horrifying terms, 'starvation', 'famine' and even 'hunger', that actually refer to what happens to a body that is regularly devoid of sustenance.[61]

Aside from a fear of being unmannerly, this use of 'distress' to signal devastating and ongoing hunger seems also to speak to a fear that the supplicant's lack of manners might signal that they were not the deserving poor. For example, in 'An Address From the Framework-Knitters to the Gentlemen Hosiers of the Town of Nottingham', at one point the writer notes that he will 'forbear' from describing the want the poor are experiencing 'as we think it would be insulting both to your judgments and feelings, were we to attempt a description of all our Calamities, which you so well know, and which we so much experience'.[62] In any case, the terms 'misery', 'distress', 'calamity' and 'want' are used repeatedly across the century to describe a constellation of signs indicating suffering, with hunger as the primary source in contradistinction to the lesser-used direct terms of 'hunger' and 'starvation'. 'Misery', 'distress', 'calamity' and 'want' also include the notion of the lack of proper clothing and shelter, especially when facing the harsh winter elements. Together, starvation, lack of shelter and lack of warm clothing describe the disenfranchised, poverty-stricken British citizen. This constellation of words describing lack must be set alongside a growing political sense that a British citizen deserved a modicum of comfort, not luxurious, but, certainly, a feeling that one's very life was not always on the brink.

Etymologically, there is a double sense to the word 'distress'; its ancient meaning has to do with 'distraining or with one's goods and chattel being taken away; older meanings also suggest 'The overpowering pressure of some adverse forces, as anger, hunger, bad weather'.[63] The lower classes experienced both these older meanings of 'distress' in that through the enclosure acts, game, wood and corn laws and resulting mass move from agricultural to factory labour they were 'distrained' of their economic lifestyle, with their bodies literally and symbolically rent from the fabric of a feudal society and thrust into that of the market economy. This event, if you will, was ongoing and traumatic for the masses as a whole and for the individuals who directly experienced it. As the Hammonds note, 'labour continued to find its own level of starvation' under the aegis of capitalism.[64]

Another rhetorical feature must be seen in light of the conflict between those who put a premium on property as sacred and those who argued that the human sufferers of hunger should be prioritised by the government. The lack of connection and understanding between these voices is often jarring. The radical *Black Dwarf* engages in this rhetorical contretemps, saying that a bill to revise the Poor Law put forward in 1821 by MP Scarlett was a 'cat's paw' that should have been called a 'Bill to *exterminate the wretched,* instead of *removing* their *wretchedness!*' because, 'under the false pretense of *protecting property,* it will *hazard life!*' and only give the poor a 'vegetable existence'.[65] This seems to be an argument between those who viewed Elizabeth 43 as the ur-text for a governmental response to starvation as opposed to those for whom Edmund Burke's (1729–1797) powerful essays on the sacred rights of property resonated. On one hand, then, there is the suggestion by those supporting the poor that the rich were the true idlers and paupers who were supported by government and by the labouring classes. For example, in 'Acts of the "Collective Wisdom" of the "Thunderers"', *The Black Dwarf* comments of Lord Grenville that 'one of his family of *expensive public paupers'* was 'eating the bread of the public' and 'devou[ring] as much as would maintain a thousand families in plenty'. Hence, 'He has no right to complain of being compelled' to 'give a bare subsistence to the destitute of his parish, while he is enjoying the plunder which has made so many destitute. *He* should be silent, until he had disgorged his share of the spoil'.[66]

On the other hand, the genuflection to property can be cringe-worthy. One newspaper remarks of a factory owner that he is a 'Gentleman' of 'the first respectability', and then adds that his 'fortune is a sufficient guarantee against his motives'.[67] Likewise, in an article entitled 'State of Public Feeling in Scotland', the journalist derides 'the ignorant thousands who petitioned for Reform' because they do not understand that 'their landlords, employers, their teachers, their benefactors' are those 'whose benevolence had saved them from starvation'. Further, he assumes that 'if a great body of wealthy and influential persons' would stand 'forth at once, their wealth, character, and connexions' would 'overawe and subdue the turbulent', 'mere' labouring class and their 'brute violence'.[68]

An article titled 'Machine-Breakers and Stack-Burners Against the Boroughmongers' attempts to parse out why in attacks against property, 'thievery' seemed justified in certain morally questionable situations and reverts to demands that the rich be held accountable for actually taking the property of comfort and existential livelihood from the poor. Strategically beginning with the assumption that 'The right of property must be admitted on all hands' as 'the very basis of all civil society', the piece quickly moves to explaining why lower-class workers might end up turning to thievery instead:

> These unhappy men were all labourers; and, like every individual of their class in the country, they found their usual comforts not only diminishing, but actually gone, and themselves and their families reduced to a state of the most abject misery. They [...] could see no reasonable prospect of improving their condition; but, on the contrary, a *moral* certainty of becoming worse. They saw their only *property,* their labour, depreciated in value by reductions in their wages, or the total want of employment. They saw machines employed to perform the labour by which they and their families had hitherto subsisted. Thus destitute, with no friend to fly to, and no hand to relieve them, shunned or scorned by the great and affluent, and insulted even by the very men whom the law had appointed to shield and shelter them in the house of necessity,—the parish overseers; if they went to beg a crust, they were threatened with the tread-mill; if they uttered complaint, they were denounced as disorderly and insolent.

Then comparing how these men faced 'their own helpless, succourless, starving offspring' in 'a state of actual starvation' the petition argues that 'if the existing laws against the poor are to be enforced, shall we not also insist on the execution of those which are violated by the rich?' Thus he asks, why should not the law be 'enforced with the same rigour against' the 'Dukes of Newcastle, Devonshire, Buckingham, Norfolk, and Northumberland, the Marquises of Hertford and Cleveland, the Earls of Lonsdale, Grosvenor, and Fitzwilliiams', who 'alone return 54 members of the House of Commons, contrary to the express law of the land'.[69]

Similarly, another rhetorical and political contestation occurs around the meaning of the term 'combination'. 'Address of the Relief Committee of Stockport to the Public', written 13 weeks after the beginning of the cottonworkers' strike in 1831 and describing the Stockport workers' situation, illustrates a brilliant *double entendre*, as it were, when using the term 'combination'. In contrast to the sinister meaning some members of the upper classes found in it, the writer asserts that,

> we maintain that every Government and Law is, or ought to be founded upon the PRINCIPLES of *defending the weak and the honest, against the powerful and the unjust*; and every well regulated community is a *Combination* for that purpose.

Thus exclaiming that all members of a State should expect the government to 'combine' for the good of the whole, he continues:

> Now that so much indescribable misery exists, in the districts of the cotton manufacture, in consequence of successive reductions being forced upon the Operative for years: we boldly affirm, that the present opposition to this reduction is no other than a *Combination for life,* against those who would sacrifice our laborious people to their avarice [....] combination [is] the only check under heaven in the work-people's power [....] Every comfort of life, and life itself is [,...] the object of the present contest. Let no man tell us, that there is a point, on this side of starvation, where blood-sucking avarice will cease to grasp the vitals of the manufacturing labourers.[70]

This suggestion around the meanings of 'combination' beyond its purpose of describing the unionising of workers is that 'combination' refers to a society that is concerned with the care of all its people.

Likewise, an exchange between MP Joseph Hume and the Secretary of the Manchester Weavers illustrates the disconnect between classes but also how the meaning of words was being fought over in a heightened fashion. After the weavers had sent the MP a petition for redress of their state of starvation, Hume responded in a smug letter illustrating his complete obliviousness to his own position of privilege and comfort. Says Hume,

> I can assure you, that I am fully sensible of the state of deprivation and distress to which the weavers are reduced; and it would afford me the highest satisfaction, if I could in any way assist in improving your situation.

Ultimately, his point is that 'It is the interest of all manufacturers, to get their work done as cheap as possible' and that 'The real cause of the distress of the weavers to be a diminished demand for labour, in comparison to the number of workmen that offer for the work'. How these obvious and cold-hearted comments were to help the workers is utterly absent. The Secretary for the weavers answered with sarcasm, reminding him that 'Our powers of description, Sir, will fail of giving any adequate idea of our situation to any person except those who feel it'. He then turned to the deprivation Hume could not find it in his vocabulary to address, noting that 'the greatest number of us cree[p] about like living skeletons, habited like scarecrows'. He continues:

> We are without every thing that makes life desirable, and without the means of purchasing any thing. Great numbers of us are even unable to get a sufficient quantity of the cheapest and coarsest food for ourselves and our families.

He ends, saying,

> Thus we are clearly marked out for legislative protection or starvation; of the latter we are in full possession at present, whether we are to have the former will depend, Sir, in some degree, upon your exertions in our behalf.[71]

Another rhetorical debate featured across all levels of society concerned whether poverty was the fault of the individual or what some would now call systemic classism and a capitalist economy. Many conservative venues assumed that the lower classes were not only lazy and lacking in thrift; they also decried them for not saving towards a pension as well as not showing the proper obeisance to their betters. This was in competition with a strong growing theoretical sense on the part of many of the poor and their supporters that poverty was the result of political dynamics brought about by repressive and inhumane governmental actions. Certainly, the lower classes did see a systemic new form of economics cutting their bonds with the earth, seasonal cycles, former familial and work patterns as well as the feudal relations with the master. The rhetoric illustrates the understanding that capitalism was not only changing their connections with the body politic but also with their own suffering bodies.

An uncomfortable and mistaken comparison of labourers with slaves often occurs in the writings of those who supported the lower classes. For example, in a meeting of spinners in Glasgow the argument was made that labourers would become like 'abject slaves' if their right to have 'Combinations' [trade unions] was abrogated.[72] In 'The Infernal Act', the anonymous writer complains of the 'white slaves' in the agricultural districts of the South of England and 'the general distress occasioned by an almost denial of relief, joined to a depression of wages to the starvation point'[73] Similarly, in another letter to the editor, 'Currency, Corn Laws, and Crime, To the Editor of *The Morning Chronicle*', the writer, 'Probus,' remembers the 'halcyon days' before landlords raised the rent and labourers 'refuse[d]' the essential slavery of working 'for 5s per week', which would result in the labourer 'd[ying] for want of food' and was thus, according to Probus, worse than slavery.[74]

The comparison of the lower-class worker to a slave also is iseen in discourse that invokes 'manhood' as the opposite of slavery. Thus, for example, an 'Address to the Much-Injured Part of the Community, the Cotton Weavers' laments the fact that the weavers had repeatedly put up 'no resistance' to wage cuts, a response seen as 'scandalously shameful and degrading to the human character'. The writer points to the weavers' 'half-starved children' and questions if 'the last spark of manhood' had been 'extinguished in your bosoms'. Asking why 'should such a numerous body remain in slavery, misery, and want', the piece concludes:

> Consider your dignity; consider that you are men, and that you stand in the first rank of beings in creation [....] No, no; there is bread enough and to spare in the store-house of Nature, and many of our fellow-sufferers have, within the bounds of the last ten years, perished with hunger. Arise, then, you who have been hitherto inactive [....] throw off the galling chains of slavery [....] the God of Nature never intended man to be a slave, but to confer on him happiness.[75]

The archive also includes documents with the repeated refrain that, in the new economy, being poor was tantamount to being a criminal. In the reform-minded journal *Figaro,* 'The Reform Egg' (26 October 1833) wittily complains that 'under the guise of the Reform Bill' the 'awful crime of starvation is increasing daily, and magisterial malignancy has full employment in the punishment of the fast-spreading enormities of hunger and homelessness'. Hence, 'Persons are perpetually being brought to the police-offices under the awful imputation of daring to be seen in the public thoroughfares unfed'. Likewise, the writer scolds, 'the prisons teem with wretches sufficiently depraved to permit the eye of affluence to be offended by the sight of their own wretchedness'.[76] As will be seen below, writers often resorted to such dark jocularity either to force understanding upon the upper classes or deconstruct the apparatus under which the State allowed mass hunger and starvation.

To conclude this section, but certainly not to suggest that there are not other rhetorics being used around this topic, there is a constant theme that the nation had never before experienced anything like the starvation and distress at hand in the beginning decades of the nineteenth century, and that the grinding poverty resulting from capitalist doctrine made for the worst situation the country had ever faced. This sense of rupture is found in the repeated title of many topical articles on the 'distressed state of [the] nation'. For example, in the House of Commons, Liberal MP Sir Francis Burdett (1770–1844) remarked the 'distress and famine which now afflict the land', while a speaker in a radical meeting exclaimed that though Parliament was aware of 'the distress of the country', the 'House was either unable or unwilling to remove this general calamity'.[77] Such language feels apocalyptic, and one senses that the nation was overwhelmed by the dynamics of the new capitalist economy. In keeping with this fear, many writers, upper and lower class, worried that the new economy, with its goal of protecting property, was requiring them to negate their Christian duty to help the suffering.

The following selections are organized under six sub-topics: 'War, taxation and the end of the social contract'; 'Responses to Malthus, the Poor Laws and the Corn Laws'; 'Distress of the Nation'; 'Labour petitions and reform meetings', 'Dietary: real and imagined'; 'Violence, revolution, crime'.These topics arise out of the mass of documents researched.

Part 1

SELECTIONS

War, taxation and the end of the social contract

One of the longest conflicts faced by the British, the French Revolutionary Wars lasted about twenty years, from 1793–1815. The country went into enormous debt to fund the wars and lent enormous amounts to other countries as well as to many of the French people who were expelled by the radical Jacobins. Coming just after the War with America in 1776–1783, and followed by another war with America in 1812, the Napoleonic Wars forced Britain to begin a new form of taxation in 1798 to subsidise this new normal of seemingly endless wars. Indeed, Julian Hoppit notes that after the Napoleonic wars, three things were certain regarding needed changes in the state: that 'massive retrenchment would be essential', that rapid population increase led to 'significant local pools of under- and unemployment', and that 'prolonged war had structurally altered the economy'.[78]

In the following set of texts, we hear how the war, in one form or another, affected society. Further, predictions of and fears about the fraying or destruction of the social contract between citizens of the State became paramount, along with anger at ever higher taxation. These representations usually see the working classes as being pinched by all three of these trajectories.

DOI: 10.4324/9780429198052-1

1

ISAAC EATON, *THE TOCSIN. THE BRITISH TOCSIN, OR PROOFS OF NATIONAL RUIN*

4th edition (London: Daniel Isaac Eaton, 1795), pp. 4–18, 23, 27–28, 31–34, 38, 53

The Tocsin (a tocsin being an alarm bell), a self-published pamphlet by Daniel Isaac Eaton (1753–1814), is an anti-war, anti-tax rallying cry against state corruption and profligacy under the scandalous Prince Regent (George IV, 1762–1830). Railing against what was happening to the 'starving peasant', Eaton was a radical author and activist who describes how the bonds between the classes were rent apart when the self-indulgent aristocracy was blind to the famine ravaging the poor. In apocalyptic rhetoric, he warns that Britain was on the 'brink' of 'ruin' because of the prince's policies and decadence, that the lives and contributions of the poor were being degraded and that hunger, whereby the poor must eat the 'rudest trash', would cause a revolution. It appears that in 1793 the Crown brought the same Daniel Isaac Eaton to trial for publishing a pamphlet entitled *Politics for the People, Or, Hog's Wash*, because it was '*scandalous, malicious, inflammatory*, and *seditious*' concerning the king. Eaton was found not guilty.[79]

Other instances in the archive illustrate this anger against a prince who had no care for his people. In '*Letter from a Briton*', dated 27 May 1812, the writer calls George IV 'My Dirty Prince' and claims that 'you have shown yourself a damned unfeeling brute witness the tens of thousands starving without the hope of relief'.[80] It ends with the caustic caution, 'No more you damned rascal of hell from a few lovers of this Country and haters of you as long as you do nothing for its welfare'.

The Tocsin is set against a country now 'eternally' at war under a corrupt prince.

DOI: 10.4324/9780429198052-2

1. Isaac Eaton, *The Tocsin. The British Tocsin, or Proofs of National Ruin* (1795)

[....] I write from the heart—and the warmth of feeling may exceed the boundaries of prudence—but as a Man, I have a right to enjoy my native sentiments, and as a Citizen, it is my duty to communicate them[....]

Britain is on the brink of ruin—it is not the vain dreams of politicians, or the idle malevolence of parties that vociferate, or create this idea; it is found on fact, and the daily contemplation of men corroborates the assertion. Deceitful pictures have been drawn by the dependants upon power of the flourishing state of our country, notwithstanding the effects, unavoidably produced by a continuation of war, but experience is the best reply to their insinuations;—the soldierized mechanic, the starving peasant, and the deserted widow, are living protests against the veracity of their reports.

What are the symptoms of national ruin? Corruption and distress, walking hand in hand through the country; and war eternally completing the triumvirate of despotism. In arbitrary governments, the people may be slaves before they are corrupted; but in countries, which once were free, the people must have been corrupted before they were enslaved: corruption is always the companion of misery, and both are in their turns the produce and the cause of war. Kings, corruption, and misery, too often originate from national dissentions, and too often repay the obligation with the false gratitude of loyal suffering, and glorious destruction.

The government is near its end, when having once depended upon the free temper of the people, they endeavour to reign by their own extent of power; it is much easier for the people to serve the king with cheerfulness, than for the king to restrain the people with distrust;—this jealousy is the watchword of tyranny's dissolution, it is the token of disunion between the monarch and the nation, and in the termination of the affair the nation generally acts for itself.

[....] Other circumstances have accelerated the downfall of the British system, and the abuses of a constitution have been the causes of its ruin.

Perhaps no country in the universe ever presented to the observation of the citizen a more melancholy picture than Britain at this present moment; but the ruin of countries which pretend to be free, is not visible upon the surface of affairs; it lies buried in the heart of the land, amid the obscure circles of existence, where aristocratical oppression and association smothers in secret the honest indignation of the rustic soul[....] Great men, and aristocratic splendour, are vapours which conceal the prevalence of misery; disperse the cloud, and you will find the peasant cheating his appetite with the rudest trash which nature can digest; and the mechanic deploring in secret the insufficiency of his industry to supply the necessities of his being.

Proud of their borrowed luxuries, the rich may libel the patience and resolution of the poor; but the index to national dissolution is the inequality of enjoyment. Starvation will bring those to their senses on whom this principle has no effect.

The simplest feelings of nature teach men, that luxury is criminal wherever famine is known; and these feelings tempt them to terminate the abuse[....]

Individuals may be hushed into silence, rich men may be coaxed by honours, but when the great body of a country feel, no *hush-money* or *honours*, can quiet their murmurs or steal from the heart of a nation, those dictates which nature has engraven on it. Men learn from necessity the blessings of liberty, the sensation of hunger, enquires from whence that hunger originates, and the continuance of toil obliges man to enquire, who reaps the produce of his labour; thus tyranny itself is the herald of freedom's felicity, and by suffering the evils of famine, pride, and toil, the peasant and slave, are exalted into men.

Wars in a commercial country may be carried on, and supported for a series of time, by the methods of funding, which have been adopted by the ministers of the three last reigns; but this is only a protraction of ruin, and it is an injustice in principle—it protracts our ruin, because one time or other[...] the profits of national industry will not equal the increase of national indolence which this system occasions, for all funding destroys its own purpose, it swallows up those sums of wealth, and terminates that industrious exertion in the individual, which would otherwise be employed in renovating the exhausted powers of the country[....] Whatever is unjust, must be ruinous, and the injustice of funding is one of he principal evils, which shakes the British empire to its base.

Thus having briefly and loosely stated what I conceive to be the causes of the apparent decline too flagrantly witnessed in the stability of our constitution, I proceed more largely to expatiate on their effects[....] I see my country in a perilous situation, and I consider it my duty to point out the causes of that peril, lest in the crisis of the disease, a remedy should be applied to a wrong part, and the guilty not only be released from the vengeance of insulted justice, but also exult in the unmerited sufferings of the virtue which opposed them[....]

Chapter I.

A PRODIGAL King is the most criminal being upon earth, for no other criminality can be so extensive in its effect, or so universally felt[....] if his wars and nonsensical quarrels cost the nation near two hundred millions—where is his frugality, and what can authorize the boasting eulogiums of his reign? Alas, the people (could they speak their sentiments), would say—O, king, view the distresses which you inflict upon the nation that supports you; *your crown is a burthen, and your reign a ruin*[....]

if a king *can do no wrong* in his actions, I am certain, I can do no wrong in speaking of them.

Let the courtly caterpillars, who swarm about the factotum of royalty, hear for once in their lives an humble individual echo the dictates of truth. Stubborn facts have arisen, which will not bear the illusions of sophistry, and every intellectual quality of man combines to validate the evils, which for the last twenty years, have scourged the inhabitants of Britain.

In the year 1763, when the nation was released from the war it was engaged in[,..] the national debt amounted to one hundred and forty-eight millions; and the interest of it was not less than five millions annually: at the present period the national debt amounts to three hundred and thirty-one millions, five hundred thousand pounds; and the interest of it is not less than twelve millions and one eighth: subtract the difference, and we shall find an increase of one hundred and eighty-three millions in the grand debt, and an increase of seven millions in the interest, which is yearly obtained from the profits of our agriculture and commerce[....] The present reign has caused an addition to be made of one hundred and eighty-three millions to the national debt; and a subtraction of seven millions from the annual exertions of the starving peasant and the laborious mechanic; the present reign has been a reign of taxation; and the blessings derived from it—defeat, ruin, tyranny, and distress.

[....] the British people have suffered misery through patience; they will now learn the lessons of justice, and necessity will be their tutor[....]

All unnecessary wars are systems of extravagance invented by kings and ministers, no matter which, to rob the people and enrich themselves. The contest with America was begun by avarice[....] The system of taxation was so firmly riveted on Britain, that certain persons imagined they might also extend it across the Atlantic, and open another source of tyrannical swindling[....] the project failed, and after thousands of our countrymen, and millions of our wealth, had been lavished at the desire of hypocritical dispositions, the King of England concluded a peace with Congress, and the British people paid the expences of a war, in which they had neither interest or will.

[....] The last twenty years have been nothing but a continuation of loans and funding. The government's appetite has risen in a duplicate proportion to national industry, and the drained purses of the country will testify the fact.

[....] and why the British Nation does not erect the scourge of censure and criminality over the posteriors of an offending debauchee, I can assign no reason whatever, when a prince whines and cries to have his wild impudence supplied by the mother-like bounty of a nation, he deserves the rod of correction, and the treatment of a child.

Chapter II.

[....] The excess of this reign's *extravagance* has produced a universal famine, both in the subsistence, and the felicity of society.

[....] [T]he British people have not resources sufficient to bear oppression, which only grows heavier by duration; and profligacy, which encreases in a due ratio with our patience[....]

When princes gamble with the gifts of their people, the people should snatch the national property from the power of the gamester, and not permit the *black legs of royalty*, to stake the felicity of man against their unprofitable ambition. If ever a King should so far forget the bounty of the people, who placed him on his throne, as to make their credulity the means of his extravagance, and their industry the supply of his obstinacy and ambition, that King wherever he may exist or reign, will one day or other find public justice succeed public forbearance, and the sanctity of the throne will be no barrier to the vengeance of an insulted nation[....]

Chapter III.

[....] The landed property of a nation cannot be productive of much revenue, because it produces little more than is necessary for the immediate sustenance of man; it is commerce, that supports the exorbitant income of the British Government. The people are slaves, who labour and toil for a certain pittance of existence, while government exact the fruits of their industry[....]

[....] Famine is an evil which our governors must immediately remedy—hunger is not a grievance which the contempt of tyrants may adjourn from day to day, the necessaries of life must be obtained, or man will be unable to bear with the oppression, which his indolence would otherwise neglect to notice.

This dreadful misery is to be derived alone from the wickedness of the present ministry[....]

But this is a famine likely to continue and increase, unless national vengeance burst at once, and make tyranny its food. Throughout Europe the same scarcity extends; and unless the soldier be returned to his cottage and plough, the earth will remain uncultivated, and man unfed. Circumstances are come to a crisis—kings must either disband their armies, or else the famine, which those armies produce, will prove the compressing signal of universal revolution[....]

[....] It is not likely that kings will disband their armies—it is not likely that Russia and Prussia will resign their booty; and yet these being the causes of famine, will continue and increase the evil, till starvation operates as an universal restorative, and nature herself, neglected and oppressed, sounds the Tocsin of Revolution and Revenge[....]

Chapter IV.

[....] The evils we complain of are, *ruin*, *famine*, and *war*—and our requisitions are, *reform! liberty*, and *peace*[....]

Appendix

[....] Detested monsters! inhuman parricides of nature's faculties! The very means of tyranny are its downfall! for you have driven us from the temples of Reason and Justice—it is your fault if we open the gates of Janus, and found the war-hoop of retribution.

2

ANON., 'THE GRUMBLERS'

The Town and Country Magazine, or, Universal Repository of Knowledge, Instruction, and Entertainment, 27 (1795), pp. 200–201

The Town and Country, a posh publication founded by Archibald Hamilton, features a tongue-in-cheek response to how war affects the table. It is unclear what class is being represented in this rather generic characterisation, but the sentiment speaks to the alimental lack that follows upon the ongoing prosecution of war and concomitant increased taxation.

DOI: 10.4324/9780429198052-3

2. Anon., 'The Grumblers', *Town and country magazine, or, Universal repository of knowledge, instruction, and entertainment* (1795)

THE GRUMBLERS: A Conversation [....]

A. Poor Old England! 'Tis all over with her—She has seen her best days!

B. Starvation is the word now: What will become of her once happy subjects? Eating begins to be out of fashion in this country.

C. Some people are never satisfied! Have we not plenty in this island?

A. Yes, of taxes.—How few among us can procure the necessaries of life!

C. It is not necessary that we should. Gluttony, a vice of the most detestable nature, has formerly made great havoc among us; but, thank Heaven, people will now learn moderation. We cannot now make beasts of ourselves.

B. A *little* bread and meat, now and then, would certainly be acceptable.

C. A *little* may still be had if that would satisfy us. But we are a dissatisfied race, and cannot be contented with a *little*. Bread and water will allay the cravings of some people; and, among all the imposts hitherto so loudly complained of, those articles are still exempt from taxation. It is a comfortable thing that we enjoy the liberty of making use of our eyes, upon all occasions but that of looking through a window.

A. That indeed is a consolation: neither do we pay any duty for our mouths, unless the tongues within them happen to be riotous or licentious. I wish, however, we had a little more employment for our teeth.

C. I shall conclude this conversation with an elegant phrase, which I borrowed from a certain noble duke—'Hold your Jaw!'

Exeunt

3

SIR FRANCIS BURDETT, SPEECH, COMMONS SITTING

Hansard, HC (12 November 1800), Volume 13, Images 11, 4, 15, 6

Sir Francis Burdett (1770–1844) was an upper-class reformer and MP in the House of Commons for Westminster. He believed that the war with France caused the 'distress' and 'ruin' of the country, and he saw a direct relation to the worsening condition of the poor. In this speech to Parliament, Burdett complains that for frivolous reasons the government could not successfully engage in peace negotiations with France in 1800 and then bluntly asks for an end to the 'calamitous war' with France because it had caused the 'famished' condition of the 'public'. Prior to Burdett's speech, MP Mr. Robson avowed that 'a distressed people have been petitioning for, and anxiously waiting our meeting, in full expectation that we could give them relief'.[81] In his speech, Burdett disparages the Treasury Secretary William Pitt, the Younger (1759–1806), the famous Tory politician and prime minister in 1801, and 1804–1806. Pitt was reviled by many for his conservative politics and for raising taxes and also for helping put into place the repressive Acts against seditious activities. The speech also references Conservative MP Lord Greville (1762–1832) and diplomat and MP Lord Malmsbury (1746–1820). Burdett's speech aligns with many of the positions Isaac Eaton takes in *The Tocsin* in the first entry of this section regarding corrupt princes and their ministers and the results of endless war. It is time, says Burdett, for the country to turn to its own 'starving condition'. 'Bread', then, is the universal cry. Burdett derides the imperial motivations behind England's forcing of Union on Ireland in 1801 and its concomitant land grab in colonies afar, implying that such aggrandising ambitions abroad only hurt the ability to feed the poor at home.

DOI: 10.4324/9780429198052-4

3. Sir Francis Burdett, 'Speech', Commons Sitting (1800)

I must confess I never heard any thing with greater surprise than the speech I have heard this day from the throne. How dare Ministers put into his Majesty's mouth that which themselves and every man in this kingdom know to be false?—that they have been uniformly actuated by an ardent and sincere desire for peace!—The right honourable gentleman may possibly be afflicted with a shortness of memory, similar to that which manifested itself upon a very remarkable and interesting occasion in the year 1794; but, can it be obliterated from the memory of this House, that the right honourable gentleman, in a tone of exultation, and with fervent thanks to Divine Providence, expressed his heartfelt satisfaction at the prolongation of the horrors of war, on failure of Lord Malmsbury's negotiation at Lisle? Can we forget the still more recent instance of the hostile disposition of Minister to the French Republic, exhibited in that curious specimen of statesman-like wisdom, foresight, and moderation—the answer of my Lord Grenville to the peaceful overtures of the First Consul of France? I cannot consent to re-echo such falsehoods to the throne; nor indeed can I agree to any address, unless it were to remove his Majesty's Ministers, and put an end to this calamitous war.

Sir, the Chancellor of the Exchequer, regarding only the immensity of his receipts, his patronage and influence, and totally disregarding the consequent burthens and misery of the people, has from session to session been vaunting to us, in pompous strains, the prosperity, the triumphs, and boundless resources of the nation. At length, however, this triumphant nation is compelled, by imperious necessity, to turn its sorrowful eyes to its own starving condition. Administration have indeed triumphed over our unfortunate friends and allies the Dutch; they have flogged, tortured, massacred, and finally subjugated our fellow-subjects the Irish; they have wrested from a company of our own merchants the East Indies; they have annihilated the dearest rights and liberties of our countrymen at home; these are their triumphs—but the people want bread. Will it satisfy a starving Englishman, to be told that the Treasury-board sends its own members and creatures to enrich themselves as governors of Ceylon, the Cape of Good Hope, Madras, Bengal?—that they have bought out the proprietors of Irish boroughs, and made a hollow, because constrained union, and formed an Imperial Parliament?—that, at the expence of the miserable inhabitants of this country, they have indemnifed the American loyalists, rewarded the Corsican royalists, and supported the French emigrant clergy and the French emigrant noblesse?—that, with millions upon millions, the hard-earned substance of our industrious poor, they have prodigally and profligately subsidized the Russian, the Austrian, the Prussian, the Hessian, the Hanoverian, the Bavarian, the Sardinian, the Neopolitan, and even sent troops to protect and support the Pope? Will these triumphs, and their bounties, satisfy a famished public? No, Sir, the universal cry is for bread!—or that bread the scarcity of which is singly owing to these triumphs and bounties of our Ministers. They are the real monopolizers, forestallers, and regraters; a corrupt and wicked system of Government monopolises the wealth and prosperity of the country, and starves one part of the inhabitants to bribe the other. In announcing these harsh truths, I am discharging a sacred duty. We are called upon, at this time, to inquire into and point out the cause of that distress and famine which now afflict the land. We, Sir, of this House, have not far to look for it; it stares us in the face. There, Sir, it sits on that Treasury Bench! Sir, we have been long accustomed, and with too little attention and emotion, to go on voting millions upon millions, year after year, at the requisition of that right honourable gentleman. Sir, I am persuaded this House would not have proceeded so far in this career, if they had not believed they were merely voting so much money, and so many banknotes, which might be increased at pleasure as easily as they were voted.

Had the right honourable gentleman proposed to us the necessary though hidden consequence, instead of the specious and unsuspected cause; had he put to us the unmasked question, and bid us in so many words vote the starvation of our country, I dare not believe that any confidence in Ministers, any connections or dependence, any hopes, titles or emoluments, could have procured him a single vote in this House. And yet, Sir, that has been the real question on every one of his budgets. We do not eat money and bank-notes—money, and bank-notes are nothing but as they are representatives of the produce of man's labour. The Minister would not thank us for money and bank-notes, but as they are tickets entitling the bearer to so many heads of cattle from the graziers, or so many quarters of corn and grain from the cultivators of the earth. If this, Sir, cannot be denied, (and I am sure it cannot be denied,) let this House look attentively at the real situation of the country, and know the full-grown cause of our distress and ruin. Sir, let any man who understands arithmetic take his pen and ink, and see what remains to the cultivator, or other producer, after having satisfied all those who have tickets against him, as the reward of all his sweat, labour, and thirst employed upon his capital. Let us divide his produce into ninety, or nine hundred parts; perhaps we should have rather taken nine thousand, for it will be found that a very small fraction of a nine hundreth part remains to the producer.

From 900, the tythes, which must be paid, first	90
The rent,	300
The interest of the national debt, now equal to the rental of the kingdom	300
Income tax, at least	50
	740

These four articles alone take from the producer 740 parts from the 900, leaving him 160 parts, with which to satisfy the other ticket-bearers, such as, the king, and all the branches of the royal family:

For the civil list;
For the expences of government;
For the monstrous expences of the war;

For the increased and increasing poor;
For the militia;
For raising seamen and landmen;
For parochial and county rates.
Besides all these, there are
Tickets for those who invent the taxes;
for those who collect the taxes;
for those who receive the taxes;
for those who pay the taxes out again;
for penalties to spies and informers.

To this situation of the country, brought on by the politics of Ministers, I ascribe the present distressed state of the people; and as the address to approve the conduct of those to whom the public owes all its calamities, I certainly shall most strenuously oppose it.

4

THE WEAVERS AND TOWNSPEOPLE OF ROYTON, 'HANDBILL ISSUED BY THE WEAVERS AND TOWNSPEOPLE OF ROYTON IN MAY 1808, AFTER PARLIAMENT REJECTED A BILL TO GUARANTEE THE WEAVERS A MINIMUM WAGE'

(30 May 1808), NA Catalogue Ref. HO 42/95 f.375

With a sense of pride in their profession of weaving and confident in their patriotism, the weavers of Royton suggest that not everyone saw the decades-long war with France as being important to the nation's well-being. Instead, they note repeatedly the 'distress' the war was causing to the nation's labourers.

DOI: 10.4324/9780429198052-5

4. The weavers and townspeople of Royton, 'Handbill issued by the weavers and townspeople of Royton in May 1808, after Parliament rejected a bill to guarantee the weavers a minimum wage' (1808)

ROYTON.

At a Meeting of the Weavers and other Inhabitants of the Township of ROYTON, it was agreed to submit the following Statement of our Sufferings, and the Case thereof, to our Fellow Countrymen:

As we have been called upon to take part with you in your present proceedings, we the said Inhabitants feel it our indispensable duty to address you at this important crisis, upon the subject of our mutual distress; a subject that demands the most serious attention of every one of us, and upon which depends our happiness or misery. While we lament the general distress we beg leave to suggest that it is our opinion your proceedings are not likely to obtain you relief; for that distress can only be removed, by removing the cause;—which cause we have no hesitation in pronouncing is the WAR:—to prove which we need only refer to our dependence upon Commerce, and how it is obstructed by the War;—and it is our humble opinion that it is impossible for either the Legislature or commercial characters to remedy the evil by any other means than that of the restoration of Peace.

Fellow Countrymen,—We have been misrepresented and treated as enemies to our King and Country; but we can safely say, that our only wish has invariably been, a determination of the contest in which we are unfortunately engaged; and are now convinced, that it is an object equally the wish of the major part of the Country; and which we believe has been withheld from us by those whose Counsels have too long prevailed in this Country. Yet notwithstanding, we are ready at all times to forward, in any constitutional manner, that which is likely to be productive of the good we all aim at. But will never lend our aid to any illegal measure; therefore, by your permission, we will advise you to desist from our present proceedings—return to your families and respective employments; as the neglect so to do, will we fear, only tend to your misfortune and distress.

May 30th, 1808.

5

'A SUFFERER', 'LETTER TO PRINCE REGENT', 23 MAY 1812

Letters and Papers (MS Home Office Papers and Records, May 1812), Part Five: HO 42, Box 123

The early 1810s saw the rise of Luddism. The Luddites were famously known as machine-breakers who fought the reduction of wages and loss of employment due to the rise of the machines that replaced them. During 1811–1812 the Luddites committed breaking of machines and even murder to protest their conditions.

In 1811 merchant John Bellingham (1769–1812) murdered the British Prime Minister, Spencer Percival (1762–1812). As seen in this letter from 'A Sufferer', it was hoped by some in the lower classes that this assassination would lead to better conditions for the poor.

The Six Acts, with their repression of press and individual free speech as well as the prohibition of meetings, caused an outcry. One lower-class speaker complained of 'a large Army of 20,000 Men marching into the North of England', not to do battle with Bonaparte, but 'to subdue your own starving Countrymen, who are said to be in a state of insurrection, open rebellion against laziness for the want of employment, and consequent want of Bread'. Exhorting the tax-gatherers, or 'muck-workmen, these enemies of your rights and liberties, these hell-hounds who rob and plunder the people', the writer suggests these armies would eventually go after the 'half-starved, half-famished Army of wretched frame breakers', the Luddites.[82] Avowing that the lower classes saw no point in the war with France, the 'Sufferer' writes as follows.

DOI: 10.4324/9780429198052-6

5. 'A Sufferer', 'Letter to Prince Regent' (1812)

The Nation, Sir, has heard with indignation & no small portion of contempt the cobbled manner in which the old shoes of administration has been mended— The removal of the late Premier by the Patriot Bellingham created hopes in the breasts of Millions of Starving Tradesmen and Mechanics that a change of Men and consequent <?> measures would have ensued—that honest enlightened Men, Men in & on whom the country could have relied would have been called into the councils of the Nation—but their hopes are disappointed,—the Gauntlet is thrown down—they hestate not to take it up—The worst of Deaths stare them in the face—Starvation!—what man willing to work to support the cravings of an Infant family, will longer endure the prohibition of his Industry, whilst an unprincipled Prince surrounded by Whores & Rogues—whilst a profligate corrupt & obstinate ministry—shut their Eyes & Ears to their distresses—whilst Inquisitors under the appellation of Commissioners & Surchargers & their rapacious followers are let loose on them—his not the Work houses, his not the paupery about the public Streets, that denotes, that depicts the greatest scene of distress,—NO—his is the dwelling of the half famished Mechanic, his the house of the Honest Industrious Tradesman, accustomed to see better days tis there you must look to find real distress, tis there you must look to find misery in Perfection—look if you could into the minds of Thousands nay tens of Thousands of Fathers of Families—who have nothing but Despair in View—What say they, are the Berlin & Milan Decrees to us,—repeal them or we starve—We cannot Dig, for nobody has employ for us—We are ashamed to beg!—What must we do—Rob, Murder!—why then say they let us look first to those who whose wicked <causes>, to the infatuated Men & their more than infatuated Patron who has brought us to this deplorable State—

These are nice Sentiments,—What then must the Prince expect, who can without a struggle look down on the sufferings of a generous people with apathy, who shuts his Ears to every thing but what pampers a vitiated appetite, whose minions & mistresses engross all his thoughts,—who can spend at a feast a Sum that would make Hundreds happy—but this spending we do not think so much of—give us trade, give us an opportunity of exerting the Talent God has given us & that is all we ask—& then his Highness may honor the <?> of all, his Sycophants by planting Horns on every one of them—

You will not be pleased to observe, & which you are not only desired, but ordered to convey to the ear of your Master—that there are ten Thousand at least in this country equally daring, equally resolute, & equally determined as the Man branded with the name of Assassin—men who decry the doctrine, 'that to Murder Millions make a Hero, but to rid the World of one makes 'a villain'—Tell your Master (as you will answer for your neglect) to remember the Fortitude of Bellingham, Tell him that to starve is the worst of Deaths—that if he has no affection for his Wife

& Child, we have enough for ours to lay down our lives for them, even tho' ignominy be attach'd thereto—Tell him, that without a speedy alteration of measures, the gathering Storm will burst with irresistible force, as will not only shake the already tottering House of Brunswick to the Foundation, but will not even leave on Stone upon another—above all tell him to place little reliance on the fulsome addresses—for he may be assured that Thousands of those who have been compelled to sign them will be the first to gain the Red Flag when hoisted—

This letter Sir, is dictated by many, who are all ready to perish by famine—but who have united in this town & throughout the Country in Swearing that they will not perish alone—whose confidence in each other, Death has not terror to shake—Finally I do on their & my own part, conjure you as you value your life to communicate this to the Regent—I am—Sir,

A Sufferer

6

ANON., 'ART. XI. 1. *AN INQUIRY INTO THE CAUSES OF GENERAL POVERTY AND DEPENDANCE OF MANKIND; INCLUDING A FULL INVESTIGATION OF THE CORN LAWS*'

The Quarterly review, 16 (1816), pp. 225–278, on pp. 225–227, 229, 239, 244–245, 247–249, 251–253, 255–256, 259, 262–263, 272, 274–278

This article illustrates a strong aristocratic and monarchical bias, defending the Prince Regent and seeing the war as the only means to keep the nation secure and prosperous. The anti-democratic rhetoric glorifies and extols the sacrifices made by the country during the long war with France, and urges the people to see this period as one of England's legendary, even mythic, heroic ages. The writer assumes that everyone in the country was in agreement with this assessment, though the article is written to deride the 'anarchists' who were making the 'easily deluded' masses become dissatisfied with the government, in the belief it had caused their 'distress'. The writer seems to believe that the glory of winning the war after arduous years of fighting should be enough to fill the stomachs of the poor.

The piece refers derisively to the leaders of the masses as 'Mr. Examiner Hunt' and 'Mr. Orator Hunt'. Examiner Hunt was the famous poet Leigh Hunt (1784–1859) who published the radical journal *The Examiner*; Orator Hunt was Henry Hunt (1773–1835), an upper-class radical who was a powerful speaker at such events as Peterloo, for which he was arrested and jailed. Referring to the poor and their agitators as the so-called 'worst' parts of the British community, this article can also easily be seen as a response to *The Tocsin*. The famous and quirky agitator against the Corn Laws who published the weekly *Political Register*, William Cobbett (1763–1835), is also mentioned as one of the rabble-rousers trying to lead the masses to revolution. In an insulting blunt assessment, the text ultimately asserts that the constitution did not make the people hungry and thus it could do nothing about their hunger. Spence's Plan is a reference to Thomas Spence (1750–1814), a radical who believed in a form of communism where land would be commonly owned. Perpetually poor, he spent long periods of time in prison for his radical writings.

DOI: 10.4324/9780429198052-7

6. Anon., 'ART. XI. 1. *An Inquiry into the Causes of General Poverty and Dependance of Mankind; including a full investigation of the Corn Laws*'. *Quarterly review* (1816)

[....] Never before had the country been engaged in so long or so arduous a struggle; never had any country, in ancient or modern times, made such great and persevering exertions; never had any country displayed more perfect magnanimity and scarcely ever had any contest been terminated with such consummate and transcendant glory:—this at least is universally acknowledged;—it is confessed as much by the rage and astonishment of the ferocious revolutionist[....] Yet at this time when the plans of government have been successful beyond all former example—when the object of a twenty years war—has been attained, and England, enjoying the peace which she has thus bravely won should be left at leisure to pursue with undistracted attention those measures[,..] can [...] provide for an increasing and stable prosperity;—at this time a cry of discontent is gone forth, the apostles of anarchy take advantage of a temporary and partial distress, and by imposing upon the ignorance of the multitude, flattering their errors and inflaming their passions, are exciting them to sedition and rebellion[....]

It is boldly asserted that the late war was undertaken and carried on against the wishes of the people, and in support of despotic governments against the liberties of mankind; that it is the cause of the existing distress, being itself a consequence of the corrupt state of the representation; and that the remedy for all our evils is a Reform in Parliament[....]

[....] That the French were in a state of madness, is what all Frenchman of every party have confessed since they came to their senses after the reign of terror,—[....]

[T]he contest [...] loaded England with an enormous debt[....]

[....] Even now it is delightful to look back upon that exhilarating time, when after so long and unmitigated a season, hope came upon us like the first breath of summer;—when we met with gladness in every countenance, congratulation in every voice, sympathy in every heart, and every man felt prouder than in all former times of the name of Englishman, of the part which his country had acted, and was still called upon to act. These very men who now tell us that the present distress is the effect of wars unjustly commenced and pertinaciously persisted in, when no rational object was to be obtained—these very men who tell us that the war was not popular, that it was the work of a corrupt Parliament and not of the people,—these very men belie themselves as well as their country.

In reality, as Great Britain never before had been engaged in so long or so arduous a war, so never was any war so constantly approved by the great body of the people, because none was ever more unequivocally just[....]

[....] It was shewn in our last Number, in what manner the transition from a state of war to a state of peace produces, inevitably great embarrassment and extensive distress. The war, a customer to the amount of more than fifty millions annually, left the markets[....] Add also the consequences of a season which has been unfavourable to agricultural produce of every kind than any within the memory of man; and whatever difficulties and distresses may exist either in the agricultural or manufacturing part of the people, may be explained without referring them to corrupt parliaments, profligate ministers, and the Prince Regent[....]

We have before us the resolutions of sundry meetings held in the city of London[....] The resolutions from Bishopgate assert that the people are 'goaded with an army of remorseless tax-gatherers, urged on by the cravings of a rapacious, oppressive, and imbecile administration:' they remind us that our history exhibits the patriotic sons of England as 'dismissing and chastising those kings and counsellors, whose profligacy and arbitrary attempt had rendered them obnoxious;' they say that 'the most profligate expenditure among the people's servants, from the lowest to the highest rank, and an unfeeling disregard of the people's wants and miseries, are among the lightest subjects of complaint'[....] They say[,...] 'We claim, we demand and insist that we may have a constitutional voice in the House of the people'[....] The resolutions[...] complain of 'the long, desolating and profligate war against the French people, a war whose object, character, and consequences they both reprobate and deplore'[....]

'We asked bread', says an orator at one of the mob-meetings in the country, 'and they gave us a stone'[....] the men who invent or repeat every kind of calumny against their country have neither ears to hear, nor understanding to comprehend[....] these distempered times, when men[,.,] are continually addressing the worst passions of the worst part of the community for the purpose of bringing the worst of all imaginable calamities upon their country[....]

[....] Mr. Examiner Hunt does but blow the trumpet to usher in Mr. Orator Hunt in his tandem, with the tri-color flag [French] before him[....]

The circumstances which render the multitude more dangerous and more apt instruments for madmen and villains to work with than they ever were in other ages, have been indicated in this Journal on more than one occasion. We are treading upon gunpowder, and if we suffer the insane or the desperate to scatter firebrands,—it will be but a miserable consolation to know that the explosion by which he perish, will bury them also in the ruin which they produce[....]

[....] At present it is the influence of the democracy which has increased, it is increasing, and ought to be diminished[....]

[....] The multitude being ignorant are at all times easily deceived, and therefore sin through simplicity[....]

Our constitution has arisen out of our habits and necessities; it has grown without growth, and been gradually modified by the changes through which society is always passing in its progress. Under it we are free as our own thoughts; second to no people in arts, arms and enterprize; during prosperous times exceeding all in prosperity, and in this season of contingent, partial and temporary distress suffering less than any others, abounding in resources, abounding in charity, in knowledge, in piety and in virtue. The constitution is our Ark of the Covenant;—woe to the sacrilegious hand that would profane it[....]

[....] The representatives would still be what they are and what they ought to be—men of large landed property, whose families are as old in the country as the oaks upon their estates, having hereditary claims to the confidence of their constituents,—in a word, true English gentlemen[....] Such are the men whom the counties must always return upon any plan of representation: unless the frantic scheme of universal suffrage were adopted, which would inevitably and immediately lead to universal anarchy[....]

a mob-government [...] is much worse than anarchy, as the vilest ruffians of a civilized country are more wicked than rude savages[....]

[....] Those persons who tell the credulous and deluded people that taxes are levied for the good of administration, and who represent our statesmen as living and fattening upon the public spoil, must either be grossly ignorant, or wicked enough to employ arguments which they know to be false[....]

tavern-orators and mob-orators tell us 'a crisis is at hand,' [..] and stimulating the people to bring into practice what the Oracle at this precise time, with its usual felicity, calls the *sacred principle of Resistance*[....] 'every mechanic in the country'[...] who has legs to carry him, is invited to [...] 'hoist the flag of general distress'[....]

[....] It is fit that our readers should have their political confession of faith before them.

Spence's Plan.

For Parochial Partnerships in the Land
Is the only effectual Remedy for the
Distresses and Oppressions of the People[....]
For the LAND is the PEOPLE'S FARM[....]
'The Profit of the Earth is for all'[....]
Yet how deplorably destitute are the great Mass of the People![...]

It is then impudently false, as well as egregiously absurd, to charge that war [Napoleonic] as a crime upon the Government, and arraign Government for the distress which is unavoidably felt upon withdrawing from circulation the war expenditure, and the other changes incident upon a transition from the state of war to the state of peace[....]

We have shewn also that as the constitution of Parliament has not been the cause of the existing distress, so no change in that constitution could in the slightest degree possible degree alleviate that distress, or otherwise benefit the people[....]

No city in the kingdom is at this time experiencing such difficulty and distress as Birmingham; for this obvious reason, that no other place received so much direct employment from government during the war. This great annual expenditure was suddenly withdrawn, and there are now nearly a fifth part of the population receiving weekly relief; the masters being no longer able to employ the men, very man indeed having been ruined themselves This is a deplorable state of things, but it has not been occasioned by any misconduct or impolicy by [the government]; it is the plain unavoidable consequence of events over which no man or body of men could have any controul. In such a case what is to be done?[...] to mitigate the evil by giving as much temporary relief as possible, till new means of subsistence can be provided, by opening new channels of employment[....] There are above an hundred guardians of the poor, who go through the town[,...] and see where relief is wanted[....] And it is to the journeymen and poor of this town at this time that Mr. Cobbett addresses himself, seeking to irritate and inflame them, by the most seditious language, and the most calumnious falsehoods, and telling them that they are 'coaxed and threatened [by the government], with a *basin of carrion soup* in one hand, and a *halter* in the other!'

Why is it that this convicted incendiary, and others of the same stamp are permitted week after week to sow the seeds of rebellion, insulting the government, and defying the laws of the country?[...]

Of distresses, such as now pervade the mass of the community, small indeed is the part which parliaments or governments either create or cure. The causes of them, as we have abundantly shewn, either lie without the limits of human controul, or have been carried beyond our reach by the tide of time. We cannot command the seasons whose unkindness has aggravated the pressure bequeathed us by a long and exhausting war[....] In passing from a state of war to a state of peace, the shock of the revulsion might not improbably have been lessened to all orders of society somewhat graduating the transition. The die is now cast—the results, be they what they may, must be abided[....]

If stagnant manufacturers, and languishing agriculture, and a population suddenly turned loose from the military or naval services of the country, produce a supply of hands for which there is no work, a partial and temporary remedy might perhaps have been found in undertakings of public utility and magnificence—in the improvement of roads, the completion of canals, the erection of our National Monuments for Waterloo and Trafalgar[....]

The revision of the Poor-Laws—a work now of crying necessity—may lead to such corrections in that system, as shall at once extend its efficacy and lighten its almost intolerable burden[....]

In the midst of all these difficulties, however, one duty there certainly is which Government and Parliament are competent and called upon to discharge. They cannot stay the pestilence; but they can take care that, while it rages, the city is not plundered. They cannot (would to God they could!) charm away the embarrassments of the rich, and the privations of the poor; but they may, and they MUST, save both the poor and rich from the common curse and misery of a Revolution.

7

'PATRICIUS', 'TAXATION AGAINST POPULATION. *TO THE EDITORS OF THE LIVERPOOL MERCURY*'

The Liverpool Mercury (13 December 1816), p. 190

The Liverpool Mercury was a reformist newspaper, which can be inferred from the opinions of the letter writer below, who praises Cobbett and reviles Malthus. In incendiary prose regarding 'child murder', the writer, using the pseudonym 'Patricius', blames taxation and Malthusian malevolence for the starvation of the children of the poor. The piece refers to the government's abrogation of a former law that reduced taxation on those working-class families with two children or more. In other words, says the writer, once the war was over, government no longer needed the poor to produce more men to fight in the war.

DOI: 10.4324/9780429198052-8

7. 'Patricius', 'Taxation Against Population', *Liverpool Mercury* (1816)

To the EDITORS of the *Liverpool Mercury*.
GENTLEMEN:

I beg leave to commend to your notice the arguments contained in 'Cobbett's Address to the Journeymen and Labourers of England, &c.' which is calculated to do a vast deal of good, as it shows the origin and cause of the evils and privations now suffering by a great portion of the people.

I was much struck with that part of it which refers to the hints thrown out by Malthus to prevent the increase of population, from which we might infer that we shall not hear of any more prosecutions for child murder, particularly as the *Courier* of the 9th October says, 'we must be cruel only to be kind,' meaning, I suppose, that we must be guilty of the cruelty of killing our children, in order kindly to prevent their suffering the torments of poverty and starvation, to which they appear to be doomed through taxation.

Although I believed this Malthus was their scribe, and the Courier their tool and organ, it did not occur to me as at all possible that such doctrine could be sanctioned by the government of England.

But I have found that notices have appeared in the newspapers, that an act of parliament was passed on the 22d June, 1816, specifically for the purpose of repealing or omitting the allowance of 4 percent. (for each child above two years old) hitherto made out of the assessed taxes, not exceeding £50 per annum, paid by those who had and maintained more than two of their own lawful children.

This allowance, by being confined to those whose assessed taxes for a year did not exceed £50, was evidently intended to show that government was previously disposed to encourage population, and, as in justice they were bound, to equalize the burden of taxation, by such abatement to those who had to maintain a family of children.

I do therefore think, that by taking away the allowance, the ministers have identified themselves with Malthus and the *Courier*; and thereby proclaiming that population ought to be checked, they have virtually said to those who are now struggling to maintain their family of children, 'when we wanted men for the army and navy, to fight in the war by which we profited, we were glad to encourage children; but now we have ruined you by the taxes to support that war, we shall be glad to get rid of you and your children'.

Can any thing more fully prove the vassalage of the House of Commons than their having tamely passed such an act? No: and it adds another proof, if any were wanting, of the positive necessity of a reform in the manner of electing the members of that House, in order that the *British* people, who pay the taxes, may be fully and fairly represented therein, which they are not unless they resume the privilege of voting which by *birth-right* they inherit under the original constitution of their forefathers.

I am, Gentleman,
Yours, &c.
PATRICIUS
Liverpool, 2d Dec. 1816.

8

'ARISTIDES', 'RADICAL REVOLUTIONISTS AND MODERN WHIGS. TO THE EDITOR OF THE MORNING POST'

The Morning Post (24 December 1819), np

1819, the year of Peterloo, was a dangerous year for the labouring classes, particularly in the manufacturing districts. This letter to the editor is from an upper-class point of view in that, though it recognises the distresses of the people, it ultimately argues that such distress makes it even more important for the masses to rally round the government and resist radical agitators who would lead the people to rebellion and sedition. Said sedition, the writer remarks, is caused by the ignorance of the masses and would not put bread in their mouths. Negating those who blamed the war and taxation for the prevailing misery, the writer asserts in an odd conclusion that all of the money of the country ends up in the hands of the poor anyway. The writer reserves particular contumely for upper-class men like Burdett who supported the cause of the lower-class 'miscreants'. Hardly 'miscreants', the protestors at Peterloo were peaceful. In an article entitled 'Folly and Villainy of the Ministry—Manchester Meeting' in *Sherwin's Weekly Political Register* of 14 August 1819, just two days before this famous event, the writer excoriates Parliament for its acts against the people that 'crush the progress of political opinion'. The writer notes that the government and its loyalists

> are struck dumb with amazement to see forty or fifty thousand men assemble together, and though many thousands of them are literally in a starving state, conduct themselves quietly during the discussion of their grievous injuries, and at the conclusion proceed to their respective homes, without a single breach of the peace. It is vain that they seek for a pretext to call in the military.[83]

This piece, then, acts as a haunting plaudit for those who would die just two days later.

DOI: 10.4324/9780429198052-9

8. 'Aristides', 'Radical Revolutionists and Modern Whigs. To the Editor of The Morning Post', *Morning Post* (1819)

Sir—There never was a period when it appeared more important for every honest, honourable, and virtuous man to rally round the Government and Constituted Authorities than at the present. It is a melancholy fact, that at this moment of general distress in manufacturing quarters, there are many individuals wicked enough to take advantage of that distress, and to urge on ignorant and weak minds, by falsehood and seditious speeches, to acts of open rebellion and anarchy, with intent to rob and murder the loyal, honest, and peaceable people of the country; and ultimately, if in their power, to demolish the Government, and carry on a horrible state of savage disorganization and debasement. How much those vile teachers of sedition, of the wished-for scene of murder and robbery, are deserving of the severest punishment—of at least a removal from the country which they seek to embroil in the most shocking and deplorable state of revolutionary crimes and calamities, it is unnecessary to dwell on; suffice it on this head to say, that it is to be hoped for by all, both the deluded and those whom they seek to overwhelm with death and destruction, their punishment and day of retribution is not far off. It is to be remembered, that they are not practising on French ground, and that every man who has 20l. to lose, and a principle of Christian virtue to maintain, will be found more than a match for the horde of infidel miscreants, who trample on all law both divine and human. Moreover, to hear of men styled Nobles and Gentle-folks (*alias* gentry) thrusting themselves forward uncalled for, to countenance such wild and anarchous proceedings, and in fact rebellious movements, as they must be called, is beyond my comprehension, when contemplating that they would likely fall the first victims of that rebellious spirit, which their countenance, by upholding the false clamours against the Government and Parliament of the United Kingdom, tends to support and encourage. This is a lamentable fact, not so much on account of the mischief they do, as the circumstance that men of supposed sense, honour, and honesty, and who should be full ready to support the laws and crush disorder (so hurtful to all), are to be found wanting in the duty, which, in their respectable and exalted stations, they are bound to *exert*, in a state of civil society. Are they mad?—Are they desirous of conflagration?—Do they wish to divide their properties among the rascals, who would, but for the laws and the strong arm of Government, plunder them of it[?...] Far more wise and amiable would it be [...] to point out the real causes of distress, and the groundlessness of the pretended grievances, as held forth by both knaves and fools, and to unite with the supporters of the true interests of the country, and friends of Government, in proposing modes of relief unmixed with indigestible materials, for the truly distressed in the manufacturing districts, than to pursue their plans of starvation, by throwing out bones of contention that can do no good to none, but must increase the wants and calamities of those poor people[....] And as to their seditious meetings, they will never put bread in their mouths. I would certainly advise the true Whigs to propose meetings for the purpose of exploring the extent of the distress, and adopt, speedily, plans of relief. By this mode, the honest-minded and virtuous members of the distressed bodies from the loss of trade, would be withdrawn from the resolutely wicked, whilst the worthy and peaceably disposed would be provided for. If, on such occasions, any inflammatory or indigestible stuff were to be thrown in to injure the wholesome materials, I would pick them out and fling them over my shoulder[....] All paltry *party-spirit* and squabble should be unheard on such occasion. Benevolence and humanity should direct the proceedings. One thing, however, is to be borne in mind, which is, that the whole wealth of the nation constantly finds its way into the hands of the labouring populace of the country, and merely stops in the hands of the rich, until dispersed, whilst millions go to support the very poor and helpless part of the population. At the same time I should like to know, in what respect the grievances alluded to by the modern Whigs, as well as Radicals, are founded in fact? I should like to have them pointed out. They are *imaginary* and *fictitious*. Those fancied grievances are also brought home to Government, in as unfounded a manner as their existence. They are said to have proceeded from the measures of Government, and the loyal, for the last 25 years. The *War*, during which riches and every thing increased is said to be one. The very effect of the War, our then great prosperity, confutes the assertion. Next, we hear of the *Taxes*, but I will defy any man to prove that these have not been distributed, directly and indirectly, among the mass of the labouring classes of the community, and of course cannot have caused any distress in that quarter, but quite the reverse. Indeed, the taking off 20,000,000 of the taxes, has caused much distress, to manufacturers in particular, as well as in various lines. Where then are the grievances on these accounts, except in the imaginations of weak and knavish minds[?...]

9

T. WILLIAM, 'ADDRESS TO THE INDUSTRIOUS CLASSES OF BRITAIN AND IRELAND, PARTICULARLY TO OUR NEIGHBOURS, THE DISTRESSED SPITALFIELDS WEAVERS'

The Co-operative magazine and monthly herald, 1 (1826), pp. 333–337

In this radical venue (that only lasted a year), the author complains that the labourers produced the wealth of the country and yet still were relegated to starvation by the government. Calling for a system of communism, it urges the Spitalfields weavers to reject the politicians who would dupe them. Outlining the strategy of 'starvation wages', in which wages were pushed down through using the desperate Irish as scabs, the address appeals to the working classes to become conscious of the systemic biases that keep them at subsistence levels. This tirade against capitalism and the starvation wages it brought the poor ends up being an advertisement to break out of the systemic injustice of capitalist competition and join the London Co-Operative Society, where, according to this advertisement, labourers could work for each other and invest together to own land instead of having their lives destroyed by the landowners and manufacturers who currently owned the means of living. Only in this way would the worker find the 'comfort and happiness' they deserved by becoming their own masters. I have been unable to find further references to this group.

DOI: 10.4324/9780429198052-10

9. T. William, 'Address to the Industrious Classes of Britain and Ireland, Particularly to our Neighbours, the distressed Spitalfields Weavers', *Co-operative magazine and monthly herald* (1826)

The system of labor, by which your productive powers have been hitherto misdirected, is fast coming to its close. All kinds of labor, agricultural and manufacturing, Irish and English, are rapidly approaching their fated equality, the level of competition, or the starvation price, the lowest that, even in times of average employment, will support a miserable existence. The first years of the lives of those of you who are esteemed the most fortunate, are spent, at an absurd sacrifice of time and wealth, in acquiring a peculiar species of manufacturing skill: scientific improvements, mechanical, chemical, or otherwise, render in a moment all this skill useless. Peculiar circumstances give activity to some branch of trade, and your wages begin to advance: your employers, speculating every man for himself, as you are working every man for yourselves, invite by bounties and premiums of conveyance poor laborers from Ireland and Scotland to bring down your advancing wages: this temporary activity ceases: the strangers are left to perish, by those who invited them and by all the world, from diseases brought on by poverty; and your superior lot is that of a pauper starvation-preventing maintenance, or starvation-preventing wages. You produce all the wealth yearly consumed in the country, as well as that of a more permanent nature; and yet you, the producers, are in constant peril of perishing from want. Are not these things true? Look around you. How long shall these things be thus? *Ought* these things to remain thus? How long will you *permit* them to remain thus? It is in your power, without violence, to reverse this state of things, once and for ever.

Yet remain thus for ever they must, as long as you all continue, every individual working in opposition to every other, laboring for you know not what consumers in all parts of the globe; and as long as every trade and every individual in the same trade, whether living in the same or different places, continue the rivals and foes in competition of every other trade and of every other laborer. In vain, while this system of divided and jarring interest lasts, will you struggle against the evils that oppress you. Even your peaceable voluntary combinations or unions, legalized as they are, will not bear you up out of poverty and want, out of ignorance and vice, out of continued or encreasing wretchedness.

You struggle in vain against capitalists and landowners, who besides the overwhelming influence of their private wealth, are necessarily the makers of the laws, which regulate and tax your labour and control all your actions, even your words and opinions, to their supposed advantage. You struggle in vain against the competition of scientific power, which is every year rendering useless the acquired skill of your lives and rendering larger masses of your labor uncalled for, and thus in both ways bringing down the wretched renumeration of your toils. You struggle in vain against the free intercourse of persons and goods, which are necessary for the equal diffusion of knowledge and of mechanical and other species of scientific skill, throughout the globe, and for the purpose of raising, at the least cost of labor, the varied products of the earth for the use of its whole inhabitants—a freedom which not the united power of yourselves and any rulers you might appoint, could now restrain. Poor laborers or cheap goods, will, whether you or your rulers consent to it or not, continue to bring down to their own level your always decreasing wages. Not even the benevolence of your employers, unless that benevolence extended all over the globe, could remedy the evils that arise to you from this source.

How long, then, will you be the dupes of politicians and speculators, themselves the sincere dupes of their own want of knowledge and acquired habits? Each of whom is only looking forward to make what is called his fortune, that is to say, a large yearly command of the products of your labor for his exclusive use, by some of the thousand expedients of individual competition?

Did they not long ago and often promise you that *peace* [the end of the Napoleonic Wars] would make you comfortable and happy? Did they not promise that those who were *prudent as to marriage*, would infallibly be comfortable and happy? Did they not promise that *free trade* would make you comfortable and happy? Are they not now promising you that a *free trade in corn*, will make you comfortable and happy? Do they not tell you than an abolition of tithes, a reduction of taxation, a fixed metallic currency, a real representative system of government as affording the only solid foundation for the hope of these and other useful measures and a continuance of them, will make you comfortable and happy?

None of these measures will make you comfortable and happy, while the three paramount causes of your degradation, individual exertion and competition, scientific improvements superseding labor, and free intercourse of poor men or cheap goods, remain *in union*. Of these three obstacles, which now united oppose your happiness, the first, your only real foe, the misdirector of the others, individual exertion and competition, your own voluntary agreement may remove: but happily, no human power can now arrest the progress of scientific improvement and freedom of intercourse.

None of the above nor any other proposed measures, though all in themselves very useful measures, will, in any degree worth your consideration, amend your situation, until you yourselves adopt, in conjunction with these measures, *or even without them*, other and more efficient measures, which are in your power, without real injury to any, but with an ultimate increase of real happiness to all, which will together banish the wretched higglings and antipathies of competition, and will not only surmount the evil effects which you now experience from scientific improvements and free intercourse, but will at once convert them for you into the greatest blessings.

Who now consume—they do not enjoy—the products of your never-ending cheerless toils? Those who are in the actual possession of the land which supplies the basis and raw materials for all labor; those who are in possession of the machines, clothes, food, and articles to work upon, necessary to put your labor in motion and to support you while employed; factors, carriers, wholesale and retail dealers; those who contribute to your amusement by word, writing, or gesture;

those who take the trouble to do what they are pleased to call instructing you, and those who take the trouble of ruling and taxing you and distributing to those whom they think proper, with or without services, the amount of such taxation.

Would you get out from a wretched contest with these classes, who are now preying upon your labor, without any discussion or quarrelling with them? Would you like to be your own masters and your own employers? Would you like to be secure of employment, and of abundant remuneration for that employment, every day of your lives? Would you like that the labor of your wives should be in as constant demand, and while employed should be made as productive and as well remunerated as your own? Would you like that your children's labor, from the age of five to fifteen, should support and educate them more happily and better than the children of the richest are now supported and educated? Would you like that your hours of labor should be limited to the time compatible with health and daily enjoyment of social and intellectual pleasures? Would you like to be freed from all employments consuming your health, and cutting short your lives, and to enjoy an alternation of labor inside and outside of doors? Would you like to be provided for and taken care of, when accident, disease, or old age overtakes you? Would you like that your children should, during your lives and after your deaths, enjoy all the same advantages that you would enjoy? Would you like that your orphans should be provided for as well as if you lived? Would you like, yourselves to be the possessors in a few years, of the land from which your labor extracts food and materials, of the houses in which you live, of all the machinery and raw materials necessary to render your labor productive? Would you like, by these means to enjoy yourselves the whole products of your labor; and to obtain from that labor every means of comfort and enjoyment which rational beings deem it worthy their while to take the trouble producing?

If you would like to acquire these things, you have nothing more to do than simply to *alter the direction of your labor*. Instead of working for you know not whom, *work for each other*. Instead of all of you making silks, or shoes, or cottons; let some raise food, let some make and keep in repair your dwellings, manufacturing buildings, machinery, and furniture, let others make your clothing of linen, woollen, and cotton cloths, shoes, stockings, hats, &c. and let some of you continue to make silks or other articles in general demand, for acquiring by exchange those articles of convenience or comfort, which our climate or soil will not permit to be produced at home, or for the payment of necessary charges; or dispose of the surplus articles of your ordinary consumption for these purposes. Or let a competent number of your silk-weavers join a much larger number of agriculturalists and other artizans, and thus *supply each other's wants*, being producers and consumers, masters and employers, to each other.

For this purpose you must take land, at a perpetuity, or for a very long lease, or with liberty to purchase, within a given time, at a per centage on the rent, sufficient to afford, by your labor, food in abundance to support the whole of you and supply the most of the raw materials requisite for the making of the various articles of your clothing. Some of you must on this land erect your buildings, first for the most necessary manufactures, then for dwellings beautiful as your judgment and fancy may desire them; while the rest of you will be employed in raising food, making machinery, and providing for every one all the comforts, and ultimately all the desirable elegances of life. You must honestly and equally distribute to every member of your community all the means of happiness at your command, particularly all the means of happiness arising from wealth produced by your united labor, the faculties of all being equally cultivated and directed in the way most conducive to the happiness of all.

You are called upon, in order to accomplish these great objects, to no greater exertion than to contribute or gradually to save and accumulate, at the rate of five shillings down to sixpence a week, five pounds for every adult individual, and fifty for every child under ten years of age. The rest of the funds, but a few thousand pounds, necessary to make your labor productive, and ultimately to secure to yourselves the whole of its products (taxation excepted) will be contributed by those who now live, vexatiously to themselves, on the products of your labor, but would wish to cease so to live and to join with you in a scheme of equal and universal justice and happiness, or will be advanced on simple loan to you by benevolent persons who may possess them. Pay therefore either into a saving bank, or to a treasurer of your appointing, or to the secretary of the London Co-operative Society, 36, Red Lion Square, (who will attend for this and other purposes every Tuesday evening and Sunday morning) such subscriptions as you can afford, entering your names, with your occupation and residence, as members of a community for the supply of each others wants, and mutual and permanent insurance and independence. Should you wish in a few years to retire, you will be entitled on retiring to your full share of the encreased value of the establishment, which even in three or four years, though the first and most inefficient years of production, cannot be less than one hundred pounds each individual.—It is intended that a tract of land will be taken during this winter of some hundred acres, in proportion to the number of individuals contributing, and that early in the ensuing spring operations will be commenced on the ground. A community on these principles will be begun in the spring of 1827, with any number of the industrious classes who may come forward, from 200 to 2000 individuals. For details apply to the secretary, 36, Red Lion Square.

All your affairs are now managed by those whose immediate short-sighted interests—the only interests that the circumstances of their situation permit them to comprehend—are opposed to yours. *Take into your own hands the management of your own concerns.* Let the management and the interest go hand in hand. Look amongst yourselves; cast off the opinion of your own degradation, and you will find amongst yourselves skill of the head as well as of the hand. Let these two, henceforth, be equally cultivated and support each other.

Resolve; make a beginning. Persons having skill in every line of exertion will aid you. You own happiness and that of your descendants will be secured: and the selfish principle of competition will soon every where give way to the benign principle of mutual universal co-operation. In this great work you will have the happiness of leading the way in England.

(Cork, September 22, 1826) Wm. T.

10

D. W. HARVEY, SPEECH, 'STATE OF THE COUNTRY', COMMONS SITTING

Hansard, HC (12 June 1829), Volume 21, cols. 1781–1791

Daniel Whittle Harvey (1786–1863) was a radical returned to the Commons from Southwark. In this speech, he makes absolutely clear what caused the distress of the labourers—taxes. His contempt for his dithering colleagues, who thought endless looking into the matter was the proper course of action, is withering. Harvey captures how bureaucracy works, or, as Dickens, would later put it in *Little Dorrit* when famously describing the 'Circumlocution Office', 'How Not To Do It'. In this case, Parliament opted to avoid any action in response to the distress through 'prorogation', or the official ending of parliament for the season. The parliamentary record summarises the speech in the third person.

 DOI: 10.4324/9780429198052-11

10. D. W. Harvey. Speech, 'State of the Country', Commons Sitting (1829)

Mr. D. W. Harvey, said, he could not suffer the present occasion to pass without entering his protest against the extraordinary doctrines advanced from all sides of the House. Great distress was allowed by all to exist; some asserting that it was fearful and appalling, yet all seemed to concur in the impracticability of any remedy: now this for one he unequivocally denied. Oppressive and cruel as were the sufferings of the people, and aggravated as were their nature and endurance, he contended that the remedy was obvious, simple, and just. Inquiry was the fashionable cant of parliament; but the country was wearied with the sound, for inquiry was only another term for delusion and delay. If hon. members were ignorant, or rather affected to be ignorant, of the cause of our distresses and of the true remedy, the people were not: every man of common sense and common honesty well understood the national disease, the sole cure. The truth must be told: the country demanded, was entitled to, and must have, relief from the grinding oppression of taxation. All other plans and schemes were hollow shifting and worthless pretence. It was utterly impossible that the affairs of the country could move on with such a pressure. War taxes contracted through the agency of a paper currency could not be sustained when the currency was superseded, and consequently contracted, by metallic money[....] The plain truth was, that no man suggested the real remedy, and the people were made the instrument of their own undoing. All the petitions they presented and all the long and elaborate orations we heard upon corn, currency, ships, and free trade, were so many schemes of delusion. That House was quite satisfied with things as they were, and all that was aimed at was, to keep the public mind in a divided and distracted state upon matters which they little understand, and of little consequence if they did. If his voice could be heard to the remotest parts of the kingdom, and his advice were taken, it would be to proclaim one subject, and one subject only, and to petition for one object only namely, an honest deduction of taxation[....] For his part, he would far rather that 10,000 parsons should be a little inconvenienced than that millions of industrious citizens should be borne down with sorrow and starvation. The country ought to know how honourable members-those who talked long and loud upon corn and currency-acted when any question of practical relief was suggested. They either walked out of the House in troops, or remained to swell the ignoble triumphs of the Treasury bench. He was astonished at the plea which had been urged, that it was too late to do any good this session. When could it be too late to do good? Did we find it was too late to do evil? Unhappily, no[....] When private interests were to be promoted, or a Scandalous job confirmed, no period was too late; but to talk of relieving the people, or to care about them, was to touch the sensibilities of honorable members to the highest pitch of anguish, for which there was no cure but in prorogation. He had thus briefly spoken his sentiments, as a protest against the ungenerous doctrines which were advocated, and would conclude by declaring it his deliberate opinion, that nothing was easier than to place the affairs of the country in a sound, healthy, and prosperous position; that under able and honest councils this country might rise pre-eminent over all her difficulties, and become as distinguished in arts and peace, as she had been glorious in arms.

11

ANON., 'DOMESTIC POLICY. NO. III. *THE CONDITION OF THE LOWER ORDERS*'

Blackwood's Edinburgh magazine, 27 (1830), pp. 90–96, on pp. 91–96

Blackwood's (1817–1980), a Tory magazine, acted as the alternative magazine to the *Edinburgh Review*. The author of this article is extremely perceptive about the cultural and economic shifts brought about by the war, including the end of the social or moral compact between the classes. Noting that as long as the upper classes needed the labourer the labourer would be safe and comfortable, the article finds that the Napoleonic Wars had changed this relationship and led the masses to wretchedness and hunger. This text also participates in the argument discussed by many that England had enough unused land (called 'wastes') for the poor to live on and grow crops and thus achieve subsistence, the conclusion being that there should be no need for emigration, a remedy touted throughout the century when the poor were faced with economic disaster. The Latin phrase *pari passu* means 'on an equal footing'.

DOI: 10.4324/9780429198052-12

11. Anon., 'Domestic Policy. No. III. *The Condition of the Lower Orders*', *Blackwood's Edinburgh magazine* (1830)

[....] Our condition is the result of a new form which the industry of the country has assumed, greatly aggravated, as we must continue to maintain, by a monstrously erroneous policy with regard to trade and currency. This new form of industry, which made such rapid progress during the war, was, in consequence of the peculiar circumstances of the war, not felt by the common people, except in the alteration of their employments; but since the peace, while its progress has indeed been felt by them in the dreadful and appalling certainty, that as the world goes, it has no longer any need of them. The most important of the old relations of society have been changed, and that by a process, which although rapid, has been sufficiently gradual to bring the event upon us without our having taken such notice of it as would have led to our making due provision for the change. When society grew into its present form, of the few possessing much, and the many possessing nothing, the multitude dwelt safely, in security, that those who had possessions could not turn them to account without their aid—that wealth was nothing except in so far as it gave the power of accomplishing work—and that work could not be done without their assistance[....] It was true that labour was the portion of one part, while idleness, or at all events, exemption from bodily exertion, was that of the other[;..] and it was cheerfully submitted to, because it was the sure and always current value for subsistence. It is no longer thus; and it might melt the sternest heart to contemplate the hopeless wretchedness of thousands, almost millions, of their fellow-creatures, willing, eager, to give their labour for bread, and well able, too, until 'sharp misery had worn them to the bone', who yet cannot touch a particle of the abundance which teems around them[....] there is [...] a certain delirium reigns at the present time, about this thing, 'cheapness,' which having been taken up as a public principle, is, without hesitation, used as an excuse for individual selfishness. In vain the manufacturing towns throw off the surplus of their multitudes to the country—the poor have no land of their own—the rich, who have land, think it is very well as it is[;...] a much more perfect system of cultivation [would be] carried on, and a much greater number of people be supported thereby, in happy, though laborious, comfort[....]

London itself, with all its gorgeous show—with all its prodigious reality of wealth—with all that is magnificent in costliness, and all that is exquisite in art, yet teems with the direct miseries of actual want. Not merely that kind of want which must necessarily be found to some extent in all great cities, where disease and crime get huddled together in dark corners, and even common charity is scared away from those foul recesses in which all that is loathsome in degraded humanity rots and dies, in obscure despair. Not such want as this we speak of; but the decay of laborious decency, the misery of semi-starvation from want of employment of those hands which have never been employed in anything but honest industry[....]

[....] Why such distress should exist, and be in a progressive state of aggravation, *notwithstanding the immense accession, which has confessedly been made to our means of producing all those things of which 'distress,' as we have used the word, signifies the ABSENCE?* Why is it that want, and new and extraordinary means of producing abundance, proceed *pari passu*, and that those improvements which wear the appearance of a general blessing, are fraught with curses to the poor? It is because the process through which the advantages of industry were formerly obtained have undergone a change, and that change has taken away the *necessity* which did exist that labouring classes should have their share from the capitalists, of all these advantages. The only security which the labourer had at any time for his support was, as has been mentioned, the necessity for his assistance in order to make an advantage of the possessions held by his more fortunate brethren. If these possessions could be turned to profitable account without him, he would have been left to starve; and now that by our 'improvements' they can be turned to account without him, or with a great deal less of his assistance than formerly, he is accordingly left to starve. But had these means which are now 'improvements,' existed from the beginning, society would not have taken the form which it now has; laws would not have been suffered to accumulate one upon another, securing the property to a few, and leaving to the mass nothing but what their power of labouring gave them the command of, if, as now, that power was little or no security for support. If, then, we become satisfied that the great machine of society went well and smoothly hitherto, only in consequence of a connexion of its parts, formed by necessities and powers which adapted themselves to one another, it is not to be wondered at, that one side of the connexion, namely the necessitous, being in a great measure worn away, and one part of it work exceedingly to the disadvantage of the other. If the people are to live, if this kingdom is not to become merely the habitation of masters and machinery, with the few necessary to manufacture and attend upon those laborous and long-lived pieces of mechanism, some change must take place in the forms in which property and society are disposed.

If the people are to live, and machines make their labour of so little value to others that they cannot get the means of living in exchange for it, they must be provided with something upon which they can labour for themselves. If the world were all as one family, wherein each individual benefited according to the addition which could, by any means, be made to the common stock, then should we join with the political economists, and rejoice in the freedom of trade, and in every new device by which human labour could be dispensed with in the production of desirable commodities; but as that state of society has not yet come, we must, during the advent of such a happy consummation, resort to means adapted to the selfishness of mankind, and the new powers conferred on that selfishness, by the inventions which dispense with the labour of working men[....] Of what advantage to *us* these prodigious means of extending our manufactures without the aid of men, when so many of our own population are thereby left to idleness and starvation[....]

It is high time that the Parliament should look to this matter[....] Difficult as it is to force upon the attention of those who live in continual plenty and immoral indulgence the severe distress of those whom it is a trouble to them to think of, yet they can hardly be blind to the necessity of acting[....]

Without professing much respect for the wisdom generally displayed at extensive meetings of the lower orders, it must be allowed that at several of the many meetings lately held by the working people for discussing the subject of their distress, a rough and vigorous intelligence has been displayed, a readiness of speech and vehemence of expression, which indicate powers of mind that are worthy of some attention. We mean, that they give evidence of the existence of a description of men, who, with sense enough not to rush into a frantic and desperate tumult, can yet keep strongly alive in the minds of their companions the hardships which a state of things, subsisting only by the force of conventional law, entails upon them; and it is almost needless to add, that no duty of the legislature of a free country is more obvious than to examine, with even deferential attention, any cause of grievance which large bodies of the people firmly and calmly put forth as worthy of redress[....]

[....] Again, we say that the people know very well that the means are within the country to make them all comfortable; and let the Parliament beware how it drives them to take their own method of acting upon that knowledge[....] Parliament should take the earliest means possible of shewing the country that the distress of the people is felt, and that they will endeavour to remedy it[....] The disciples of Mr. Malthus are provided with an answer to this, by saying that the country has not resources for the comfortable support of the population, and, moreover, that the law of God is, that the condition of man inevitably leads to an abundance of people beyond the means of support[....] We are content to remark, that, as things are, nearly as much food is raised in these kingdoms as the population has need of [...] and [...] twice as much in England, and thrice as much in Ireland, could *easily* be raised.

Now the business of Parliament is, to consider *how* the resources of the country may best be made available or the people's support [...] we hold to be equally agreeable to reason, and to the spirit of the British Constitution[....]

[....] The evil is, that with respect to large bodies of the people, the means of exerting all beneficial industry are taken away; they want something *to work upon*, so as to provide for their necessities[....] The changes in the forms of industry having brought it to pass, that the industry of men will not exchange for subsistence in the ordinary traffic of the world, there is no resource, but that men shall be allowed to raise subsistence for themselves, out of the land[....]

[....] There is, undoubtedly, much to blame in our present system of provision for the poor[....] We cannot see why establishments of agricultural [...] villages, may not be adopted, connected with the parishes, to which the poor may be drafted, and where, under due regulation, they may be made to dwell very much happier than they have hitherto been[....]

[….] Our belief is, that some such things as we have mentioned, must be done for the prosperity, if not for the existence, of the state. Who can expect the governed to submit, if the protection which is the bond of their submission be not given them as far as it can be given? Let us then obtain that hold over them which a salutary guardianship will give us.

Part 2

RESPONSES TO MALTHUS, THE CORN LAWS AND THE POOR LAWS

Responses to Malthus, the Corn Laws and the Poor Laws were abundant across the first half of the nineteenth century—they were also intense and often dogmatic, dealing as they did with the distress—hunger—of the labouring poor.

In the following section we see that the radical journal *The Black Dwarf* was right in its assessment that the fight for the rights of the poor (Elizabeth 43) was against the rights of property, which were being asserted even more strongly as capitalist ideas gained ground. Malthus, James Mill and Parliamentarian Scarlett opposed any form of poor laws.

DOI: 10.4324/9780429198052-13

12

MP MR. SAMUEL WHITBREAD, 'POOR-LAWS BILL', COMMONS SITTING

Hansard, HC (19 February 1807), Volume 8, cols. 865–875

During the first three decades of the nineteenth century, Parliament attempted rather half-heartedly to revise or all but completely abolish the Poor Laws. One draconian measure put forth by Tory MP James Scarlett was clearly influenced by Malthus. Samuel Whitbread was an MP for Bedford. His speech represents a desire to revise the Poor Laws as though he was sympathetic to the poor, but ultimately he gets bogged down in vague means of reform, that is, suggesting that the poor be educated out of their poverty and distress. Implying that Elizabeth 43 and the social contract might no longer be legitimate and that the Poor Laws produced a lack of independence and a turn to idleness on the part of the poor, Whitbread still suggests that Christian charity should be adhered to. His proposal was eventually rejected. William Godwin (1756–1836), of course, was a famous Romantic writer and husband to Mary Wollstonecraft; when writing his tome on population, Malthus was responding against Godwin's utopian ideas. Robert Wallace (1697–1771) was a thinker whose work illustrated ideas Malthus would use in his own publications on population; those opposed to Malthus often made fun of him for ostensibly cribbing his ideas from Wallace.

Contrary to Whitbread's claims about the idle poor, the majority of the poor during the nineteenth century seemed to have expressed strong resistance to going into the workhouse. In addition, Whitbread does not acknowledge that the steep rise in population overall would have allowed and provided for higher levels of taxation to meet the increased demand for assistance by the lower-classes. He does, though, recognise that if the Poor Laws were abandoned altogether mass starvation and/or violence would be the result. Whitbread's speech is one of the first to lead the attack on the Poor Laws because, he irrationally noted, there were too many poor people who needed help, and, leading the charge that would see much use as an argument against the Poor Laws, they supposedly induced laziness in the poor.

DOI: 10.4324/9780429198052-14

12. MP. Mr. Samuel Whitbread, 'Poor-Laws Bill', Commons Sitting (1807)

Speaker; I rise to submit to the consideration of this house, one of the most interesting propositions which ever occupied the attention of any deliberative assembly on earth. I wish to engage you in an attempt at the solution of the most difficult of all political problems; namely, how to reduce the sum of human vice and misery, and how to augment that of human happiness and virtue amongst the subjects of this realm.-Sir, this attempt has been often and fruitlessly made; nevertheless I do not think the success of it impossible. However great the difficulty, it is our duty to endeavour at least to overcome it.-Sir, I will not now detain the house by an investigation of the original constitution of society; or enter into the abstract right of man to the succour and support of his fellow creatures. Whether that right exist or not; as individuals, we could never refuse relief to innocence, or even to guilt in distress; neither, as part of a legislature, could we ever be brought to say that such assistance shall not be attainable through the medium of the law. More than two centuries have elapsed, since after a succession of efforts, tending to the same end, there was embodied upon your statute-book, the great Christian principle, 'that you should do unto others as you would that others should do unto you.' What theory could be more delightful? As a state, you undertook to feed the hungry-to clothe the naked-to visit the sick-to protect the fatherless-to assist the widow-to find employment for the healthy and necessitous-and to compel work from the dissolute and the idle.-Sir, these plans were devised during the reign of Elizabeth; the glories of which are still vivid in the annals of our history. They were projected and carried into execution under the auspices of some of the wisest statesmen that ever presided in the councils of any country. They were not the sudden production of one particular period. They had occupied the attention of the legislature during the whole of that long and prosperous reign. From the 5th to the 14th-to the 18th-to the 39th down to the 43d of the queen, we find a constant succession of statutes, bearing testimony to the constant direction of the care of the government towards that object: till, at last, the work was complete.-But, sir, as if it were to confound the speculations of human wisdom, and to humble the pride of man, these schemes, reared upon a foundation apparently so solid, by workmen so able, have been inadequate to the object they had in view. It is an assertion now pretty generally made, that the system of our poor-laws has served to degrade those whom it was intended to exalt, to destroy the spirit of independence, throughout our land; to hold out hopes which cannot be realized; to encourage idleness and vice, and to produce a superfluous population, the offspring of improvidence, and the early victim of misery and want. That which in speculation ought to have been our glory, has been turned to our reproach. A committee of this house, appointed to enquire into the state of the poor of Ireland (where great wretchedness is said to prevail) and to suggest some remedy, have solemnly rejected the system of your poor-law, as likely, not only to be exceedingly oppressive to the land-owner, but to aggravate the distress of those for whose relief they would be enacted.-Sir, there has been a great revolution in the public mind. Till within a very few years of the period in which I am speaking, the 43d of Elizabeth was, if I am allowed the expression, considered as the *bible* on this subject. Many persons observing the rapid increase of the burthens imposed by that statute, have projected plans of reform, and the legislature has adopted many new acts; but they have all proceeded upon the same principle[....] But, sir, the period is arrived, in which I think it seems, by common consent, to be admitted, that some steps must be taken. You have lately had severe visitations from the hand of Providence, which have roused your attention to the state of your community. It has been said, that those calamities have been greatly increased by the depression they have occasioned of the character of your labouring poor. It has been said, that necessity having overcome the honest pride which formerly withheld a man from resorting to parochial relief, he no longer cares to recover his independence, but now voluntarily resorts to that assistance which he would before have indignantly avoided.-That such was the effect during the continuance of scarcity (and even since it has ceased) no man can deny: but, sir, I am willing to believe, and not without ground, that that effect is gradually wearing off; that the mind of the labouring class is recovering its elasticity, and that the proper pride of independence has, in a degree at least, resumed its place.-Sir, by the accurate returns which have of late years been laid before parliament, your situation is exposed to your view. The spectacle is indeed fearful, but it must be contemplated. In order to cure any wound, we must know its exact situation and depth. By the abstracts then upon your table, which were made up in the year 1803, it will appear, that upon a population in England and Wales, (exclusive of your army and navy) of 8,870,000 souls; not less than 1,234,000 are partakers of parochial relief. That is, that nearly one seventh part of your population is indebted to the rest wholly, or in part, for their support: and by far the larger part of that number is wholly subsisted without any exertion of their own. Sir, it is also proved that, exclusively of all collateral expence, such as army, militia, &c. which is raised at the same time with the rate for the relief of the poor, and paid out of it; there had been raised, in the year ending at Easter, 1803, for the maintenance and relief of the poor alone, the sum of 4,267,000*l.*; being almost double the sum raised for the same purpose, on the average of the years, 1783, 1784, 1785, and nearly treble the sum raised in 1776.-Sir, that a remedy for an evil so great and so rapidly increasing, ought immediately to be sought, all will be ready to agree: and I stand up before you, under the persuasion that I shall be able to propose to you improvements, regulations, and modifications to effect that end, which will not be found wholly unworthy of your attention.-However, small my personal claims to consideration may be, I am sure in the contemplation of my task, I shall meet with the favour of this house[....] I believe man to be born to labour as the sparks fly upwards; that a certain portion of misery is inseparable from mortality; and that all plans for the lodging, clothing, and feeding of all mankind, with what may be called comfort, are quite impossible in practice[....] One philosopher in particular has arisen amongst us, who has gone deeply into the causes of our present situation. I mean Mr. Malthus.

His work upon Population, has, I believe, been very generally read; and it has completed that change of opinion with regard to the poor-laws, which had before been in some measure begun[....] I am desirous of doing the most ample justice to his patient and profound research; to the inimitable clearness of his demonstration, and to the soundness of the principles on which he proceeds. I believe them to be incontrovertible. But in many of the conclusions to which he comes, I materially differ from him. Although I believe the design and intention of the author to be most benevolent, and that so much is to be collected from his writings, I think any man who reads them, ought to place a strict guard over his heart, lest, it become hardened against the distresses of his fellow creatures; lest in learning that misery and vice must of necessity maintain a footing in the world, he give up all attempt at their subjugation.-Sir, this philosopher has delivered it as his opinion, that the poor-laws have not only failed in their object, but that they have been productive of much more wretchedness than would have existed without them: that 'though they may have alleviated a little the intensity of individual misfortune, they have spread the evil over a larger surface.' [Malthus, v.ii.p.149.] Many persons agreeing in this position, have wished that the whole system was well expunged from our statute book; and perhaps I should not go too far in saying that such is the prevailing sentiment.-But, sir, I think no one has been bold enough to propose a total and immediate abrogation of the poor-laws. Sir, I need hardly say, that no man could be bold enough to propose that, which must in its operation generate a most formidable political convulsion, when the good to be obtained would be at best problematical and uncertain. But supposing the ultimate good to be certain: could we, to obtain it, give our consent to a measure which, in its dreadful execution, would be more widely fatal than any edict which ever proceeded from the hand of any tyrant conqueror upon earth; which would spread desolation, famine, and death throughout your land; and consign to a premature grave, infirmity, age, infancy, and innocence. Sir, the immediate abrogation of these laws is absolutely out of the question. I will dwell no longer upon it[....] The next plan we have to consider is Mr. Malthus's own: 'He proposes a regulation to be made, declaring that no child born from any marriage taking place after the expiration of a year from the date of the law; and no illegitimate child born two years from the same date, should ever be entitled to parish assistance' [vol. ii. P. 396]. It is unnecessary to state the details wherein he gives an account of the method whereby he would have such a law promulgated. By this measure the poor-laws would absolutely cease, after the expiration of a very short period, as to the rising generation[....] Sir, I am perfectly certain, that if the legislature could be induced to pass a law pregnant with such cruelty, within two years after the commencement of its operation it must be repealed. Neither of these plans, then, in my estimation, hold out any rational prospect of success towards the gradual abolition of the poor-laws[....] We ought, therefore, to consider, before we consent to its destruction, what the probable consequences would be[....] You could not condemn them to starve, and therefore you must allow those in need to beg. Are you prepared to encounter that host of sturdy and valiant beggars, who under the cloak of the distresses of those who were compelled to beg in order to preserve life, would extort from you wherewithal to indulge their profligate idleness? If you should absolutely deny their right to support out of your property, they might have recourse to the original right of occupancy. For each man born has surely a right to occupy a spot of ground, which may have been left unoccupied by those who had come into the world before him[....] But if all the land be occupied, so that those who are born can settle no where in order to maintain themselves, and you deny their right to assistance, your metaphysical positions may be unquestionable, but you would create a set of dangerous enemies. Might not they become a most formidable body? And what step could you take to cure or correct the evil you thus improvidently created?-Sir, I cannot look forward to such a situation without great dread and apprehension, nor can I consent to break that chain, which, with all its imperfections and disadvantages, binds the different classes of society so indissolubly together, and which I hope to preserve undissolved, and to be able to render light.-if then, sir, a total and immediate abrogation of your poor-laws is out of the question, and if no practicable plan presents itself for their gradual abolition, what remains to be done?[...] Sir, my wish is not to get rid of the poor-laws, but, I think, by taking proper steps, they may hereafter become almost obsolete. And I am sanguine enough to hope that if what I have to propose should meet with the concurrence of parliament, in the lapse of half a century they would be little used; but I would have such a code always remain on your statute book, in order that there might be a sure and legal refuge under any change of circumstances, or society, for indigence and distress.

13

ANON., 'LIBER SINE TITULO; OR, COPY OF A MANUSCRIPT-FRAGMENT FOUND AT A CERTAIN MOUNTAIN IN DERBYSHIRE, WHICH TAKES ITS NAME FROM THE DEVIL'

The Scourge, or, Literary, theatrical, and miscellaneous magazine, 9 (1815), pp. 277–281

This piece in the radical northern journal *The Scourge* satirically uses a common trope of the Devil speaking as the leader of governmental attacks on the poor; in this case, the Devil is a Malthusian who gleefully uses war as a means of population control and of overturning the rights of the poor to life itself. The author indulges in the beloved rhetorical tool of including a guessing game or fill-in-the-blank with a noteworthy name of the time. Not all of these references are possible to decipher. Note how this devil makes fun of the poor for asking for bread to live. The 'learned divine' is Malthus.

DOI: 10.4324/9780429198052-15

13. Anon., 'Liber Sine Titulo; or, Copy of a Manuscript-Fragment found at a certain Mountain in Derbyshire, which takes its Name from the Devil', *Scourge, or, Literary, theatrical, and miscellaneous magazine* (1815)

For as hunger tameth the lion, even so shall lack of bread enervate man. Therefore, listen unto me, ye rulers of the earth, and ye kings and princes, hearken to the counsels of the first subduer of men.

And the multitude crieth—give us bread—that we may live. And why must the multitude live? Verily, as was aptly observed by one of my most approved ministers, I see no necessity why they should live!

Hath not a learned divine proved to demonstration, that the power of population in man, and the power of the earth in producing sustenance for his support, is proportionate and commensurate to the difference between a geometrical and an arithmetical series? What will ye then with peace? Is not war necessary, to prevent your dying by starvation?

Again, has not a very learned and famous professor of political economy published a most marvelous and masterly work, in which he proveth to you, that whoever amongst you, be he man, woman, or child, who can not suffice to his own support, by his own manual labour, hath no right to live? yea, verily so doth the learned Doctor M___s write! And shall the multitude then be permitted to grumble and repine? Why do they not march? and why should starving wretches rail against a standing army?[...]

A late learned and right reverend divine has publicly told you, that the multitude have no right to reason, or to think about the laws; all that they have got to do, is to obey them[....]

Ye complain likewise of the scarcity of money. What is it, I ween, makes an article rare and valuable, but its scarcity? Ought ye not then to thank the rulers, who effect so valuable a scarcity among you. And in what country do the rulers, and the mighty men co-operate more strenuously, more efficaciously towards the *increase* of this *scarcity*, than in your own?

Ye pretend, that all men are, by nature, equal; that they have a right to equal laws and equal justice. Fine doctrine this, in very truth! Wot ye not, that the several members of society are like unto the notes of an instrument, even like unto the keys of a *piano-forte*. And have ye not, amongst these several keys, some which are *sharps* some which are *flats*, and some which are *naturals*? Or, if ye will liken yourselves unto a fiddle; so are ye subjects the *cords*, and your ruler the *fiddle-stick*, that plays upon you—or rather, your rulers are the *fingers*, which *pinch* and attune the *cords*!

Peradventure, were I to tell you my name, and who I am, you would imagine that I am the enemy of all religion[....]

Behold, I tell you a parable:—Where mushrooms grow, there must be soil. Now, the mushroom is of speedy growth, and waxeth amazingly. And so do *toad-stools* likewise. Now if a man have a bed of mushrooms, and it so happeneth, that toad-stools spring up among them, what doth this man do? Doth he not root out the toad-stools, which suck up the nurture of the soil, and impede the wholesome growth of the mushrooms? But which, ye will say, are the mushrooms, and which the toad-stools? That question must ye decide yourselves.—Ask not counsel of the rich, nor of the mighty—for then will ye be the toad-stools, and the hand of power shall root you up.

Again, I no longer speak in parables, but I will hold you up a mirror, even a reflecting glass, in which ye may discern at once, your own wants, and the quarter, from which those wants may be relieved.

Doth any man want virtuous example, and moral pattern to regulate his conduct, let him look ......*to the P*_____ [the Prince Regent?]
For munificence, liberality, and generous feeling *to the Q*___[Queen?]
For unfeigned piety......................*to a certain Reverend Baronet* [Francis Burdett?]
For true and genuine patriotism.........................*to the INS.*
For disinterested politics...................*to the OUTS.*
For ability............. *to Ministers.*
For modesty............*to Lord C------h.* [Whig MP Castlereagh]
For candour, and for justice.....................*to Lord E-----------.* [Chief Justice King's Bench, Ellenborough]
For economy..............*to the Dispensers of the Public Purse.*
For wisdom and shrewd talent..........*to a worthy Alderman.*
For patient resignation.........*to Lord Cochrane.*
For the counter-part to the matron of Ephesus *to Mr. C-----tts.* [Sir Francis Burdett Coutts]
For untasted fruit------------*to the late Miss M-------.* [Miss Martineau (1802–1876) writer, philosopher, and supporter of Malthus]
For the most flourishing country in the universe *to his own.*
For happiness.....................*elsewhere.*
For the blessings of peace...........*to a starving Population.*
For patriotic zeal and sacrifice........*to the Landholders.*
For an ass.................*to John Bull.* [fictional name for the English people]
For mildness......................*to his Drivers.*
For wit..................*to our modern Play-wrights.*
For unassuming worth..........*to our Actors and Actresses.*
For deference to public opinion.......*to the Managers.*
For heaven................*abroad.*
For hell....................*at home.*
For the devil.........*to his Wife, or any person except myself.*

14

GEORGE ENSOR, 'AN INQUIRY CONCERNING THE POPULATION OF NATIONS; CONTAINING A REFUTATION OF MR. MALTHUS'S ESSAY ON POPULATION'

Monthly Magazine, or, British register, 45 (1818), pp. 640–650

A prominent Irish journalist, Ensor (1769–1843) calls Malthus to account for his lugubrious and all-consuming belief in the misery of human life, but further derides him for making the poor the premier group for such distress. He particularly lays waste to Malthus's claim that God made a mighty feast for his children but not everyone was allowed at the table—some mighty feast, as it were. With vigorous sarcasm, he examines what he sees as Malthus's hypocrisy and contradictions. Ultimately Ensor finds the fallacy of Malthus's thought in the fact that one-fifth of the population (the rich) consume four-fifths of the food. Ensor mentions William Paley, the educator and thinker (1743–1805). *Hanc deus et melior litem natura diremit* means 'God or a better Nature'. *Est operae pretium duplicis pernoscere juris Naturum* means 'It is worth twice the understanding of natural law'.

DOI: 10.4324/9780429198052-16

14. George Ensor, 'An Inquiry Concerning the Population of Nations; Containing A Refutation of Mr. Malthus's Essay on Population', *Monthly Magazine, or, British register* (1818)

[....] Mr. Malthus says, 'It is an utter misconception of my argument to infer that I am an enemy to population,—I am only an enemy to vice and misery.' In what religion, in what state, in what age, does he not exhibit the misery of mankind? What is the burthen of his theme?—That population 'presses so hard against the limits of their food, that their population pressed so hard against the limits of their means of subsistence,' which he frequently repeats. Does he not involve all savage and civilised societies, all states ancient and modern, every European nation now existing[,..] as labouring under this pressure? Distress so clings to mankind in his system, that the sum of his philosophy is,—man and misery, no matter whether many or few, whether thronged in cities, united in towns, cultivating the earth, pasturing herds of cattle, hunting nature's commoners,—in every variety of life, in every shade of being, mankind exceeds the subsistence which the earth affords:

> No living thing, whate'er its food, feasts
> there,
> But the chamelion, who can feast on air.

[....] Yet what is more broadly advanced by him?—is it not his primary position; is it not the aim of his argument; does it not intervene in his details—that man by nature tends to increase beyond the increase of subsistence, and this with accelerated progression? He states in the beginning of his treatise, that *population has a constant tendency to increase beyond the means of subsistence.* To the same effect, he says, 'the *tendency* to early marriages is so strong that we want every possible help that we can get to counteract it.' Here this natural tendency [of sexual desire] is so strong, that it requires, according to him, a double check. Is this tendency natural or not? Will he say it is unnatural?—Yet it is to be counteracted by every possible means, he says, because it is pernicious. And yet Mr. Malthus also says, 'We cannot but conceive that it is an object of the Creator that the earth should be replenished; and it appears to me clear, that this would not be effected without a tendency in population to increase faster than food: and, as, without the present law of increase, the peopling of the earth does not proceed very rapidly, we have undoubtedly some reason to believe that this law is not too powerful for its apparent object. The desire of the means of subsistence would be comparatively confined in its effects, and would fail of producing that general activity so necessary to the improvement of the human faculties, were it not for the strong universal effort of population to increase with greater rapidity than its supplies.'

Mark this passage. What becomes of his praise of population when it follows its natural order? which order, in the last quotation he insists is not the order of God's providence; for God impressed a tendency to population faster than food;

and that this advance of population was necessary to improve the human faculties and people the earth.

Hanc deus et melior litem natura diremit.

The contradictions of Mr. Malthus multiply on every topic. He talks of the wisdom of the Author of nature, 'which is apparent in all his works;' and again, 'the laws of nature which are the laws of God.' Yet how grievously he charges with evil these same laws in the following words: that, 'though human institutions appear to be, and indeed often are, the obvious and obtrusive causes of much mischief to mankind, they are in reality light and superficial in comparison with the deep-rooted causes of evil which result from the laws of nature and the passions of mankind:'

Est operae pretium duplicis pernoscere juris Naturum.

This is truly a new way of reasoning from nature's law to nature's God. But it certainly proves one position of the Professor of Political Economy in the East India college,—that the subject of population is *yet in its infancy*, if he be the master of the art.

These contradictions and repugnances of Mr. Malthus I here mention to justify for the present a passing observation on his defects; for I shall hereafter, when I investigate his theory, exhibit numerous inconsistencies in his essay. The reason of this sad deficiency in this writer has proceeded from different causes. Having originally, as appears to me, no commanding mind, with moderate learning, and, by his own avowal in respect to this particular subject, very limited knowledge; he fastened a theory on a dispute, and thus advanced opinions which he had not ingenuousness to retract, and dared not defend. Finding, on consideration, that his original doctrine was narrow, and false, and hideous—for what could be more false and monstrous than that population was only controlled by vice and misery?—he attempted to restore its credit by adding moral restraint to the insolvent form of his philosophy. And, in order to keep these partners in tolerable society, he laboured to reconcile antipathies and harmonize discord. Thus his contradictions have increased with every new edition; till, in some instances, as in that already noticed, of increase and supplies, tendency and natural, and nature and God, they resemble a certain glorious creed[....]

It is a dogma of Mr. Malthus, that there is a tendency in nature to increase beyond the means of subsistence[....] as if breeding were condemned and not commanded. He says, 'in the moral government of the world it seems evidently necessary that the sins of the father should be visited upon their children.' I do not perceive the evident necessity of any punishment undeserved. We are, however, obliged to Mr. Malthus for discovering that 'increase and multiply' is original sin and its punishment also.

This is among the rare inventions of Mr. Malthus[....] he considered neither children nor parents, but full-grown men meet at *nature's mighty feast*, at which a straggler obtruded, who is thrust out, for *there is no cover for him*. A mighty feast truly, which could not afford food for one casual visitor. Yet here he holds to his text; for even at nature's feast, to which Mr. Malthus is the purveyor, population presses against the means of subsistence, and the banquet of nature shrinks into a short allowance ministered by a miser[....] By what law of nature do some feast, and many want necessaries—nay, want necessaries, that others may feast in spite of nature? By what view of nature, or God, or man, do some rejoice in all the delicacies of the season—that is, all unseasonable things; and others suffer the privations of grain and roots planted in due time, and gathered accordingly. There are questions on this subject that have escaped Mr. Malthus. Paley's *Philosophy*, which is the text-book in our university, and of course not jacobinical, speaks of another feast, from which, he says, 'you would hardly permit any one to fill his pockets or his wallet, or carry off with him a quantity of provision to hoard up, or waste, or give his dogs, or stew down in sauces, or convert into articles of superfluous luxury; especially if, by so doing, he pinched the guests at the lower-end of the table.' Yet, this is permitted by Mr. Malthus; and the guest so pinched, is reviled for not obeying the repeated admonitions of God and nature.

Mr. Malthus says, no one has a right to subsistence when his labour will not fairly purchase it. If so, a portion of this man's property is more sacred than that man's life. But suppose the position turn, and that a right to subsistence depends on the labour of the individual:—who labour? the rich, the aristocracy, the proprietors of land, the holders of stock, heirs in their own right, and princes by right divine?—Here again Paley interposes: 'It is a mistake to suppose that the rich man maintains his servants, tradesmen, tenants, and labourers: the truth is, they maintain him.' Mr. Malthus may have heard that the strongest spirit is drawn from the poorest grape; but he has not heard that the greatest wealth is produced by the poorest men.

Mr. Malthus considers that attributing in any way the distress of the poor to the higher classes of society is a vulgar error, and asserting that they suffer by the mismanagement and prodigality of rulers, is the greatest wickedness: nay, that those who impeach human institutions, for numerous evils to society, are the most successful supporters of despotism;—to which he adds something about *revolutionary horrors*. These are astounding dogmas. He thinks that governments are comparatively inoperative respecting the wants and unhappiness of the people, and *that it depends upon the conduct of the poor themselves*. Does it depend on the slaves themselves? Did it depend on the people in France that the nobles were exonerated taxes?[...] Does it depend on the poor of England that they pay for salt a tax thirty times the original cost of the article? Did the British people war on France in defence of the old monarchy and of its priests and nobles? Do the people who pay the taxes incurred in that war understand *legitimacy*?

Mr. Malthus abuses the people; and against none has he been unmeasured in his slanders than against the British people. He says of them, 'Even when they have an opportunity of saving, they seldom exercise it.' Yet, amidst aggravated taxation and distress, eight hundred thousand labouring Britons are now enrolled in benefit societies [to save money]. The fact is, the poor have increased, because the wages of labour have not at all advanced proportionably to the enhancement of the articles of subsistence, and that much capital has been extinguished. As tastes augmented, the necessaries of the people—their bread, beer, cheese, tobacco, soap, salt, &c.—were surcharged: and, as the taxes pressed unequally, some had their comforts curtailed, others were reduced to a stint; and many, from the crowd forced down into the lowest order of labourers, have been rendered miserable. The poor-rates (I speak of course generally) simply return in alms part of those sums which unfeeling landlords, griping priests, the state money-changers, and a rapacious prodigal government have wrested from the pittance of the laborious.

[....] And mark his contradictions. He states that 'the principal and most permanent cause of poverty has little or no direct relation to forms of government *or the unequal division of property*; and that, as the rich do not in reality possess the power of finding employment and maintenance for the poor, the poor cannot, in the *nature* of things, possess the right to demand them.' I tell you again, from Paley, that it is the poor who support the rich; and it is contrary to *the nature* of things, for the rich to demand more from the poor than they can conveniently grant. The question between the rich and poor is not whether the rich should give or maintain, but whether they should take and impoverish[....]

MR. MALTHUS'S HYPOTHESIS.

He says, 'population has this constant tendency to increase beyond the means of subsistence.' To make this statement very imposing, he avers that population increases in a geometrical, and food in an arithmetical, ratio, which might be summarily denied by the oracular answer[....] This perversion of the terms of an abstract science has deceived many. He proceeds, 'The rate according to which the productions of the earth may be supposed to increase, it will not be easy to determine. Of this, however, we may be perfectly certain, that the ratio of their increase must be totally of a different form the ratio of the increase of population. A thousand millions are just as easily doubled every twenty-five years, by the power of population, as a thousand; but the food to support the increase from the greater number will by no means be obtained with the same facility.' Suppose so; what fact is told, what truth is taught, what conclusion is realized or approached, in consequence[....] Should we follow Mr. Malthus in *supposing*, we might invert the terms, and assume that food increased beyond the people by a transcendental geometry. If Mr. Malthus supposes that a thousand millions may be doubled every twenty-five years by the power of population, I may suppose that the food of man may be doubled a thousand times in the same period: a herring has 40,000 eggs, a cod fish ten times that number. But without resorting to the icthyophagi, or going beyond the earth, it appears that in 1788 two bulls and three cows strayed away in New South Wales, who in seven years increased to a heard of a thousand[....] I say, I may suppose on these suppositions, that the food of man may multiply far beyond the possible multiplication of man[....]

The arithmetical and geometrical ratios are jargon. Where property is equitably divided, and labour free, there will be no tendency but to supply what is wanting. Mr. Malthus pleads for discord: yet, where is neither force nor justice, all things will repose when rest is necessary, and all will move with the general impulse. This order the ancients called the harmonical.

TRUE CAUSES OF MISERY.

[....] Let us consider the question of pressure under another view: let us dismiss the operation of misgovernment entirely from the argument, and let us make England the ground-work of this study. First, I must state, that I do not say there is no misery in England; on the contrary, I am satisfied that it is urgent and extensive. Yet I say, there is no grievous pressure by population against subsistence. When we talk of population and subsistence, we should consider all the people and all the food. Then, if the sum of one does not exceed the sum of the other, there is no deficiency. If, however, one fifth of the people take five portions of food, leaving the other four parts of the population short by so much of their proportion, this is not properly a pressure of population against food. In like manner, if one part of the community force another part to labour, while they themselves are indolent, this is not the pressure of labour on population[....]

How in this country it can be said that population presses against subsistence, I cannot understand, when so much is destroyed; for one half of the food on such occasions is burned, exhausted, evaporated—divided between the fire and air; and then, of that which escapes culinary consumption, twice as much is eaten as health requires. Compare then in England those who waste and eat and drink inordinately, with those who live sordidly through necessity,—and the pressure on subsistence will be greatly relieved: nor have I any doubt but many more die by satiety than privation. The poor man has complaints, but they are limited by his means; while the retinue of a rich man's disorders equals the extent of his fortune.

[....] But what are lapdogs and the sportsman's dogs—from king Charles's spaniel to the king's buckhounds led by the duke of Montrose—to the studs of hunters and racers, and the rabble of pampered idle horses which swarm through the land? Do these not press on subsistence? How much do the savage animals corrode and consume of man's food[....]

Nothing, however, is said by Mr. Malthus on these topics: a lady's pug-dog, or a hound, or a pointer, is unnoticed; but a child too many obtrudes on *nature's feast*[....]

LIBERTY.

Though I do not say that no free nation can become too populous, I presume that when the government is essentially vicious, the cause of the people's misery is more decisively referable in the first instance to the badness of the government than to the improvidence of the people. This is strictly just; for we know that nations, formerly poor and thinly inhabited, have, with a better government, increased in numbers and comforts; and, on the contrary, that nations populous and opulent, have with the debasement of their laws and constitution, declined not more in people than in their enjoyments of life. Yet am I ignorant of any nation, which, possessing confirmed liberty and equal laws, has become miserable merely by the excess of its people.

Having reviewed the state of population in different countries and in dissimilar situations, I conclude that neither the populousness of a nation, nor the paucity of its inhabitants, is alarming. It is bad governments and unequal laws and disproportioned property that are dreadful;—these render the few and the many miserable: while a nation well governed, or rather not misgoverned, increases in people, and enlarges their store and their comforts[....]

STATE OF ENGLAND.

The people are poor, and growing poorer. The cause of this seems to me no mystery. Some say, the more you give them the more they want. The misapplication of funds may increase the mendicant order, I admit; but the poor in England increase not by what is given, but by what is subtracted from the people. The wealth of states was derived from labour, and by labour it must be sustained. It seems equally clear, that a certain profit is necessary to support capital, and certain wages to support labour. Thence it follows, that, after a certain charge on capital, it will escape abroad or perish at home; that this will affect the wages of labour, as it curtails the means of employment; and should wages, beside their depreciation in consequence, be lessened by direct or indirect charges, poverty must ensue. That this has happened, I shall evince by a recital of the repeated and enormous impositions on the people of England.

The waste of the people's money by the House of Commons is almost incredible[....]

It is wonderful how any nation could support such universal waste. The British subsidized almost every nation in Europe with many millions [during the Napoleonic Wars]; and she alternately fought and subsidized the same nation; she became security also for some, and of course liquidated their debts. She bound herself for Austria to her own money-lenders; and she pays them, and must continue to pay them. She remitted ten millions sterling to the French, due for the maintenance of their prisoners, as part of the bonus for their submission to Louis. She pensioned the emigrant French priests, and continues to pay them. She paid Ferdinand's travelling expenses from Valencia to Madrid; Louis the Eighteenth's from London to Paris; the Pope's from Bologna to Rome. She, to please the prince, raises a monument to the last of the Stuarts. Yet all these were but the outward flourishes of the waste and prodigality of our sad government.

CONCLUSION.

[....] Populousness is good, if the government be good; and, as Hume says, 'every country will abound with people and their comforts as it is well governed.' Under a well-organized constitution, authentic laws, and their prudent administration, the people will improve their intelligence; and this will regulate their number, by ascertaining their wants and conveniences. That constitution is best which effects the greatest good to all without injuring any. If one obtains more than his usefulness merits, if one obtains less than his usefulness deserves, society is disturbed, and in proportion to the amount of the iniquity. Every one should possess absolutely his time and the profits of his labour: and, as the pains to obtain things teach prudence in their use, he who earns will best employ the produce of his industry. In like manner, those who contribute to the public should not merely determine the necessity and quantity of the supply but superintend its expenditure:—therefore, that representation is most secure which is most popular; and that administration is most efficient which introduces domestic economy into the management of public affairs[....] In consequence, whatever lessens expense is good: for expense is supported by labour, labour is onerous, and the burthen is the people's. Utility should be regarded in all political concerns, and utility can only be learned of the people, through the people;—the people are the eye, the light, the object, and the mirror.

Far be it from my philosophy to adorn one with the attributes of all, and to starve the board of many, that whom supports a *royal servitude* may sicken with plethora and kill sense with enjoyment. Still further be it from me to prefer the few to the many: for this multiplies a single mischief, transforms the dog to Cerberus, and the snake to Hydra. The people, the many, the commonality—these are the only legitimate objects of philosophical legislation. What are patricians contra-distinguished to the people? Parentage. What nobles? The will of one man [the king],—of one weak man, made weaker by flattery and dominion. It is that monstrous perversion—counting the many as ciphers, and one or the few as millions—which has occasioned disaster, distraction, revolutions in states and societies, and which has confounded, outraged, overwhelmed mankind in all countries and ages. The wickedness and infatuation of ambitious individuals to move a great weight by an inferior force, and to continue the extravagance, may be called the *great war*. It contravenes the principles of matter, of mind, of the earth, and universe.

15

'POOR RELIEF BILL', COMMONS SITTING; CONTINUATION OF DISCUSSION 'POOR RELIEF BILL', COMMONS SITTING

Hansard, HC (24 May 1821), Volume 5, cols. 988–999; (2 July 1821), cols. 1480–1485

In an embarrassing admission, MP James Scarlett states in this speech to the House of Commons that he could provide very few details about his plan for revamping the Poor Laws; he also rather shamefacedly seemed to understand that his bill would not see the light of day. Nevertheless, leading the charge against the assumptions inherent to Elizabeth 43, he attacked the Poor Laws for engendering the idle poor. He received in good measure some complaints about his plan from Liberal MP Robert Thomas Wilson (1777–1849). MP F. Lewis (the famed writer Matthew Lewis, who wrote the salacious gothic novel *The Monk*; 1775–1818) came down on Scarlett's side. MP John Bennet (1772–1852) asserts that if the Poor Laws were abandoned the people would starve. MP Hudsen Gurney (1775–1864) also furiously contested Scarlett's deleterious assumptions. Some roundly savaged him for saying Elizabeth 43 did not require the government to provide relief to the poor in times of distress. Scarlett seems mainly fearful of providing relief for the so-called 'indolent' poor rather than finding measures to help the so-called worthy poor. Discussion revolves around many of the indignities manifest in using the Poor Laws to subsidise inadequate wages, support married as opposed to unmarried men, and impose rules about which of the poor would be allowed to marry.

DOI: 10.4324/9780429198052-17

15. 'Poor Relief Bill', Commons Sitting; MPs James Scarlett, Robert Thomas Wilson, F. Lewis, John Bennet, Hudsen Gurney (1821)

[....] Mr. Scarlett, in rising to move the second reading of his bill, commenced by observing, that he wished at the outset to state, that it never was his intention, even when he first proposed the measure, to incumber it with many matters of detail. He was desirous rather to point out to the House the principles upon which he thought the present system of our poor-laws a vicious one, and one which required correction. He had been desirous of putting it in the most simple form, and of calling the attention of the House to what he conceived to be the grand sources of those evils under which we now laboured. He would shortly recapitulate the three great causes of all the various mischiefs and inconveniences which are found to result from our present system of poor-laws. They were to be found, first, in a compulsory and unlimited provision for the poor; secondly, in the administration of that provision, not to support industry, to encourage good conduct, and to be a relief for those who might be disabled by infirmities, but to cherish the vices and the indolence of that class of the poor who are disposed to exist rather on the charity of others, than to depend for their bread upon their own exertions: thirdly, (which was the grand and principal source of all those evils, as compared to the others), in the restraint that now existed upon the free exercise of labour. No one was more aware than he was that there were some evils which did not arise out of the principle of these laws, but were rather connected with the character and habits of the poor themselves; and such evils were modified by the benevolent attention and patriotic exertions of individuals, by the activity of magistrates, and by other circumstances affecting the character of the population of the district; but, whatever the evils were, they were ultimately referable to one or all of the three grand sources which he had enumerated. It had been urged as an objection to the bill, that it was a measure affecting the rights of the poor. He acknowledged it did affect the rights of the poor; but then it went to put them on a better foundation. It went to relieve them from their present state of dependence and calamity; but if his learned friend opposite said the poor man had a right to relief who was not labouring under old age, sickness, or infirmity, he would be glad to know in what book he found that law. He challenged him to produce it. The mistakes of individuals and magistrates had put an erroneous interpretation on the statute of Elizabeth. The decision of no court of law confirmed that interpretation, or authorized any such existing right. On the contrary, the courts had held that an order of the magistrates for relieving a poor man was not valid, unless it stated him to be incapable of labour. He would ask, then, in what way the present system operated? Was it not rather to the prejudice of the poor, than to their relief? There was one way in particular. The farmer, finding that he was called on to pay heavy poor rates, resorted to the practice of diminishing the wages of labour. They thought it best to employ only men who had families, which must receive a certain sum from the parish, and allow them only such wages as would barely allow them to exist. The farmer said, if the parish pay five shillings, and he could get his work done for nine, why should he give more than nine?[...] Thus the poor man, who was working; almost his blood out, had only before him the melancholy prospect of terminating his life in a workhouse—had no other refuge. How different was such a man in point of moral existence and affinity to the state, from him who was enabled to make some acquisitions of property by his own labour, and to lay up for his old age an independent provision In every point of view, moral, political and religious, the man who hoped to lay by something from his own earnings, was more valuable to society and to himself, than he who was doomed to present labour and prospective wretchedness, without any hope whatever. Another evil was, that a single man, when he found that the farmer employed a man with a family in preference, would be induced to get married, and thus burthen the parish with another family. If the House would consider the effect of the present compulsory and unlimited provision, they would find that it tended to create idleness, misery, and accumulated distress[....] They offered a bounty to pauperism, and consequently must lamentably augment the number of paupers. Those laws had the effect of preventing many a man in the labouring classes from earning his own subsistence, because they laid up a provision to which idleness might give him a claim; while those who worked, had to endure the mortifying reflection, that even out of their scanty pittance a portion was to go to the support of idlers and vagabonds. There was a great difficulty here; and it was the first duty of the legislature to remove that difficulty; but such difficulty could never be removed, as long as the class of persons who were reduced to dependence and misery, was multiplied by a compulsory and unlimited provision, and by the continuance of the restraint on labour[....] but he would ask, what gentleman thought such a case probable, or that landed proprietors could have such a short-sighted view of their own interests? He would propose, that where rates might become very oppressive, other places in which they were not so should be taxed in aid[....] He agreed that the calamities under which the poor were suffering had been produced in a great measure by the increase of taxation. But why had those sufferings been so produced? Because increase of taxation, and the consequent increase in the money price of almost every article of consumption, had not be attended by a proportionate increase in the rate of wages paid to them. The labourer was now paid, not by wages, but by charity: he was demoralised, enslaved, deprived of that independence and self-respect which alone could make him a good man and a useful citizen. All this took place without a single shilling be saved to his employer; nay, the employer, in the end, was a loser by the system[....]

Sir R. Wilson said, that before the House consented to abrogate the laws of Elizabeth, those laws which Blackstone had described as founded upon the first principles of civilized society, they should look at the artificial state in which, from circumstances, the country was placed. When labour was in many places an unmarketable drug; when corn laws and excise laws prevented the lower orders from obtaining at a low price the necessaries of life; when the poor were many of them absolutely unable to obtain a livelihood, surely they had a right to look for the means of existence, to those who had the power of affording them those means. Let the House beware how they touched that statute of Elizabeth, which was the Magna Charta of the poor, and might be called the palladium of their rights. Men would live; and it was better that they should live by charity than by rapine. The statute of Elizabeth provided that the lame, the blind, and the indigent poor, unable to work, should have relief in money; and that all persons, married or single, who were able to work, should have labour, and the means of exerting it given to them. That they must have at present immediate subsistence was clear. The hon. and learned member seemed to think that only the sick, the blind, or the impotent were entitled to relief; but how long would it be before the poor who could work, but were unable to find work, fell into that situation?[...] In truth, the *maximum*, would do harm; for it would always be looked upon as a *minimum*. Such a scheme was incompatible with all the legal, moral, and religious institutions of the country. How could the House check marriage by law, and yet seek to maintain those laws which rendered illicit intercourse a crime? Did hon. members hope that they could control the impulses of nature, and subject human beings to such unnatural restrictions? He would not speak of men only. In what situation did the House place the female part of the community? They were to be shut out from the resource of marriage; and they were liable to ruin and disgrace, if not to absolute punishment, for adopting an intermediate course. They were not to be permitted to marry; and their illegitimate children, if they had any, were to be starved to death. Would any man who had looked into the labourer's cottage say that parish relief was a bounty upon idleness?—that an allowance of a shilling or eighteen-pence a week for a man's second or third child was a premium upon population? Even if this anti-population scheme succeeded, would it not go to increase the very evil of which the landlords complained?[...]

Mr. F. Lewis could not refrain from offering a few words on that part of the gallant general's speech in which he seemed to consider the statute of Elizabeth as the Magna Charta of the poor, and the palladium of their rights. That he utterly denied.

He denied that the House ought to consider that or any other law on the subject as one which they were not perfectly justified in amending, according to the demand of the time, or their altered view of the circumstance of the case. The basis of the constitution was, the security which it gave to all persons in the enjoyment of whatever property they had honestly come by. If it could be shown that the principle of the poor-laws was subversive of that by which property was protected, then it would be evident that such an antagonist principle ought not to be allowed to prevail. The meaning of the statute of the 43rd of Elizabeth was, to inflict compulsory labour by way of punishment, not to afford labour for the mere purpose of maintenance. It was any thing but in the nature of giving the poor personal property.

Mr. Bennett, of Wilts., observed, that the greatest evil of the poor-laws was, that it rendered the poor man dependent on his superior, and made him so abject a wretch, that he had no object in acquiring property or maintaining a character in society. But, although that was a great evil, yet by its removal there would be danger of inflicting a still greater cruelty on the poor. There could be little doubt that if the existing poor-laws were suddenly repeated, the effect would be general starvation[....]

Continuation of Discussion, House of Commons, 2 July 1821

Mr. Scarlett said[,...] He was aware that many inflammatory and calumnious misrepresentations had gone abroad on this subject. He assured the House that his motives in meddling with the matter were of the most pure description. He felt that the existing system of Poor-laws was most oppressive on one hand, and that it defeated its own end on the other. He had no motive but to restore the ancient system to its primitive state and intention[....] He proposed to renew this measure next session. If he should meet with encouragement he should bring forward another bill for the greater discrimination of the moral claims of those who sought relief, to prevent the profuse expenditure of the Poor-rates in some respects, by taking away some provisions, which acted as a premium for pauperism[....]

Mr. H. Gurney said, that as the hon. and learned gentleman threatened them with a renewal of these most dangerous discussions in the ensuing session, he could not allow the bill to be withdrawn, without the strongest protest he was able to make against all the principles on which it was founded. He maintained, that the understood right of the poor to reasonable support was as old as the law of England; that up to this time it had been the boast of England, that no man could be left to starve; that the learned gentleman's bill went to the reversal of the law of the land, the laws of nature, and the law of God, and that its only possible tendency would be, to make the country a scene of rapine and violence and utter confusion, from one end to the other[....] As to the clause impeding the marriages of the poor ['No no!' from Mr. Scarlett.] Mr. Gurney said he could hardly trust himself to speak on it. But it was an attempt to bring the detestable system of Mr. Malthus to bear upon the legislation of the country, a system which every chapter of sacred history condemns, every page of civil history confutes, and every map of a half-unpeopled world, after a duration of near 6,000 years, proves the absurdity of[....] But he hoped and trusted that that House would never be led to legislate on the theories of such philosophers as these; and least of all, to give any countenance to a doctrine which in this country should recognize a right in the rich, to say to the poor, that they had no business to be born; that it was in the order of nature that they should starve; and that whatever might be the abundance of his superfluities, from him they could demand nothing.

Dr. Lushington said, that he would certainly oppose such a bill, if he believed that it tended to degrade the poor; but his settled conviction was, that the increase of Poor-rates was an increase of misery. If he failed to express this conviction from any unpopularity to which it might expose him, he should prove himself destitute of moral courage. The effect of the present laws, was, to oblige the industrious and prudent to support the improvident and thoughtless; to mulct the single individual for the support of the married[....]

16

ANON., 'PROPOSED REFUSAL TO SUPPORT THE POOR, AND TO ABOLISH THE POOR LAWS'

The Black Dwarf, 6 (1821), pp. 773–778

This article is from one of the most important radical journals of the time and might act as a gloss to the debate in Parliament started by Scarlett and noted in the previous section, as the text goes through the arguments of all the MPs and their speeches on the subject. Scarlett, of course, is found to be indefensible. There is an interesting reference here to 'social justice', a precursor, perhaps, to modern ideologies inherent to this phrase.

DOI: 10.4324/9780429198052-18

16. Anon., 'Proposed Refusal to Support the Poor, and to Abolish the Poor Laws', *Black Dwarf* (1821)

[....] Mr. Scarlett, or somebody for him, has called his outrageous proposal, the 'Poor's *relief* Bill!' It ought rather to be called, a Bill to *exterminate the wretched, instead of removing* their *wretchedness!*' We cannot conceive with what feelings a man could coolly propose such a measure. Of course, the feelings are conscientious, but we cannot enter into their spirit, or account for their nature, by any impulse that could impel ourselves on any such occasion. We disliked the ministerial approbation of a measure so proposed by an opponent. We remembered an often expressed wish of the ministry, to get rid of the poor laws, if it were practicable. We recollected all the bush-fighting of the official members on the subject; but we saw they were afraid to meddle with the fabric, lest it should tumble about their ears. They knew themselves to be unpopular—that such a proposition, fabricated in their workshop of national delusion, would have been more than suspected, and a clamour excited in defence of the right of the poor to live, which, though they might have conquered, might have left fatal effects behind[....] It is, in its nature, a most terrible outrage on the principles of social justice: and we care not who devised, or who support it. The result of its adoption will be an *interminable* and *exterminating* warfare between rich and poor; and under the false pretence of *protecting property*, it will *hazard life!* We thought we had clearly demonstrated this; and that dearly as a certain portion of the community value their beloved wealth, they set a still greater value on their personal security; yet, it seems, the case is so desperate that a desperate measure must be tried; but while we can resist its progress, we will; and if in despite of all warning, it is determined to drive the wretched to desperation, those who wake the sleeping passions into madness will bear the responsibility on their own heads[....]

His [Scarlett's] reasons are, *first*, the *compulsory* and *unlimited* provision for the poor! This we again repeat is a *delusion*. There is no such thing as an unlimited provision for the poor. Their provision is LIMITED to *less* than any medical man would state as competent to support a mere vegetable existence. We are bold to state that '*unlimited*' provision does not amount to *half a-crown a week*, on the average of men, women, and children, who are maintained on parochial charity. Mr. Scarlett means by his unlimited provision, that parishes are not allowed *absolutely* to *starve* to death all whom they may not choose to support in the most scanty manner!

Secondly, this legal philosopher, objects to '*administration* of that provision:' which he adds is devoted, 'not to *support industry*, to encourage *good conduct*, and to be a relief to those who might be disabled by infirmities:—but to *cherish the vices*, and the *indolence* of that class of poor, who are disposed to exist rather on the charity of others, than to depend for their own bread upon their own exertions.'

[....] This is all a fallacy—all a dream—all a fanciful invention of an imagination much more volatile than we should have expected to find in so experienced a lawyer[....] This, however, is an equal libel on the different parish authorities, and on the people who are classed as poor! Oh, we most heartily wish the learned gentleman could send *all* the *vice* and *indolence* of the country, to be *pampered* and *cherished* as the *poor* are *pampered* and *cherished.* No, no, Mr. Scarlett, you are here most egregiously mistaken[....] The *pampering* and *cherishing* of parish bounty, is what the *indolent* would spurn. There is not a beggar, in ordinary good fortune, who would not obtain from casual charity in one day, more than from parish bounty in a week. That class of the poor, which prefers to live on the alms of others, instead of personal labour, would never choose parish *pampering!* Of which it is rather a misfortune that some of our legislators should not have a more intimate knowledge. A residence for a few days, in a parish workhouse, or in a cottage upon parish allowance, would give Mr. Scarlett more feeling idea of the cherishing, and pampering, to which he so ludicrously alludes! and we dare pledge ourselves he would never be jocular on such entertainment in future! But what says his new bill to the administration of poors rates? Does he propose to devote them to the *support of industry?* Or to encourage *good* conduct! No! Directly the reverse—for he requests parliament, (the wisdom of parliament) to tell the labourer who cannot obtain work, that it will not give him a morsel of bread!—that he may live upon his industrious disposition, and sleep upon his good conduct! He proposes to refuse relief to all but *the infirm!*[...] for says the learned gentleman '*beyond a specified proportionate amount.*' *The church-wardens would have but a short answer to give to the* parties—they would be empowered to say, '*You must go elsewhere, for we cannot afford* to maintain you!'' *Where* ELSE, save to the Devil, if Heaven were no kinder than the learned gentleman, would this *short answer* send the miserable applicants? The *highway*, or the *hen-roost*, would be their only resource; and, then, indeed, the learned gentleman might have a professional opportunity of *terminating* all their sorrows!

His *third* ground is, that the present operation of the *poor laws*, is what he, more quaintly than intelligibly calls, 'the restraint that now exists upon the free exercise of labour.' We take it for granted, though the words so reported do not necessarily imply it, that he means they depreciate the value of labour. However, this is equally fallacious. The poor laws do no such thing. They have not reduced the price of labour, any more than they have raised the price of provisions. This has been done by *the system*, to which the poor laws have been rendered subservient. To abrogate the poor laws will not raise the price of labour any more than it will raise the price of produce; but will most probably reduce both still lower. Labour is no where YET at so low an ebb, as parish charity; but it will speedily become so, if the wisdom of parliament should sanction the proposal of the learned gentleman.

One of the *professed* objects of Mr. Scarlett is to restore the labourer to *independence!* While a taxation proposed to be left undiminished robs his children of nearly half the bread his earnings may procure! The crying philosopher would have burst his sides with laughter at this odd reason for shutting the door of relief to a man in the fear of starvation! This is a means of assisting those who, as the learned gentleman admits are 'working almost their blood out, without any prospect but a poor-house in their old age!' This is true, though it agrees but ill with that *cherished vice*, and *pampered indolence* of the labouring poor, of which he speaks in a prior part; but, bad as the prospect of a poor house is, it is better than *none*, which is the remedy proposed.

Mr. S. admits that a maximum might be occasionally *inconvenient!* Is this a fit term to apply to the misery attendant on the accumulated horrors of starvation? But let that pass. It is admitted a case of *inconvenience* may occur; but that may be remedied by 'calling a parish meeting of all the inhabitants, and 'they should have the *power*, (not be compelled) to make an additional allowance!' This would have one *convenience* possibly not contemplated by the learned proposer. The *inconvenience* might have been abated by the *death* of those who were inconvenienced, before the remedy could be applied; and thus the parish might save its money! 'What signifies a *few gunners*, more or less,' said a Turkish Minister, 'provided the Grand Seignior be we served!" An impertinent gunner had the audacity to reply, 'What signifies a few ministers, provided the Grand Seignior be well served!'

[....] Mr. Scarlett admits 'the calamities under which the poor are labouring, have been produced in a great measure by the *encrease of taxation!*' Then, why not propose a *reduction* of taxation as a remedy?[...]

Mr. F. Lewis declared the poor laws, 'by far the *most serious evil* that pressed upon the country!' This would have surprized us, could we have been surprized at any absurdity; but it is trifling to the climax which he afterwards reached:—for 'he was *astonished* to hear it asserted that the laws of Elizabeth had *given irrevocable rights* to the poor!' Now, as nobody did say this, it is astonishing the honorable member should have heard it;—for every one who has a spark of common sense, or an idea of common justice must know that it was not Elizabeth, but GOD himself, who have rights as irrevocable to the POOR as to the RICH!

[....] The legislators of the reign of Elizabeth only made a transcript of the laws of God, when they enacted that none should starve amidst the abundance with which he had blessed the earth. Has the deity commissioned Mr. F. Lewis, to reverse that summary of the law and the prophets, which commands us to do to others, as we wish they should do unto us? Mr. F. Lewis, has not yet done. He took 'the *right of property* to be one of the first principles of the British Constitution, of which the poor laws were subversive.' We ought to apologize to our readers for noticing such *reasoning*[....]

[....] Mr. Scarlett did not think a man who was *obliged to beg*, because the parish had shut the door in his face, ought to be treated as an incorrigible vagrant; so that beggary, it seems, is one of his remedies for inevitable poverty[....] We will venture to add, that it would be monstrous for the legislature to refuse relief to the distress occasioned by the measures it sanctions, and the system it continues to sanction.

17

‘PROBUS’, ‘CURRENCY, CORN LAWS, AND CRIME. LETTER TO THE EDITOR OF *THE MORNING CHRONICLE*’

The Morning Chronicle, 6 (6 December 1825), p. 4

This writer, under the pseudonym ‘Probus’, makes a rousing call to end the paper currency and the Corn Laws, which raised the price of bread out of reach of the poor. The dispute about using paper currency as opposed to gold currency was a longstanding nineteenth-century issue, which is used here to say that paper currency increased inflation. This writer implies that something had changed profoundly in the way the poor were viewed and treated in terms of wages so that, with the loss of the social contract, they no longer could afford a ‘comfortable’ existence without fear of destitution. Claiming that the rise of crime was due to poverty, Probus calls Luddism criminal. He also uses an ingenious argument collating slavery with the wages of the poor.

 DOI: 10.4324/9780429198052-19

17. 'Probus', 'Currency, Corn Laws, and Crime. Letter to the Editor of the *Morning Chronicle*' (1825)

Sir—The present melancholy and ruinous state of trade induces me to offer[,...] a few remarks on the causes of these disastrous events; I say *events*; because those destructive and extraordinary depressions have, for the last fifteen or twenty years, been of frequent and alarming recurrence, accompanied not only with severe loss of property, but, what is still worse, inducements to the commission, and consequent increase of crime. The two main sources of these evils, unquestionably are, an uncertain and variable circulating medium, and the high price of provisions resulting from our present system of Paper Currency and the Corn Laws which have already pauperized the agricultural labourers and are reducing those of the artisan and mechanic to the same condition, and will, if continued, ultimately divide the whole mass of society into two classes—very rich, and very poor.

Previous to the year 1797, when the Bank of England stopped payment in gold [...] labourers of all sorts were in [a] state of real comfort—and [...] the Poor Laws were seldom resorted to except in cases of old age or infirmity. But no sooner was the gold currency substituted by paper than the sad effects of the change began to exhibit themselves, in producing a state of things the very reverse of our former condition, and amongst the most alarming were the almost universal riots of the labouring poor, occasioned by the high price of provisions; and in the year 1799, I remember armed associations were almost universally formed, by the loyal as they were designated, for the purpose of awing the poor people into good order, and compelling them to suffer starvation quietly[....]

in 1810 [...] the condition of the labouring poor became miserable in the extreme, and their fruitless complaints ('excited by the feelings of hunger') which had formerly been suppressed by the bayonets of armed associations, were now manifested in the dark and vengeful spirit of Luddism, which spread to a fearful extent through the manufacturing districts of the North, & terminated, at length, in an awful catastrophe[....]

[....] no rise took place in the wages of labour, for throughout the years of 1817, 1818, and part of 1819, they were the same, or very nearly the same, as in the destructive year of 1816, and thus arrived another distressing and deplorable era in the sufferings of the poor;—Their wages excessively low—food excessively high—the pangs of hunger were too poignant to allow them to lie down and die in silence; therefore, suppressed by bayonets and the public executioner, now sought for some new channel of relief and exploded in loud calls for a reform in the Commons' House of Parliament; and while vast numbers of them were peaceably assembled, for the purpose of concerting the best means (as they thought) of securing to themselves the enjoyment of the fruits of their own labour, their complaints were unceremoniously & heartlessly silenced by the sabres of yeoman cavalry [and thus] Radicalism was extinguished by this barbarous massacre[....]

[....] They are compelled to labour for a pittance altogether inadequate to support life in a state of vigour, by means equally coercive and equally preconcerted—the pangs of hunger. For it has been enacted by these humans sub-legislators, that if any labourer refuse to work for 5s. per week he will not be allowed any relief from the parish; and as the amount of relief depends on the will of the Overseer, the measure amounts to an absolute domination over the labour of the man. In other cases this noble officer takes the labourers of the parish into his care, and lets them out for hire (as he would his horse or his ass) to work for whom and for what price he (the Overseer) thinks fit; and the Lord Mayor declared, in the Justice-room, on the 17th of this month, that he had been offered a whole squad by the Overseers of a parish in the country where he was building, to labour for him at the rate of four shillings per week!! Now, I ask, what this is, but forcible appropriation of the labour of one human being for the exclusive benefit of another, which is the very essence of slavery?[…] If a negro slave refuse to work, he is coerced by the whip; and English slave, in the same case, must die for want of food[….]

Finally, in addition to, and in aggravation of, all the mischiefs and privations attending the paper currency system, come in aid the Corn Laws; it might have been some alleviation to our sufferings for the last fifteen years, had we been permitted to eat cheap bread, but the monopoly which the Corn Laws give the landed interest in the market till it attains instead a famine price, act as a powerful stimulus in all the advances of the price of corn […] hence, during the last 15 years, we have only had two periods of any thing like cheapness in the Corn Market, viz.,—part of 1816, 1821–2[….]

[….] Thus have these two ruthless monsters, Paper Money and Corn Laws, gone hand in hand (fit associates) through the whole space of time which covers my remarks, the fruitful parents of misery, violence, and crime. And to what other source can we trace among the labourers and lower orders, the riots, and Luddism, and Radicalism, and Combinations, but to these prolific authors of our endlessly varied ills? What were these difficult modes of insubordination which I have noticed in this letter but so many varied expressions of hunger, arising from the wages of labour being totally inadequate to purchase the necessaries of life?

18

DAVID ROBINSON, 'THE POOR LAWS'

Blackwood's Edinburgh Magazine, 23 (1828), pp. 923–936, on pp. 923–929, 933–934, 936

The writer David Robinson (1787–1849), a regular at *Blackwood's*, ends this article with a discussion of his fear that if England's Poor Laws were abrogated England would become like benighted Ireland, which, at the time, had no poor laws. Robinson goes through many reasons not to abrogate the law and he is especially good at pointing out the faults in the arguments made to override the Poor Laws. Robinson pointedly asks: Are 'labourers, when they are stripped of employment, to perish from hunger?' He also points out that if the State relied on private charity to fill the gap, it would never be 'methodical' or timely. A 'subscription' was a commitment to provide a charitable donation.

DOI: 10.4324/9780429198052-20

18. David Robinson, 'The Poor Laws', *Blackwood's Edinburgh Magazine* (1828)

The Poor Laws of unhappy Old England are at present in a state of great tribulation and jeopardy[....]

The history of these laws for many years has been exceedingly curious. Our *improvers* have almost annually, in one way or another, arraigned them before Parliament, as being most defective in form, and most injurious in operation—return upon return has been moved for and printed to give evidence against them—committee upon committee has at and reported upon them—yet, strange to say, although their defects and baleful consequences have been represented to be so glaring and ruinous, no one has been able to devise any plausible scheme for their '*improvement*.' Individual improvers, indeed, have in succession delivered themselves of new systems, ravishingly perfect in their own eyes, but these have been so manifestly inferior to the old system in the eyes of the whole, that no attempt has been made to adopt them[....]

[....] everything which can be urged in favour of the Poor Laws ought to be dispassionately, carefully, and even indulgently examined, for the sake of the many millions, who, while they are threatened with the loss of their subsistence in the hour of need, cannot make themselves heard, and can scarcely find an advocate to plead their cause against the tremendous mass of power, prejudice, and interest, which is arrayed against them[....]

[....] a comparison between Ireland and England fills us with amazement that men can be found to triumph in the hunger and wretchedness of their countrymen[....]

[....] The Englishman may be easily misled—he may be, as late times have abundantly proved, converted into a dolt or a madman—he may be taught to rob himself, and strike at his own existence—but never can he be stripped of his benevolence and humanity. To his benevolence and humanity we now address ourselves—[...] we speak for what is peculiarly English in parentage and operation—we speak, that the poorer part of HIS countrymen may not be robbed of their legal rights, may not be divested of their morals and character, may not, in their day of distress and suffering, be deprived of the means of subsistence—and we shall not speak in vain. In spite of the disgraceful admissions of this minister or that, and of the wild and destructive conduct of the house of Commons, he will hear us.

In a country like England, able-bodied labourers must often be destitute of employment, even though there be no real redundancy of population. The demand for agricultural, manufacturing, and other labour is subject to violent and frequent fluctuations. In one year, the farmers or manufacturers will employ much more labour than they will employ in the succeeding one. At one period the labour of the country is generally employed, and immediately afterwards almost half of it is for months rendered idle. If we look at the past, we find, that in almost every third year a vast portion of the labour, which had been employed in the preceding two, could not for a large part of the year find employment; and that in every year, one business or another was compelled to render the chief part of the labour idle for some months, which it generally needed. Of course the labourers of this country must frequently—in one business or another they must annually—be for many weeks, and perhaps for many months, deprived, from no fault of their own, of employment; no matter what their wishes and exertions may be, they must be disabled for earning anything.

Do the Abolitionists deny this?[...]

[....] No matter what the price, or the system of trade, may be, the sales of our manufactures must always be subject to very great variations; and, of course, the quantity of labour required for the fabrication of these manufactures must always be subject to very great variations[....]

As clearly as mathematical demonstration ever proved anything, it is proved by experience and the nature of things, that the sales of manufactures and the price of corn must continue to fluctuate, as they have hitherto done, and that no legislation can prevent them from so fluctuating. It of necessity is equally clear that the demand for labour must continue to fluctuate as it has hitherto done, and that frequently vast numbers of able-bodied labourers must be for a time deprived of employment.

Having established this point, we will now ask, are these labourers, when they are stripped of employment, to perish from hunger? No, says the Abolitionist; if they cannot obtain work in one place, they must obtain it in another. Worthy sage, this is little better than nonsense, unless you can prove that it is practicable for them to procure work in one place, if they cannot in another. If, from ruinous prices of corn, or bad seasons, a great number of agricultural labourers are thrown out of employment, to what place are they to travel to regain it? Finding it in agriculture is out of the question, for they are in excess in every village throughout the country; and as to their finding it in manufacturers and trade, we may safely pronounce it to be equally impossible. The ploughman cannot turn weaver or tailor when his own falling fails him; and if he could, he would find no one to give him work[....] Their own trade is pretty sure to need them again after the lapse of a few months; and to the country at large, it is most advantageous for them to be in readiness to attend its call, even though they have to subsist in the interval on the poor-rates[....]

[....] In every business there must always be an excess, or a deficiency, of labour; and it is more advantageous to the country at large to pay the poor-rates to a moderate excess, than to have a deficiency and be exempted from such rates[....] If times be reasonably good, still looking at the year as a whole, there must always be a great number of able-bodied labourers unable for a part of the year to procure work, however anxious they may be to do so[....]

We therefore say again, are these labourers to perish from hunger? They must do this; or they must subsist during the time they are compelled to be idle on some fund they have provided while in work, or on charity, or on robbery.

As to their perishing from hunger, it has not yet been openly recommended by the most flinty-hearted Abolitionist of the tribe; and we may therefore put it out of the question. In truth, if the House of Commons, in the plenitude of that wisdom which it has in late years displayed, should vote it to be an admirable means of getting rid of surplus population, and should legislate accordingly, the law would be inoperative. Never will men die for hunger, so long as bread can be got by burglary and high-way robbery. The matter, therefore, to be considered in the first place, is—is it practicable for these labourers to provide, while they are in employment, what will support them when they are compelled to be idle?

The Abolitionists of course reply in the affirmative; but they content themselves with general assertion: they supply none of the description, calculation, deduction, and demonstration, which are essential for preventing changers of law from being a national scourge. Now, putting out of sight a few trades, the vast body of labourers in both town and country are at present receiving wages which barely enable them to exist; they are receiving wages, from which nothing could be taken, as a provisions for the future, which would not be a subtraction from the necessaries of life. There is not the least hope of amendment; but, on the contrary, it is pretty certain that matters will be worse. The tendency and even avowed object of the new system of trade is, to reduce the price of labour to the lowest point; and everything in both legislation and circumstance, in operating to sink to this point for ever the wages of the bulk of the working classes. To expect that men, whose earnings will scarcely supply their families bread without the assistance of the parish, should voluntarily make a provision for the future, is idle; to compel them to do so, would be gross cruelty[....]

Without parish relief, then, the labourers in question must subsist on charity, or on thefts. With respect to charity as a source of maintaining them, the Abolitionists are enraptured with it. Before, however, charity be made the basis of legislation, it may be proper to inquire whether it will yield what legislation expects from it. The question, would charity support the able-bodied labourers who are now supported by the Poor Laws?[...] The mass of those who attend our churches never give a farthing at them for the poor. The money received is below notice as a means of saving the needy of each parish from starvation.

But then it is said, that public subscriptions would be formed. When would they be formed? would they start into being the instant the Poor Laws should be abolished, to keep *constantly* relieving the mass of labourers, who would be *constantly* destitute of employment? No, they would exist only in times of great and general distress. Would they be formed at the commencement of such distress, and be kept in efficient activity until its termination? No, they would not be thought of until after the poor should be brought to the verge of starvation, and no dependence could be placed upon them for affording the necessary relief. In the distress of 1826 tardy and mercenary public charity did not creep from its hiding-place to blazon forth its subscriptions, until hundreds of thousands of poor wretches were not only almost famished, but were committing wholesale outrage, and threatening the state with convulsion. The subscription had such a combination of powerful stimulants in its favour, as no future one could hope for; and still it would have been deplorably inefficient without the poor rates. A subscription was in the same year formed for the exclusive relief of the Spitalfields; silk-weavers; a short period elapsed, and then the most pathetic and urgent appeals could not prevail on public charity to subscribe what was necessary, In the same year the landholders and other wealthy persons undertook to support the distressed manufacturing population of Scotland; for a time things went on smoothly, but the landholders, &c. soon grew weary of their burden, and at length they publicly resolved to petition Parliament for assistance from the public purse.

Excepting times of great and general distress, the destitute labourers would have no other charity to look to but that of individuals. Let any man separate in any parish the benevolent few who would weekly contribute liberally to the wants of the poor, from the many who would rarely contribute anything; let him then calculate how much the poor of that parish will need weekly, and he will then discover the folly of placing any reliance on individual charity.

But how is the labourer to avail himself of individual charity? Will the charitably-disposed seek his dwelling intuitively, and administer to his needs without solicitation? Alas! no. He must beg, or be a stranger to charity. Throwing the working classes upon charity in their hour of distress, must of necessity convert them into beggars[....]

It is not asserted that the poor, when they cannot procure employment, are to be suffered to perish from hunger; it is admitted, that in their need they ought to be supported by charity. When this is the case, why not make charity general and methodical? Why not make it a rule for every member of the community to contribute to the needs of the poor according to what he possesses? The Poor Laws stand on this principle, although they do not apply it so far as they ought, and it is an unassailable one.

It is assumed, that the body of the working classes have the means of saving when they have employment, what will support them when they have none: this is demonstrably false[....]

[....] Now, here is a man who cannot work; and there is one who has strength and skill, but who cannot possibly procure work; in reality, both are equally incapable of supporting themselves by their labour. Nevertheless, the one is to be maintained by the parish, and the other is to starve. Here are two children who are alike incapable of labouring; the one is to be kept by the parish, because it has no parent to work for it; the other is to perish from hunger, because it has parents who cannot, from scarcity of employment, work for it. This distinction evidently rests on the assumption that every man who is able to work, is able constantly to maintain himself and his family by his labour; it stands upon falsehood, and it is at variance with every principle of justice and equity[....]

The country at large may rest assured, that if it will not support its poor in one way, it must support them in another; and that, if it deprive them of parish relief, they will deprive it of something far more valuable[....]

[....] If Ireland had possessed Poor Laws like England, it never would have suffered what it has suffered; the landlords would have been compelled to look after their estates, and the subletting, penury, and barbarism, would have been prevented. If it be now impossible to introduce Poor Laws into Ireland, we may at least be permitted to lament that they were not introduced when it was possible, if we may do no more. If the absence of them have materially contributed to bring on Ireland alike horrible and irremediable we pray Heaven, that the abolition of them may never bring similar miseries on England.

19

ANON., 'THE POPULATION QUESTION.—MR. SADLER AND THE POLITICAL ECONOMISTS'

The Monthly magazine, or, British register, 11 (1831), pp. 526–544, on pp. 527, 529–530, 544

Michael Thomas Sadler (1780–1835) was a Tory politician and MP who found Malthus's ideas unChristian and anathema and wrote a book to prove their premises false. Whatever issues this anonymous essay has with Sadler, it has an acute ear for the upper-class insensitivity to the plight of the starving poor; the writer accuses the upper classes of believing that they had all but the exclusive right to live. Malthus's ideas, Sadler asserts, are a direct insult to God's plan as well as being irrational, to boot.

DOI: 10.4324/9780429198052-21

19. Anon., 'The Population Question.—Mr. Sadler and the Political Economists', *Monthly magazine, or, British register* (1831)

[....] Who now advocate the Rights of the Poor? Who now stand up in the proper places to redeem by practical deeds, at the moment when the exigencies of famine and anarchy demand it of them, the solemn promises of their cheap popularity? Who are now to be found the Apostles of Hope and Messengers of Good, dispensing in the season of want the sustenance granted in prospect when it was wanted? Where are they to be found? Do the Irish landlords succour the Irish poor who starve and rot on their estates? Do the Liberals oppose the crushing, diabolical, selfish, grinding, and unnatural doctrines of Malthus? Who are the promoters of those doctrines? Who are their enemies? And who is their Detector and Exposer? The last interrogatory concerns us mainly here. The master mind that developed the ingenious sophistry and laborious artfulness of the Malthusian system was a Tory—no other than Mr. Sadler! The Malthusian system was essentially a defence of a gilded and luxurious order of hereditary families that could never experience a pang of distress, against the natural wants of the defence-less peasant-born race that cried at their gates for bread[....]

[In Malthus's argument] it appears that the natural and ordained progress of mankind is to starvation[....] Indeed[,..] we might say that this theory refutes itself, since if human beings were to be decimated after so wholesale a fashion by the inscrutable decrees of Providence, there never could arise any danger of that super-fecundity which the theory propounds, seeing that the people who were to have propagated at so fierce a rate must have died for want of food. But it does not appear that mankind has run into any such excess, for every man contrives to get enough to eat either by honesty or theft, and many men get much more than their share, which would be things impossible if it were true that the quantity of food in the world was inadequate to the demand.

But Mr. Malthus asserts that such would be the case, were it not that Providence checks against the increase of our race under the forms of moral restraint, and vice and misery. 'Only for something the sky would fall.' Grant Mr. Malthus these premises, and away he goes, whistling like a man who had just sold a spavined colt for sound wind and limb, and had got the money in his pocket.

It requires very little penetration to perceive that these checks, which Mr. Malthus assigns to the Creator of life, and the Giver of the means of living, are as direct impeachments of the goodness and mercy of GOD as they are insults to the dignity of our own nature. To add to that they are also an unequalled specimen of bad logic would be an anti-climax from which we will spare the Political Economists. They pre-suppose that GOD had miscalculated the power and operation of the machinery constructed out of His own bidding, since they assume that He has found it necessary to repress its springs and retard its motions; that He made a world which so fructified in its own vile luxuriance, as to outgrow the Original Design, deform the pure symmetry of its plan, and render imperative some mighty scourges to cure those excrescences, to the evils of which it was exposed from its formation. In this, either the wisdom or the goodness of the Omnipotent is staked. The Malthusians cannot escape from the force of this impiety. They have committed it, and they continue to commit it in their professors' chairs, in their dark lectures[....]

This system, then, with its many charms for people in high places—with all its absurdities, blasphemies, and inconsistencies, permitted the rich to propagate *ad libitum* [as often as desired], and it is even said that Mr. Malthus himself is the father of seventeen children[....]

This question is essentially a question that goes to establish the right of the poor to live. The political economists would invest the aristocracy with the exclusive right to enjoy life, and taste of all the privileges which Nature in her bounty has showered upon Man.

20

ANON., 'POOR LAW CATECHISM, TO BE LEARNED BY EVERY PAUPER PREVIOUS TO HIS CONFINEMENT IN THE BASTILE. *PRINTED NOT UNDER THE* DIRECTIONS OF THE POOR LAW COMMISSIONERS'

Northern Liberator, 4 (November 1837), p. 3

Published after the new Poor Law was enacted in 1834, this spoof on catechism as a bait-and-switch for the poor highlights the 'Starvation Law' (the Poor Laws) and its repercussions, including separating husbands and wives and parents and children; it also illustrates an understanding of how hunger might affect the poor not only individually but across generations, as current medical and scientific understandings would seem to prove. The use of the catechism genre to deride the Poor Laws is also seen in the satiric article on how the much-pampered parsons and the great Duke of Wellington and the Archbishop of Canterbury should be made to take their own medicine and reside in the workhouse based on their own wish to use the law as a means to force the poor to avoid the temptations of eating food.

The *Northern Liberator* was a radical newspaper that had a knack for powerful satire, as is here used to show the hypocrisy of any catechism of the poor that did not examine the loss of the social contract between the classes. The West Riding was a pocket of fierce radicalism in the Yorkshire area of England. Here, the catechism shows the unnatural bent of Malthusian philosophy in its view that only the upper classes had a right to enjoy the sexual pleasures of life because they could provide their children with life's necessities. 'Harry Bruff'em' is a reference to conservative MP Henry Brougham (1778–1868). The poor hated Somerset House, from which the workhouses were administered by three 'lousy' commissioners.

DOI: 10.4324/9780429198052-22

20. Anon., 'Poor Law Catechism, To be Learned by every Pauper previous to his confinement in the Bastile. *Printed not under the* Directions of the Poor Law Commissioners', *Northern Liberator* (1837)

POOR LAW CATECHISM,
To be Learned by every Pauper previous to his confinement in the Bastile.
Printed not under the Directions of the Poor Law Commissioners.

[The following curious document has been widely circulated over the West Riding of Yorkshire, and we publish it merely to show what is done in the country.]

Question.—What is thy Name?

Answer.—Pauper.

Q.—Who gave thee that Name?

A.—My Godfather Insult, and my Godmother Reproach; they gave it to me in my adversity, wherein I was made a member of want—the child of Penury—and an inheritor of extreme Distress.

Q.—What did your Godfather and Godmother then for you?

A.—They did promise and vow three things in my Name First, that I should renounce Plenty and Content,—the pomps and vanities of decent attire and wholesome food, and all the sinful lusts of comfort and delight. Secondly, that I should believe the articles of the Malthusian Faith to be separated from the wife of my bosom—to be torn from tender and beloved offspring, and each of us to be immured in cells, where we must neither commune together nor taste the sweets of life. And thirdly, that I should keep my Tyrant's unholy will and commandments, and patiently endure the same all the days of my life.

Q.—Dost thou not think that thou art bound to believe, and to do, as they have promised thee?

Q.—No: and, by God's help, I will not. And I heartily thank the defenders of the poor, that they have called me into a state of determined resistance, through absolute necessity; and I pray my fellow-sufferers to shew forth their strength, that we may not continue in the same unto our lives end.

Q. Rehearse the articles of thy belief.

Answer.—I believe in the existence of Harry Bruff'em and of Miss Martineau and of a host of Whores and Rogues, the makers of the Accursed Poor Law Starvation Act.

And in three lousy Commissioners, their pauper-starving tools; who were conceived by Satan, born in the sink of iniquity, serve under pompous pirates, have crucified charity and benevolence, are dead to every feeling of humanity, and have buried the rights of the poor in the sepulchre of the robber. They descended into Hell, received instructions from their father, and in three days rose again from the rakings of the damned. They then ascended to power on the wings of plunder, and now sit at the right hand of injustice and tyranny, from whence they shall come and be judged according to their deserts [sic].

I believe in the existence of a common house of thieves, the communion of robbers, the perpetrators of sin; the resurrection of a revolution, and the death everlasting of British slavery. Amen.

Q.—What dost thou chiefly learn in these articles of thy belief?

A.—First, I learn to believe the being of a gang of villains, who rob me and would pauperize the world. In the Poor-law Starvation Act, under which they would bring me and all my kind.—Thirdly, In a latent power within the oppressed, which when brought into exercise, will sweep away the destroyers of our rights, and save me and all the labouring people of the land.

Q.—You said that your godfather and godmother did promise for you, that you should keep your tyrants' commandments; tell me how many there be?

A.—Ten.

Q.—Which be they?

A.—The same which the Prigs spake in the damnable chapter of Starve-us, saying, We are thy Lords and thy would-be Gods, who brought thee out of the land of plenty, and out of the house of freedom.

1.—Thou shalt have none other Gods but us.

Response.—Oh, have mercy upon us, and incline our hearts to break this law!

2.—Thou *shalt* not make unto thyself any graven image or any caricature of us, or of our dearly beloved Commissioners to bring us, and them, into contempt among the people. Thou shalt bow down unto us, and worship us: for we thy tyrants are jealous tyrants; and will visit the misfortunes of the poor upon their wives and children unto the third and fourth generation of them that hate us, and shew misery unto thousands that love us not, and keep not our commandments.

Res.—Oh, have mercy upon us, and &c.

3.—Thou shalt not take our names in vain, nor the names of our Commissioners; for we will not hold him guiltless that taketh our names in vain.

Res.—Oh, have mercy upon us, and &c.

4.—Remember that thou labour hard every day. Seven days shalt thou labour, and grind corn by hand, and do all that we command thee to do. Thou shalt do all manner of servile work, thou, and thy son, and thy daughter, and be to us as men-servants and maid-servants; and be, to <rest,> a stranger within our prison-gates. For in a few days we made this accursed law and all that in it is, and rest not in the enforcement thereof, because we profit much thereby: therefore we bless the Starvation Act, and hallow it.

Res.—Oh; have mercy upon us and &c.

5.—Honour thy tyrants and oppressors, that thy days may be short in the land, our of the fruits of which we, thy Lord, will not allow thee to live.

Res.—Oh, have mercy upon us, and &c.

6.—Thou shalt in no wise murmur.

Res.—Oh, have mercy upon us, and &c.

7.—Thou shalt not commit adultry with the good things of this life.

Res.—Oh, have mercy upon us, and &c.

8.—Thou shalt not eat, but starve.

Res.—Oh, have mercy upon us, and &c.

9.—Thou shalt not bear true witness against thy taskmasters.

Res.—Oh, have mercy upon us, and &c.

10.—Thou shalt not *covet* a comfortable house, thou shalt not covet a sight of thine own wife, nor of thy children, for they shall be to us as oxen and asses, and not any thing shall be thine.

Res.—Oh, have mercy upon us, and incline our hearts to break all these damnable laws.

21

'MARCUS', *AN ESSAY ON POPULOUSNESS* (OR *ON THE POSSIBILITY OF LIMITING POPULOUSNESS*)

(London: Printed by the author, 1838), pp. 3–6,10, 13–15

This shocking pamphlet takes Malthus to the logical extreme, the killing of infants born to the poor. In making the case, Marcus suggests that infanticide by the poor under the direction of the government could be seen as a kind of noble sacrifice for the State. In the shocking rendition of self-absorbed and self-aggrandising capitalist rhetoric, the author also feels the need to explain why infants had no 'property' in themselves and that murder of infants could be done without pain to the infant. This writer published another edition with John Hill, who added remarks calling the 'proletarian populousness' the 'great ulcer of modern nations'. Based on this statement, the writer asks to 'revise the rules of morality' in order to discuss how many children the poor should have and comes to the number two, with the 'third child as a *terminus*, not quite to be reached, and never to be exceeded'. He refers to norms by which to view his approach:

> A woman in Scotland, living on the hardest fare, will bring into the world twelve children, of which ten will die in early age. And this is not merely the more frequent case; it is constant [....] For, since the number cannot but be limited at last by want of food, the supernumeraries will die off: the weakest first: and the children will be these [....] We engage to insure to each couple their two children; and of those, which we take away from them, the conciliation of humanity requires that we rear and well educate some [....] Happily but little elimination of individuals will suffice to preserve our species from degeneration.

The working classes viewed this book as illustrating that the State seemed bent on designing a way to get rid of the poor through starvation or other means. The recognition that the use of labourers might be obviated because of

DOI: 10.4324/9780429198052-23

the rise of the machine along with the passing of the Anatomy Act (1832) did not help to allay these fears. Likewise, being referred to as 'over-vegetation' that needed culling was certainly a gauntlet thrown down. Nowhere in the piece is there the common sense understanding that all people deserve food security, and that food security obviates such repugnant measures.[84]

21. 'Marcus', *An Essay on Populousness* (or *On the possibility of limiting populousness*) (1838)

Section 1

'Accept this misery!' So says to man the first author upon Population: 'accept this capitulation with your destiny.' You see that it is a necessity in a double sense. Not only is it the consequence of an unconquerable luxuriance in our vegetative growth; an inevitable effect of an inevitable cause: but the very quantity and degree of misery, as actually existing, is necessary, because wanted. Since only it can set bounds to itself. How are men ever to be disciplined into labour and forethought, if they be neither chastened themselves nor terrified by the spectacle of want in others? Moveover, it is as when we are threatened by a wasting invader: we may find, that our only security lies in forming a waste, at any expense, between him and ourselves. Some must suffer for all[....]

I dare not undertake a task, whose performance is yet greatly to be wished for; that of scrutinizing physiologically all the various methods possible, by which the over-vegetation of nature might be confined, contented, or coerced. I here take for examination one: which seems to offer an hope, that it may be rendered by art and contrivance no longer inhuman, but mild, harmless, and admissible.

Let us place ourselves for an instant in the ages of antiquity. Let us, for the purpose of inspection and inquiry, clothe ourselves in that indifference which frequency begets. Let us now contemplate the stifling of a just-born infant, and let us separate the various elements which concur to arouse within us a sense of horror and reluctance[....]

[....] Next, for the feelings of compassion we will provide by making the infant to be happy, if he live; if not, to be unpained in the act of dying. And since this **is** the great and difficult problem,—to remove altogether the hideous idea of pain inflicted, an idea which makes the principal difference between to be killed and to die, I must not omit to give herewith a brief sketch of the theory required.

Section II.

Beyond these two considerations (of the parent's loss, and of his sympathy for the infant's pain), there is another, which goes to make up the complex idea of criminally killing. It is that of the right or property in life inherent in the living person himself.

However it may be, that with the extinction of life is extinguished the wish to live, this opinion is not the most natural. We sympathize strongly with the imaginary wishes of the lifeless corse. We see hovering over us the departed shade, with indignant and imploring looks demanding of us justice or vengeance. Even of the unthinking and new-born infant we cannot help entertaining the same notions, though illusive in regard to him; and although it may be clearly demonstrated that he never can have possessed the right, any more than he has felt the wish, to live.

For change for a moment the supposition; let an estate be the object in question. Why do we respect an infant's right to the property of it? Only because it lies within the boundary of the great social convention of property, of which not a single pale can be broken without letting in general confusion and insecurity[....]

Section IV.

And last, not least, the mother's special right is to be adjudged and allowed: her feelings in gestation and in parturition are to be consulted. Unconsoled by any idea of triumph or of gain, what a dismal expectancy of torture would be hers! But happily, with well-disposed minds, a very small quantity of reality will suffice for contentment. And from this principle we may hope to obtain an accommodation between the claims of society and a sensibility above all others to be respected[....]

If our great system be realized, extreme misery will disappear, and what is now called alms-giving will have become obsolete[....]

[....] Conducing to the same great end, I will offer another piece of art, seeming small, yet not insignificant: let there be a burial-ground—call it rather a repository, for the privileged remains of those infants unadmitted into life. Let it have nothing funereal about, but all that is cheerful and agreeable[....] Let this be the infants' paradise; every parturient female may be considered as enlarging or embellishing it.

22

ANON., 'POPULATION, SUBSISTENCE, AND POLITICAL ECONOMISTS'

The Charter (13 October 1839), p. 695

The Charter was a radical newspaper that explicitly supported activism by the labouring poor, specifically in promoting the six points of their Charter, which included the appeal for universal male suffrage, vote by ballot, the secret ballot and annual elections for Parliament. The article finds the rich not only self-serving but also rather doltish and uneducated in their role as leaders of the State. The writer also brilliantly explains how the rich used Malthus's theory as evidence and support for breaking the social contract. In comparison, the article puts forward Robert Owen's (1771–1858) ideas about population as a corrective; Owen was a radical who led a movement for socialist utopian societies to combat capitalism's downgrading of the poor. Here we see, again, an argument for allowing the poor to own some of the 'wastes' or land not being used so as to have a means of subsistence.

DOI: 10.4324/9780429198052-24

22. Anon., 'Population, Subsistence, and Political Economists', *Charter* (1839)

[....] Legislation is effective only when the legislator understands what he is legislating for; and what materials are requisite for giving effect to the laws. Now what do our senators, hereditary or elective, know of the nature of human beings? Some of them know tolerably well what constitutes a good horse, sheep, or bullock; but of the nobler animal—man, they are utterly ignorant. For the breeding and government of the animals enumerated they are well adapted, but they are evidently out of their sphere when they attempt to legislate for man. The possession of knowledge fits them for the one office; the want of it equally disqualifies them for the other. It is not to be wondered at that we find ignorance and selfishness characterising the proceedings of our governors, when we look at the training they receive. How can mere fox hunters and money hunters know any thing of the important practical sciences contained in the great science of society? Of the small portion of the ruling classes, who are practically acquainted with some one or other of these sciences, few ever push their enquiry farther than the particular circle in which they find themselves placed, and the bearing of others is only studied in so far as they affect their individual or family welfare. Hence ignorance or selfishness is everywhere dominant, and the efforts of well-intentioned individuals, either by writing or acting, in consequence of the want of a few sound first principles and practical knowledge, have not the slightest effect in alleviating the mass of human wretchedness which exists around them. One of the most fertile sources of error in the minds, and, consequent, error in the practice, of the ruling classes, and many state doctors, is to be found in the prevalent belief in the doctrine that population increases faster than the means of subsistence. This silly fallacy in economical philosophy, which, like its equally mischievous parallel in mental moral philosophy, original sin, had its origin in the brain of a priest, has done more to reconcile man to, and prop up, the present irrational system of society, than any other political dogma whatever. It is difficult to account for the credence this doctrine has received; for it is, in reality contradicted by all existing facts, and is the offspring of imagination, not of practical knowledge. Mr. Owen has for the last thirty years proclaimed this truth to the world: 'That the earth is now, with a few slight exceptions, a waste, swamp, or forest, *for want of population* to drain and well cultivate it; and the great want of society to improve the world, as it is for the interest of all that it should be improved, is now, and will be for many ages to come, *a want of a well-trained and intelligent population.*' Now which of these very opposite propositions are we to believe? If we adopt Plato's test of the qualifications of an instructor, we shall be compelled to give credence to Owen instead of Malthus[;...]

[....] Malthus is correct when he says that the population of the world is ever adapting itself to the quantity of food raised for its support; but he has not told us how much more food and intelligent and industrious people will create from the same soil, than will be produced by one ignorant and ill-governed. *It is however as one to infinity.*—For man knows not the limit to his power of creating food[....]'

[....] The earth always yields an abundant return for labour and manure ... the only fear we need entertain at present is not a *surplus*, but a *deficient* population, either for labour or the consumption of its product[....] This principle of the incompetency of the earth to provide subsistence for its population as fast as the latter increase, lies at the root of all the schemes of the political economists. It is to them what the doctrine of original sin is to the clergy. Destroy or disprove either and the whole of the ingenious and fanciful superstructure they have raised upon a 'sandy foundation,' at once 'vanishes into thin air.' The elaborate tomes about Supply and Demand, Capital and Labour, Free Trade and Corn Laws, Population Checks, &c., &c., become of less worth than the paper on which they are printed. Their only tendency is to mystify a plain subject, to bewilder their readers, and to keep the population on a wrong scent. Every step which our merchants, manufacturers, and legislators make in accordance with this most fallacious theory, is a step away from the true remedy for national suffering and distress. While millions of cultivable acres are lying without the hand of labour to cultivate them, covered with weeds instead of wealth, while other extensive tracts are laid down in parks, forests, and shooting grounds, for the gratifications of an idle fraction of the population; and while even the portion of our surface which is cultivated, is in the majority of instances, merely scratched over in a most unscientific manner, without, in a thousandth degree, developing the latent riches resident in its bosom: while these things continue we may be stunned with the discordant Babel of scheming preachers and state quacks—Corn Laws may be repealed, manufactures increased, and competition augmented, but the evils will remain, and increase in the exact proportion of the activity which is exerted for the spread of a false system.

Part 3

LABOUR PETITIONS AND REFORM MEETINGS

During the early 1800s the government attempted to create terms to differentiate between the poor (who were seen as able to subsist on their earnings) and paupers (who were seen as infirm, old, or unable or unwilling to work and who were without resources to survive).

Though it is difficult to get at the many voices of the labourer, the petitions and press accounts of their reform meetings illustrate a powerful and vibrant movement, which featured influential and perspicacious analysis of the changing socio-economic landscape for worker subsistence. The petitions and speeches from the labourers in this section feature a range of tones, including attempts to decide whether they are pleading for or demanding wage increases, respect and equality from the owners or 'masters'. Sometimes the tone is grovelling, at other times indomitably resistant and self-assured. It is usually possible to discern how the term 'manufacturer' is being used from the context; at times in these readings this term is referring to the labourer who works in the factory and at other times it refers to the owner of the factory. In the address from workers in document number 23 below, which includes upwards of 36,000 signatures, the conclusion is that though Parliament would 'interfere' to help farmers through the Corn Laws, it would not 'interfere' with the economy legislatively to help the 'starving' workers; hence, the address calls for workers to seek the power that the vote would give them to influence Parliament if recalcitrant MPs refused to respond to their distress. It is important to note that the petitions from the workers more often than not included the word 'distress' rather than stronger terms of 'starvation' or 'hunger'. Note, too, in the address from knitters how they appeal to their employers for 'advice' on how to improve their condition.

DOI: 10.4324/9780429198052-25

23

RICHARD TAYLOR, 'TO THE MANFACTURERS, MECHANICS, ARTISANS, AND OTHERS, (INHABITANTS OF MANCHESTER AND ITS VICINITY) WHO SIGNED AND SUPPORTED THE LATE PETITION TO THE HOUSE OF COMMONS'

Letters and Papers Supplementary, (September to November 1811 MS Home Office Papers and Records), Part Five, HO 42, Box 117

The years 1811–1812 were very difficult for the labouring classes as a result of a bad harvest, steeply lowered wages and unemployment. This was the time of Luddism, an often violent response to the rise of the machine. Workers petitioned the government for redress for their problems but to no avail. These petitions called on the government to fulfil its duty to protect the social contract. When Parliament did not act in response to thousands of petitioners' signatures in 1811, often with the excuse that nothing could be done because it would upend the economic equilibrium if it helped workers, many labourers saw this as a sign of the need to expand suffrage to the labouring classes.

DOI: 10.4324/9780429198052-26

23. Richard Taylor, 'To the Manufacturers, Mechanics, Artisans, and Others, (inhabitants of Manchester and Its Vicinity) Who Signed and Supported the late Petition to the House of Commons', Letters and Papers Supplementary (1811)

BRETHREN,

NOW that the result of your late application to Parliament is known, your reasonable expectations for the present disappointed, and little hope remaining that any future petition of a similar nature, and to the same quarter, will in future be more successful, it becomes the painful duty of the Committee, entrusted with the management of this unfortunate business, to lay before you the leading circumstances therewith connected.

Your Petition had 36,104 signatures annexed, which was sent to London on the 25th. of May, 1811. The Petition from Scotland, presented at the same time, and for a similar purpose, had 30,000 signatures. One from Bolton 7,000; which plainly proves, that the distress experienced by the Mechanics and Artisans is generally felt through the United Kingdom[....]

In perusing the evidence given by the Delegates on this business, you will see that the ruined state of the manufactures of the country, the sufferings of the labouring classes of the community, and the different allegations of the Committee to which it was referred; and by that Committee, in their report, *fully acknowledged, and most deeply lamented*; yet no one *solitary* expedient has been proposed on their part, either for a permanent relief, or a temporary mitigation, of sufferings so candidly acknowledged, and so deeply felt for. On the contrary, in the said report, the Committee seem to consider some of the measures proposed by the Petitioners of too great magnitude for the time to which they found it necessary to circumscribe their deliberations; others of a nature hostile to the principles of individual liberty, and which would ultimately be injurious even to the Petitioners themselves as calculated to arrest the progress of national improvement, and consequently of national prosperity; as tending to circumscribe matters, which ought to be left to their own operation, and which, like water, would find their own level. Above all, the report is decidedly against pecuniary aid being granted, as hopes would thereby be created, which could never be realized; as any sum that could be given must prove altogether inadequate to the distress. Besides that, the balance of commerce, of manufacture, and agriculture, would be endangered.

We are only mechanics, of course ill acquainted with the reason why the same measures are frequently opposed, at one time, by the same arguments by which at other times they are vindicated and supported. But when we consider the extent and severity of the sufferings of which our Petition complained, with the most unparalleled patience of the sufferers—when we consider the *number* of the Petitioners, their usefulness in society, their peaceable demeanour, the respectful language in which their petition was couched, and that petition altogether unconnected with party politics, not the unseasonable clamour of a discontented populace, but the prayer of starving industry, which had relief, and that alone, for its object—was it possible that some reasonable portion of hope should not have been founded on these circumstances? But when we consider likewise, that the Legislature has already interfered in matters apparently of less moment—has enacted laws for regulating the price of *corn*, for fixing the assize of *bread*, for fixing the price of labour in the case of the Spittalfield Weavers, and Journeyman Tailors of London; for augmenting the salaries of *Judges* and *Clergymen*; for regulating commerce, and a multitude of other things, which time would fail to enumerate[....] This Committee are utterly at a loss to conceive on what fair ground Legislative interference can be improper under circumstances so necessitous. If a large mound be projected from the one bank of a river, the stream must necessarily make inroads on the opposite shore: and if laws be made to regulate the price of the necessaries of life, laws should also be enacted for regulating the wages by which such provisions must be purchased, especially when *(as in our case)* such wages have lost all reasonable balance and proportion.

We have been in the habit of considering the wisdom of the House of Commons equal to every emergency. We have seen that House triumph over the united efforts of prejudice and barbarity, of ignorance and unconscionable avarice, in the abolition of the slave trade. We have seen their arm extended for the protection of the weak and defenceless—their hand opened liberally for the relief of the indigent. We still see them able to provide the means for defending our common country against the attacks of Europe united against us; even in cases the most critical and alarming, their wisdom has never been nonplussed: but our case, it would seem, stands an exception in the general rule of Legislation; but *why* it should be so, we confess we have not sufficient penetration to discover a satisfactory reason.

On the whole, when reasonable hopes have been entertained, and considerable exertions made to realize these hopes, it becomes a painful task to relate the tale of disappointment. This the Committee find it on the present occasion; and have only to say for themselves, that nothing, which the means in their power enabled them to attempt, for bringing this business to a happy termination, has been neglected; every thing that *could* be done, *has* been done to secure success; and all the consolation remains, either to the Committee or the supporters of the Petition, is the poor reflection, that they have done their best, and that the distress of the country has been fairly, formally, and specifically represented at the proper place[....]

From the foregoing statement it is evident, that although the distress of the Manufacturers and Artisans was fully proved to, and admitted by, the House of Commons, yet it is equally evident, that that House was either unable or unwilling to remove this general calamity: in either case it proves that House (as at present constituted or appointed) to be unfit to manage your affairs. They, the Members of that House, can make arrangements which advance the price of provisions-increase your taxes, introduce such a state of things as diminishes your business and employment, and reduces your wages; but when you state to them that you cannot exist under these accumulated and accumulating evils, they can coolly tell you they *cannot* relieve you. Had you possessed 70,000 votes for the election of Members to sit in that House, would your application have been treated with such indifference, not to say inattention? We believe not. Is it not therefore high time to look to your own concerns, to strengthen the connexion between you and your *nominal* Representatives, to claim the constitutional privilege of electing those Men who are to make the laws which are to govern you; who impose your taxes, and direct your exertions. Your industry and economy no longer procure you plenty, nor have you any security they ever *will*, while your affairs are managed by Men over whom you have no check or control, and who have the power of raising the price of provisions, increasing your taxation, and diminishing the value of your labour. That such is the state of things at present, the state of the Representation abundantly proves. It having been stated, and not contradicted, that in the year 1793, one hundred and sixty-two individuals sent 300 Member into the House of Commons, being a majority thereof. If therefore you have any regard for your liberty, property, or security, hesitate not to solicit the PRINCE REGENT for the restoration of that Right, without which no other rights are available or secure; namely, the right of electing your Representatives, and extending the elective franchise as far as taxation.

Richard Taylor, Secretary,
Manchester, Oct. 21, 1811

24

ANON., 'AN ADDRESS FROM THE FRAMEWORK-KNITTERS TO THE GENTLEMEN HOSIERS OF THE TOWN OF NOTTINGHAM'

Nottingham Review & General Advertiser for the Midland Counties, 4 (1811), Letters and Papers Supplementary, September to November 1811; MS Home Office Papers and Records, Part Five, HO 42, Box 117

In a strategic move, the following petition 'humbly' asks the factory owners for advice on how to redress their concerns; in this way, they show respect for the existing power dynamics while also illustrating an increasing desire to act on their own behalf politically without presenting a revolutionary aspect that other groups and individuals exhibited. The language suggests that they just wanted to be 'comfortable' and that they were unnerved that Parliament was not responding quickly to such a large group of 'peacab[le]' people in dire straits. The similar references to distress and calamity in all these petitions speak to a crescendo of voices alluding to the existence of severe hunger and even starvation amongst a large sector of the population; the general lack of response from Parliament incurred mistrust and anger on the part of the labourers for decades to come, and hence the push to unionise and fight for the vote. It is unclear what kind of reply, if any, was received from the manufacturers.

DOI: 10.4324/9780429198052-27

24. Anon., 'An Address from the Framework-Knitters to the Gentlemen Hosiers of the Town of Nottingham', *Nottingham Review & General Advertiser for the Midland Counties* (1811)

AN ADDRESS
From the FRAMEWORK-KNITTERS
To The
GENTLEMEN HOSIERS
Of
THE TOWN OF NOTTINGHAM'

"GENTLEMEN,—At a time like the present, so big with Calamity and Distress, we think it right to solicit your Advice, Aid, and Direction, as we know no Reason why our Business, which is looked upon as the staple Trade, both for ourselves and you, and a mutual good Understanding in all our Actions, we solicit your Advice, Aid, Direction, and Support, in this time of our Calamity and Distress, and we think we have a humble Claim upon you for it. On account of the great rise of all the Necessaries of Life, a Man that has full employ, with all his industry, and a Woman, with all her care and economy, can by no means support a Family with any degree of Comfort. If this is the Case (which it really is) how deplorable must the situation of those be, that have but a small portion of Employ, and at very low Rates; but still worse, what must the situation of those be that have none at all, which is the Case with INCALCULABLE NUMBERS at this time.—Destitute of all Comforts of Life, our only acquaintance is pinching Poverty and pining Want. We wish to live peaceably and honestly by our Labour, and to train up our Children in the paths of virtue and rectitude, but we cannot accomplish our wishes. Our Children, instead of being trained up by a regular course of Education, for social life, virtuous employments, and all the reciprocal advantages of mutual enjoyment, are scarce one remove from the Brute, are left to all the dangerous Evils attendant on an uncultivated Mind, and often fall dreadful Victims to that guilt, which Ignorance is the parent of. But, Gentlemen, we forbear, as we think it would be insulting both to your judgments and feelings, were we to attempt a description of all our Calamities, which you so well know, and which we so much experience. Our request, Gentlemen, is that you will favor us with your best Advice, respecting an Address to Parliament, for the better Regulation of our Trade, and means of defence against future Impositions. Being well assured that the most suitable means lie in the compass of your breasts, we wish to pay all deference to your superior judgments, and are now waiting for your decision, which we hope you will favor us with as soon as possible; that if it meets your views, the Business may be conducted peaceably and in good order, to our mutual Comfort and Advantage.

November 28, 1811.

25

WILLIAM CRUMP, 'ADDRESS OF THE PLAIN SILK STOCKING-MAKERS TO THE GENTLEMEN HOSIERS OF NOTTINGHAM, WHO HAVE AGREED TO GIVE AN ADVANCE OF SIXPENCE PER PAIR FOR THE MAKING OF BLACK SILK HOSE'

Nottingham Review & General Advertiser for the Midland Counties, 4 (1811), Letters and Papers Supplementary, September to November 1811; MS Home Office Papers and Records, Part Five, HO 42, Box 117

This address is a short but shocking indication of the delicate rhetorical situation the silk stocking-makers found themselves in, in requesting and receiving an advance of their wages because of the situation of being temporarily unemployed or underemployed. One has to wonder about such an advance actually compounding the problem while it also would reveal that the workers were, in fact, not being paid a living wage.

DOI: 10.4324/9780429198052-28

25. William Crump, 'Address of the Plain Silk Stocking-Makers to the Gentlemen Hosiers of Nottingham, Who have Agreed to Give An Advance of Sixpence per Pair For The Making Of Black Silk Hose', *Nottingham Review* (1811)

ADDRESS
OF THE PLAIN SILK STOCKING-MAKERS
TO
THE GENTLEMEN HOSIERS OF NOTTINGHAM,
Who have Agreed to Give
AN ADVANCE OF SIXPENCE per PAIR
For The Making Of Black Silk Hose'

"GENTLEMEN,—Gratitude is an Attribute imprinted upon the Human Heart by Deity himself; and for us not to acknowledge your Favor on the present occasion, would render us unworthy of your future regard, and justly expose us to the scorn of every honest and humane Man, who might be made acquainted with your present attention to our Interest. It is therefore with peculiar satisfaction that we return you our Thanks for your ready condescension in attending to the solicitations of those Persons that waited upon you, on our behalf to obtain that advance above specified. Indeed, whoever contemplates for a moment the present situation of the Stocking-Makers, with the alarming price of every necessary of life staring them in the face, will sympathize with their sufferings, and the sufferings of their Families, and will readily join with them in giving Thanks to those of their Employers, who attend to the amelioration of their piteous Condition.

Gentlemen,
Believe me your very humble and obedient Servant,

WILLIAM CRUMP, Secretary,
In behalf of the Plain Silk Stocking-Makers

26

CHARLES PRESCOTT, 'LETTER' REGARDING THE STOCKPORT WEAVERS' PETITION TO PARLIAMENT

(21 May 1816), NA HO 42/150 f264

Often magistrates sent fawning letters to the local aristocratic landowners about the petitions they were receiving from workers about their distress. In some cases, magistrates were being paid to spy on the workers' political activities; there were certainly paid governmental spies who attempted to infiltrate reformist and radical group meetings. Magistrate Charles Prescott seems to be sincere in his efforts to help labourers find 'redress' through petitions regarding their 'starving' conditions.

DOI: 10.4324/9780429198052-29

26. Charles Prescott, 'Letter' regarding the Stockport weavers' petition to Parliament (1816)

My Lord.
Yesterday two Men delegated by the Weavers of this town & Neighborhood requested me to permit a meeting for the purpose of forwarding a petition to the House of Commons stating their grievances, & praying for such redress as the House might think it to afford. I recommended their sending the Petition immediately to the Members for Cheshire, as much time might be lost by going about for probably fifteen-thousand signatures, & the inconveniences that attend large meetings be prevented.—I trust the small number of names will not prevent the petition being attended to, or its going into a Committee.

Many families are in a starving condition, numerous are & more will soon be out of work, they are almost driven to despair, the symptoms of intended <rioting?> are stronger than, I recollect they were, previous to the breaking out of the Luddites, could any method be desirous to alleviate the present distress, the probable mischief, extensive as it may be, might be prevented.—

I trust your Lordship will excuse the liberty I take (being the only resident Magistrate in this town) in intruding myself upon you, & earnestly requesting your attention to this concern which seems materially to affect the peace of the country to a great extent—

I remain with very great respect
Yr Lordship's most Obt. Servt.
Charles Prescott.

PS I inclose a copy of the petition, & a printed paper circulated last night.—The weakly earnings of a Weaver should have been stated as four-shillings, & not five;—

27

ANON., 'ADDRESS AND PETITION OF THE DISTRESSED MECHANICS OF BIRMINGHAM'

Presented to House of Commons, Hansard, HC (28 April 1817), Volume 36, cols. 21–26

The labourers in the manufacturing districts prided themselves on being patient in times of distress, but this petition suggests that, while they were loyal to their country, they felt that conditions had become so deleterious to such a large swath of workers that it was incumbent on the State to take notice and redress their ills. The petition notes that Britain had always assumed the right of the labourer to a comfortable existence, and it implies that a society could not thrive economically or morally if such a large portion of its population was experiencing ongoing distress, including hunger and starvation. The petition also illustrates how MPs participated in worker causes; in this case, Whig MP Henry Brougham seems to take up their case by putting it before Parliament, accepting it on its own terms. Nevertheless, he ultimately states his belief that Parliament could not do anything in response to the petition because the needs of the distressed were so broad and deep that there was not money enough to relieve them. This ends up being a stunning admission that the economic system and wages themselves were not working to keep the State in a steady equilibrium, while richer members of society lived in luxury—clearly a systemic deployment of food insecurity was showing its hand in capitalist economics.

The whole system seemed to be wheeling out of any man's control and it was assumed that its detrimental effects were to be borne by the labourers. Indeed, Brougham's disquieting admission should also be set against the humble, courteous tone of the workers—they avow that they just want to earn 'honest bread' through 'honest' labour. But, as they remind Parliament, the rejoinder that they must just wait patiently like good Englishmen meant that they would die of starvation. Starvation waited on no man. Brougham's introduction to the petition notes the devasting increase of distressed workers, but his obsession with how the poor rates had increased as a result is far more telling of his position in response to their need.

DOI: 10.4324/9780429198052-30

27. Anon., 'Address and Petition of the Distressed Mechanics of Birmingham', Presented to Parliament (1817)

Mr. *Brougham* said, it had often been his painful duty to lay before the House the complaints of large portions of his majesty's subjects, but he never performed this duty with feelings so distressing as at that moment, both because the evil was so much more extensive in its pressure than at any former period, and because the prospect of relief, compared with the urgency of the case, was faint and unsatisfactory. The Petition which he had to present, was signed by nearly the whole of the labouring population of the great town of Birmingham. To prepare this petition no public meeting had been held, not even any public notice had been given that the petition lay for signatures, but three copies having been laid in different parts of the town, and the fact having become known, in less than forty-eight hours 11,000 names were affixed. At each of the places where the petition was placed, several persons of respectability attended to prevent any person from signing more than one name, and to exclude all those who were under twenty-one. In a few days more, the signatures amounted to 12,500, and to prevent a concourse of people from the neighbouring villages, it was deemed expedient not to suffer the petition to remain longer, lest tumult might be occasioned by the multitude which would flock together. It was therefore from the town of Birmingham alone that the signatures were collected, which might be calculated to represent a population of 50 or 60,000 souls, probably the whole of the poor population of that town. This petition proceeded on no theories whatsoever; it urged no arguments or views connected, however remotely, with party questions. It was a statement, in humble but earnest and impressive language of the degree of misery, approaching nearly to despair, to which that once flourishing town was now reduced. Before he [Brougham] moved that the petition be read, he should state that the misery which was felt was far from decreasing. There had, a short time ago, been an influx of orders; but that was to be found temporary, and the distress was greater than ever. The statement which he had made on the 13th of March had been too much corroborated by the accounts from Birmingham. It was then clearly shown that the misery, far from diminishing, was on the increase. The average assessment to the poor-rates during the last 12 months was 9*s.* 4*d.*; the average of the last six months was at the rate of 12*s.*, of the last three months 13*s.*, of the last week 14*s.* 4*d.*, and this average fell short of the sum actually expended in the same proportion, as 14*s.* 4*d*, fell short of 17*s.* 8*d.* The expenditure had, for several weeks, been 4 or 500*l.* above the sum actually raised by the rates, and 100*l.* per week above the expenditure of any former period of distress, however great. These facts should be sufficient to awaken the attention of the House, but he should not deal fairly with the House or the petitioners, if he did not state his opinion that the distress was, to a degree, beyond the power of the House to relieve. It was mere vanity, not to speak disrespectfully of the proposal of the chancellor of the exchequer, for any one to expect a loan of a million, or a million and a half, could produce any sufficient relief. This was manifest by the fact, that to relieve the persons who had signed the petition in his hand, near half a million yearly would be required on a moderate calculation. How was it to be expected then that the sum would spread over not only the inhabitants of Birmingham and a population three times as great in its vicinity, but those districts which, though they suffered less, still suffered dreadfully. Greatly though he lamented the necessity and their want of power to relieve it, it was proper to state that no one immediate step could afford any tolerable prospect of permanent amelioration, except that general change of policy which was the only sort of relief which statesmen should consider, though not so immediate as that of which a vain and delusive semblance was now held forth[....]

The petition was then read[....]

That the under signed Inhabitants of the town of Birmingham beg leave to approach the House, and to inform them of their forlorn and miserable situation; accustomed from their earliest infancy to habits of continual labour, they have never been forward to obtrude their humble interests upon the public attention, but they have always placed confidence in the wisdom and justice of parliament and of their country, nor should they now have been induced to prefer their complaints, but their misery is greater than they can bear, and they are compelled to make known their distresses to the House; they are in distress, and in their misery they call upon their country for relief, they ask no more than the House will acknowledge that good citizens have a right to expect, they ask no favour, they only ask to have it placed in their power to earn an honest bread by honest labour, and to receive in exchange the scanty comforts necessary for the support of life; their wants are only food and clothing and shelter from the elements; never before have they known the time when the labour of an Englishman could not procure him such humble comforts as these nor can they now believe that his labour is of less value than formerly; in all former times the labour of an Englishman could produce a sufficient quantity of the good things of life, not only for his own maintenance, but to provide an ample remuneration to his country and to his employers, and they presume to believe that the labour of an Englishman is still competent to produce a far greater quantity of the good things of life than is humble maintenance requires; that some cause which they cannot understand has deprived industry of its reward, and has left them without employment and without bread, and almost without hope; they have no longer any demand for their labour, nor any bread for their families, their life has become useless to their country and burthensome to themselves, it would be better for them to die than to live, for then they should hear no more the cries of their children, their hearts would no longer be wounded by the sight of sufferings which they indeed share, but which they cannot relieve; they implore the House not to misunderstand the expression of those bitter sufferings which they endure, hunger and poverty and distress have indeed changed all things around them, but they have not changed the petitioners, they have not changed the devoted loyalty which as good subjects they feel towards their king, nor that true English spirit which binds them to the constitution and to the House; many of them have not had any kind of employment for many months, and few of them have more than two or three days work per week, at reduced wages; the little property which they possessed in household furniture and effects, and the small hard-earned accumulations of years of industry and care, have been consumed in the purchase of food, and they are now under the necessity of supporting their existence by a miserable dependence on parochial charity, or by soliciting casual relief from persons scarcely less distressed than themselves; in the midst of these painful sufferings and privations their friends and neighbours tell them that they must wait and hope for better times; they beg leave to inform the House that they have waited until their patience is quite exhausted, for whilst they wait they die; upon all former occasions of distress in any branch of trade, it was always found that some other channels of industry existed through which the honest labourer could obtain his bread, but now the petitioners find all other descriptions of labourers equally distressed with themselves, a general calamity has fallen upon the whole nation, and has crushed the happiness of all; they would indeed indulge the hope that their sufferings are peculiar to themselves, and may have been occasioned by the cessation of the war expenditure among them, but on whatsoever side they turn their eyes, if they look to Manchester or to Glasgow, or to the crowded city or the peaceful village, from one extremity of their country to the other, they can perceive nothing but an universal scene of poverty and distress, the sighs and the tears and the convulsive efforts of suffering millions too plainly convince them that some general and universal cause must have operated in producing such general and universal misery, and they implore the House to remove that cause, whatever it may be, they cannot but think that the House can remove it, or if its roots are so deeply hidden that no human wisdom can discover them, or so strongly fixed that no human strength can remove them, they must then consider their sufferings as a visitation from Almighty God, to which they must dutifully bend; but in that case they intreat the House will adopt proper measures for the whole nation to humble itself in mortification and prayer, in order to propitiate divine justice, and avert those heavy calamities which afflict them; but they cannot but think that these calamities originate in natural causes, which it is in the power of human wisdom to discover and to remove; they cannot but think that, in a great nation like this, the means of existence must exist for all; they cannot but think that, in a country abounding with every blessing, and with every production of agricultural and mechanical industry, some means may be devised by which the blessings of Providence may be distributed and enjoyed, by which the productive powers of industry may again be brought into action, and the honest labourer may again be enabled to earn an honest bread by the sweat of his brow; and the petitioners humbly pray that the House will take into consideration their distressed condition, and adopt such measures as in their wisdom may be deemed necessary for the relief of themselves and of their suffering country'. Ordered to lie on the table.

28

ANON., 'BARNSLEY REFORM MEETING'

Leeds Mercury (17 July 1819), p. 3

Written from a conservative point of view, this newspaper account summarises a meeting of reform-minded labourers and their speakers' orations about the 'distress of the country'. It includes their statement entitled 'Appeal to the Nation'. Only a few weeks before Peterloo, this piece portends the violent role of the yeomanry and standing army in repressing such meetings. The tone of the appeal is much more contentious than others in the petitions featured in this section, showing the labourers had even lost 'confidence' in Parliament to address their needs. The speakers also refer to the 'physical force' argument, that is, that if Parliament refused to make necessary changes as a result of the workers' 'moral force' approach, the radical movement would consider violence to achieve their goals. Military hero Major Cartwright (1740–1824) took up the radical cause, and in this case, presented this appeal to Parliament.

DOI: 10.4324/9780429198052-31

28. Anon., 'Barnsley Reform Meeting', *Leeds Mercury* (1819)

APPEAL TO THE NATION

We have now arrived at the height of human misery. The labouring classes of the community are daily perishing for want; our manufacturers and commerce are destroyed; even agriculture itself appears doomed to destruction. All these evils arise from a base and profligate expenditure of the public money, which has increased taxation to such an extent, as threatens destruction to every useful member of society. The men who ought to have been the guardians of the public welfare, have betrayed the interests of the nation; they have voted away our money for the basest of purposes; they have supported a set of swindlers, who pass worthless paper under the name of money; and they have insulted our present distress by the imposition of new taxes! In short, the whole course of their conduct has shown them to be unworthy of confidence. They have clearly shown that their whole design is, by the imposition of taxes to destroy our manufactures and commerce, and prevent the labouring classes of the community from obtaining employment, and thus to ruin the middle classes of society, by the payment of taxes and poor-rates, and then to reduce the nation to a despotism consisting of nothing but lordlings and slaves. We are perfectly satisfied that the only means of averting the approaching ruin, is by obtaining a Radical Reform in the Commons House of Parliament. Under these circumstances, we call upon every man, who by useful employment contributes to the necessities of the state to join with us in forming a National Union, to demand our rights, in a voice which must accomplish its end, and restore freedom and happiness to our native country. But why does any one stand at a distance? Do you not form a part of the people? Say not that you are Reformers, but prove yourselves to be such, by using your utmost endeavours to restore the freedom of Britain. Disdain the shameful conduct of saying, 'we wish well to the cause,' whilst you never hold up a finger to forward the glorious object. Do you expect to escape the ruin which the Boroughmongers have prepared for the nation? Do you think that the voracious appetite of taxation will be satiated before it arrives at yourselves? Men of moral virtue, where are you? Ye, who profess to be christians [sic] will you see your fellow-countrymen daily sinking under their burdens, and refuse to lend your assistance? Merchants and tradesmen, what are you doing? Do you expect to acquire wealth, when your labourers and customers are pined to death? Landholders, do you think that taxation will never overtake you? What will be the value of your soil, when those who cultivate it are laid in the grave? The monster, taxation, will devour you in the end, unless its progress be speedily arrested. Corruption has arrived at its height; it threatens to overwhelm us every moment. Fellow Countrymen, will you see destruction staring you in the face, and still continue idle spectators? Every principle of virtue, honour, and justice, demands your assistance to cleanse away the filth of corruption. Then if you love yourselves, if you love your friends, or your country, come forward and exert all your powers to restore the freedom of your native land.

This appeal was adopted unanimously, and a vote of thanks to Major Cartwright was carried by acclamation.

29

ANON., 'FEMALE REFORMERS'

Leeds Mercury (17 July 1819), p. 3

Illustrating the substantive role of women in the Reform movement, a short article below the 'Appeal' made at Barnsley describes how the women in the reform movement, known as 'The Committee of the Blackburn Female Reform Society', responded to the distress. In the reporter's sexist description, the focus is on the women's appearance; described as participating in an 'enchanting scene', they are praised for being 'neatly dressed'. Nevertheless, the event is punctuated with cries of 'LIBERTY or DEATH' from the crowd, along with choruses of 'God bless the women'. At one point, the article waylays the 'canibal Castlereagh' by noting that if he had seen these women reformers in action he 'must have had a heart of brass, if it had not struck him dead to the ground. An Anglo-Irish MP, Castlereagh was much disliked' by the lower classes. He supported the repressive Six Acts that the Crown imposed when dealing with the Luddites and other labourers who began calling for reforms in Parliament in 1811–1816. In response to Peterloo, Castlereagh asks what good it would do to take from the upper classes to give to the lower classes. He ultimately committed suicide after exhibiting paranoid behaviour.

The women's group takes the tack of many oppressed groups; that is, they 'apologize' for their 'interference in the politics of our country', to '*very great applause*', but they then explain that their situation is full of such 'woes', and they feel they must speak out, particularly in support of suffrage. The women's address is summarised all too briefly.

DOI: 10.4324/9780429198052-32

29. Anon., 'Female Reformers', *Leeds Mercury* (1819)

The Address was then read, and consisted of an impassioned description of the distresses of the labouring classes, and an earnest solicitation to every man in England to join the general Union, for the attainment of Annual Parliaments, Universal Suffrage, and Election by Ballot, which, say the Addressers,—'alone can save us from lingering misery and premature death.'

30

ANON., 'CORN LAWS-PETITION OF THE STARVING WEAVERS OF BLACKBURN', COMMONS SITTING

Source: Hansard, HC (9 February 1827), Volume 16, cols. 413–414

The English working classes were accustomed to the right to petition Parliament to address their concerns, but during the first half of the nineteenth century this right became more urgent as the distress increased beyond normal bounds. Labourers used this right, but it became increasingly clear across the first three decades of the century that petitioning Parliament was simply not enough, especially when this governmental body did not effectually respond to such political actions, or when some MPs did not believe the constitution allowed for any legal recourse for addressing rampant starvation. The complaint about the sinecures held by the idle rich is repeated in many of the labourer's public documents and private letters to the royals and Parliamentary figures, suggesting, again, that it was the idle rich who were the real drones in the British beehive. Dealing with issues around a living wage and directly referring to 'hunger' and 'starvation', this petition reads in part as follows.

DOI: 10.4324/9780429198052-33

30. Anon., 'Corn Laws-Petition of the Starving Weavers of Blackburn', Commons sitting (1827)

That the starving petitioners, with the rectitude of injured men, presume to approach the House in order to lay before the House a statement of their complaints and wishes, to the end that the House may grant them that relief which their unmerited sufferings require: the petitioners, for many years, have suffered more than language can express, but within the last two years they have not had half food, of the worst kind, for their support, consequently hundreds of weavers, their wives and children, have died from absolute want of food: the petitioners, being able-bodied men, cannot earn more than *5s.* per week each, and, with two workers in each family, averaging six souls, *10s.* weekly is the whole for food, clothing, fuel and rent; and this scanty pittance the petitioners are necessitated to live upon: that the petitioners, with all due deference to the House, would respectfully ask, is the sum above stated sufficient, for the moderate wants of a man? If it is not, then are they perishing for want of food. The petitioners humbly conceive, that they cannot bear affection to the House while that House manifests no disposition to relieve them: the petitioners are human beings, and worship the same god, wherefore then should they be so oppressed in their native land? Why should they, who labour sixteen hours per day, not obtain for that labour food and clothing for comfortable existence; there is a point when endurance becomes a crime, and to that point the petitioners have arrived: the petitioners cannot do much longer; they are dying daily for want of food, and to be silent under such circumstances would be highly criminal: that the petitioners have calmly and considerately examined into the causes which have produced such calamities to the working classes of this country, and are convinced that all have originated from the people not being represented in the House; that the national debt, the enormous church revenues, all the unmerited placemen, pensioners, sinecures, a standing army to murder the people if they complain, all the bloody wars that the nation has been plunged into, are all owing to a want of a reform in the House.'

Ordered to lie on the table and be printed.

31

T. B. MACAULAY, 'DIFFERENCE BETWEEN A STATE OF CIVILIZATION & BARBARISM (*FROM MR. T. B. MACAULAY'S SPEECH AT EDINBURGH*)'

Leicester Chronicle (15 June 1839), p. 4

This piece illustrates how masterful the bluff Thomas B. Macaulay (1800–1859) could be as a speaker. A famous politician, writer and historian, he illustrates here a humourous ease in engaging with the lower classes while insulting them to their faces. His racist speech does not cover his conservative views about property trumping the needs of the poor. Warning them off from violence, he also blithely asserts that he is not responsible for their starvation. The interjections in parens are from the crowd. It is unclear who Macaulay is referencing when he names a 'Mr. Frasier'.

DOI: 10.4324/9780429198052-34

31. T. B. Macaulay, 'Difference between a State of Civilization & Barbarism' (1839)

I perceive that you have been informed that I used expressions which I never did use. (Oh, oh, oh!) I see you have been informed that I described the working classes of this country as Hottentots. (So you did!) It is false. (Cheers.) I said, and I say again, and I will give you my reasons for saying so, that if this country were to be governed on the principles on which a portion of the labouring classes are calling for universal suffrage, the attempt would inevitably reduce this country to the condition of the Hottentots. (Oh, oh, cheers, yells, and hisses). My good friends, if you wish for the franchise, these hisses and yells will not establish your right to it. (Hear, hear.) The meaning of my expression is this; I believe that the condition of the labouring classes of this island, and particularly those in the north, is far, very far indeed, from what I could wish to see it. But still I do conscientiously believe that the difference between the condition of these labouring classes, and the condition of the people who live in countries utterly uncivilised is very great indeed (It's a lie.) I can establish the fact. (Cheers.) The cottages of the labouring classes are not what I could wish to see them, but still they are very superior to the kraal of the Hottentot, or the wigwam of the Indian. (Hear.) Your clothing is not exactly what I could wish to see it, but it is better than the nakedness of the barbarians existing in many parts of the world. (We're as good as you.) I am not disputing your goodness. I am telling you how much superior you are to barbarians. (Laughter.) One of the speakers to-day talked of the labouring classes being in a state of starvation. God forbid that this should be the fact; at any rate I cannot charge myself with being the cause of it; but whatever I could do to make food cheaper, I would most willingly and gladly do it. (Cheers.) but observe, there are countries where, from want of civilization and all social order, it Is not unusual to see the whole population suffering from famine, whole families swept away in a season. (Hear, hear). When, therefore, we see the great difference between those societies where the people live in utter barbarism, and these societies where, though the people are not quite so well off as I could wish to see them, yet where they hold a comparatively high rank among the nations for civilization and comfort, and which is mainly occasioned by their deference to law and the security of property, I say to every one amongst you, if any accident should befall you, if any sickness should overtake you, you could at this moment secure far better surgical skill and medical attendance than the very princes of half the barbarian nations in the world. (Cheers.) Now, to what is this owing? Why, to nothing else than to the existence and preservation of law, order, and property. (Cheers and disorder.) Now, what think you would be the consequence of carrying into effect those principles which some of the leaders of the party who are now calling for universal suffrage have publicly avowed? They had said, that if universal suffrage is refused, a war against property will be commenced. (Cries of no, yes!) I do not impute these sentiments to you my good friends; but I say that is has been said by some of the leaders of that party and I have also read in the same quarter that if the landholders oppose the people's charter, the landholders ought to be put to death. I say, also, that doctrines subversive of the rights of property have been put forth on this occasion. Even Mr. Frasier himself, moderate as he was, and not at all sanguinary, advanced doctrines which, in my opinion, are entirely inconsistent with the rights of property; and I say, that if you once touch the security of property, property will fly from this country. (Cheers.) That which is a fixed form will perish; that which is in a passing form will be carried away; and the labouring classes will be the great sufferers. (Hear, hear, hear.) Men will carry their capital to another country. I say, that out of this great, this vast population of twenty-four millions, cooped up together in a space which was never before so thickly peopled in the history of the world—with thousands unable to emigrate to any other country—if once you destroy the security of property, the consequence will be, that you, the working men, will be the great sufferers. (Hear, hear) The capital, the property, the educated classes, will depart—('The sooner the better')—the labourers will be left to perish. (Hear.) That is what I mean when I said that, in my opinion, if the measures advocated by some of the leaders of universal suffrage were carried into effect, they would reduce Scotland and England to the state of the Hottentots. (Cheers and yells.)

Part 4

'DISTRESS OF THE NATION'

Clearly, with the loss of the long tradition of guilds that dignified and honoured the skills of so many labourers, along with the rise of Luddism and the shocking incident known as 'Peterloo', society seemed on the verge of rupture in the early decades of the nineteenth century. So devastating was the event at Peterloo that all MP Bennet had to do to signal the horrifying scene there was to merely refer to the date of the occurrence, 'August 16th' [1819], in a speech he gave soon thereafter (featured later in this Part). August 16th was a day when the government violently fired upon and killed peaceful protesters, including women and children—afterwards, there was a sense on all sides, from conservative to radical, that something was deeply wrong with England. Sights of poverty, starvation and begging on city streets increased to such a level that there was a feeling that something had to be done. A common sight in the periodical press were articles on the 'distress' of the nation. As well, throughout print culture there were discussions regarding whether the response should have been through private charity or more systematic governmental action.

DOI: 10.4324/9780429198052-35

32

ANON., 'THE FOLLOWING REPORT SEEMS TO US TO BE DRAWN UP WITH SO MUCH JUDGMENT. REPORT OF THE ASSOCIATION, FORMED IN LONDON, ON THE 23RD DAY OF MAY, 1812, FOR THE RELIEF AND BENEFIT OF THE MANUFACTURING AND THE LABOURING POOR'

Universal Magazine, 19 (1813), pp. 179–185

Written from the workers' perspective, this report is an example of the use of appeal and petitioning by the labouring poor. It also illustrates one of the responses to the so-called 'distress of the nation', and shows a forceful set of arguments and evidence to support the cause of this reform group. One compelling argument used is that a great nation could not maintain its power if its labouring population continually experienced food and job insecurity. The piece also includes a common trope used in such arguments, that is, that the animals of the rich were fed better than poor people.

DOI: 10.4324/9780429198052-36

32. Anon., 'The following Report seems to us to be drawn up with so much judgment. Report of the Association, formed in London, on the 23rd Day of May, 1812, for the Relief and Benefit of the Manufacturing and the Labouring Poor', *Universal magazine* (1813)

The circumstances and condition of so large and so valuable a part of our population as that which is constituted by the labouring and manufacturing poor must be considered at all times an object of great importance and deep interest; but when it is notorious that from peculiar circumstances, such as the stagnation of trade, and the high price of provisions, many thousands of our countrymen must be greatly distressed, if not even altogether destitute of the means of procuring subsistence; an inquiry into their situation and an attempt to relieve them become duties, the performance of which is called for no less powerfully by consideration of sound policy, than by the motives of humanity.

Under this impression the Association for the relief of the Manufacturing Poor was originally formed; and whatever doubts might have been at first entertained of the utility of such an institution, the experience of the last seven months has amply proved its necessity and importance.

The existence of this institution was no sooner known, than statements of distress and applications for relief came up from divers parts of the kingdom, but principally from the manufacturing districts; and these statements have enabled the Association to take a comprehensive view of the whole subject. Several important points, which never could have been so clearly established by any other method, were thus ascertained, and measures of relief on an extended scale have presented themselves, which could never have been carried into effect by any society more limited in its views. As the persons by whom the information was transmitted were of the highest respectability, and eye-witnesses of what they reported, the society became possessed of a most valuable body of evidence, which has been digested under the following heads: *Estimate of Distress,—Causes of Distress,—Employment and Average Earnings,—Price of Provisions,—Attempts at Relief.*

On each of these heads the committee beg leave to offer a few observations.

Estimate of Distress.

All the reports agree in stating that the manufacturing districts experience the greatest poverty and want. To have a just conception of the amount of human misery which there prevails, it is necessary to consider that commonly those districts are extremely populous. One parish alone contains a population of more than seventy thousand souls.

On the whole it appears that several hundred thousands of our countrymen have suffered more in the last year than perhaps in any former period of equal length. The paupers compared with the whole population are, in some instances, as one to five, in others, as one to four, one to three, and in some cases they amount almost to one-half.

In districts thus loaded, the poor's rates, though increased beyond all former precedent, are insufficient to supply the claims made upon them; while persons, those who were formerly affluent, nay, who may still be said to be in good circumstances, partaking in the general distress which arises from the stagnation of commerce, are utterly unable to pay the rates. A worthy clergyman in Yorkshire states, that out of three thousand families under his care, he has at present only procured his vicarial dues from nine hundred and fifty-seven, and does not expect any more, unless circumstances should alter; that he is averse from compulsion, which he is aware might in many instances extort from indigence what is wanted to satisfy the imperious calls of nature.

To detail all the cases of distress which have been developed to the committee would require a volume. The selection of a few, however, will pretty correctly show the complexion of the rest.

The situation of a manufacturing parish near Leeds is thus described:

> 'The distresses of the labouring poor are great and complicated; many have sold all their goods, some have been sent to jail for debt, and the creditors are only deterred from seizing because they cannot find purchasers.
>
> The poor's rates have become inadequate from the increase of paupers, and numerous applications for relief are made weekly which cannot be complied with. The township consists of four hundred and sixty-four families, comprising two thousand three hundred and twenty-four individuals; one hundred and eighty-five of these families, consisting of one thousand one hundred and nineteen individuals, are in a state of distress.'

In a town in Leicestershire, the distress (for want of food) was so extensively felt, that it became necessary to relieve two thousand and forty persons, being more than one-third of the population of the town.

In a township in Lancashire, where the population is ten thousand, the distress is very great, and cannot be supplied either by private charities or legal rates.

In a township in Yorkshire containing nine hundred and forty-eight families, consisting of five thousand and two individuals, three hundred and fifty-six families, amounting to one thousand seven hundred and sixty-four individuals, receive relief; but five hundred families, consisting of two thousand six hundred individuals, are in urgent need of it; the poor's rates collected from the commencement of May to the end of July amounted to *974l.6s.* and the distress is stated to be unexampled in the memory of the most aged inhabitant. 'The case is not that the wretched manufacturer [labourer in the factory] feels himself and beholds his family doomed to a scanty meal of the most homely fare; he has not a subsistence of any description, without material aid beyond his own exertions.'

The uniformity so observable in these melancholy statements render these few cases, selected from the general mass, but too accurate a description of what is now endured in a large proportion of the manufacturing districts. It needs only to be stated, that the necessity under which the manufacturing poor in general have lain of spending all their earnings in the purchase of food, has caused their families to be in a miserable state in point of clothing; but although this heightens their distress, especially at the present season of the year, the committee is prevented by want of funds from promoting plans for this species of relief.

The cause of distress is almost uniformly given in two sentences—want of employ, and high price of provisions; the want of employment is generally referred to the interruptions of our commerce from the peculiar circumstances of the times; and though in some branches of our manufactures the recent revival of demand has lessened this evil, yet the succour hereby afforded is only partial, and even where it does extend is by no means sufficient to relieve the prevalent distress.

Employment and Average Earnings.

The manufacturers of woollen, of cotton, and of hard-ware, together with those employed in the potteries, appear to suffer most severely; though the pressure is by no means confined to them. In many instances the price of labour has been considerably lowered; thus, in one township the wages are stated at not much more than half of what they were in 1800 and 1801.

In another place the weaver only receives *11s.6d.* for the same quantity of work for which he was paid *23s.* in 1805; and it appears that in many places the manufacturer by his utmost exertions cannot earn more than from 10s. to 12s. per week; a large portion have only half work, and many thousands no employment at all.

Price of Provisions.

All the accounts agree in stating the great advance which has taken place in all those articles which constitute the chief food of the poor.

In the northern counties of England the lower orders live almost entirely upon oatmeal and potatoes, while in the southern counties and near the metropolis bread and potatoes are their principal subsistence. The average price of flour has varied from *5d.* to *7d.* per lb. Oatmeal from *4d.* to *6d.* Potatoes in some places have experienced a rise of 100 per cent within a few months. Bread in the metropolis is now about 4d1/4. per lb.

From these data we may form some idea of the state of the poor, it being ascertained that 6 lb. per week of bread or oatmeal is required to subsist an individual, or, in other words, to prevent him from the effects of starvation. This, if oatmeal were at 5d. would be 2s.6d. and but little less if bread were used; therefore where a man has a wife and three children, he cannot purchase this necessary quantity of food, to say nothing of rent, clothing, and other necessary expenses; but many have families still larger. If the poor then who have work, are thus circumstanced, how must it fare with those who are only half employed, or who have no employment at all? Even at a time when provisions are at a moderate price, the wages of labour, as regards the great mass of the poor, are generally fixed as low as can well be, consistently with their existence and tolerable comfort; unless therefore the price of labour rises in proportion to the rise of provisions, inevitable suffering must be the consequence. So far, however, is the price of labour from being advanced in any material proportion to the price of provisions, that we are informed from many manufacturing districts that it is depressed far below the ordinary standard.

The population of a great manufacturing country must always principally consist of those who depend for subsistence on their daily labour; and the safety as well as the happiness of such a country depends mainly upon the habits and morals as well as the means of subsistence of this class.

On every ground therefore, whether of duty or of interest, it is incumbent on the higher orders of society to provide a suitable remedy for those evils which must arise from the stagnation of commerce and the deficiency of food. How to apply this remedy without introducing other evils, is the problem which has occupied the attention of this society.

By a law of our nature it appears that no human being will exert himself but for some attainable good, or something which at least, in his opinion, is such. This is the principle, the main spring of action; but when a poor man has no other prospect than to drudge, day after day, for what will not satisfy the cravings of nature, and has no hope of making the least provision for a time of sickness of decrepitude, the stimulus is taken away. That independent spirit which would prompt him to support his family by every honest exertion is broken down; and from the moment that he begins to accept parochial relief, he gradually sinks, in mind as well as circumstances, to the state of a pauper; he loses his independence; and having no motive for exertion, he will naturally become indolent, and finally claim support at the hands of the public as a matter of right.

The grand point then is to provide against a temporary pressure: the exertions made for this purpose during the present exigence will appear in

The Attempts at Relief.

The statements included under this head do great honour to the feeling and liberality of the country; though in many places it is not found possible, by the greatest exertions, to keep pace with the increased and urgent call for relief.

The subscriptions [donations] in about forty places, where the amount happens to be mentioned, are very near *15,000l.* but the total sum raised by private contributions, and only reported in general terms, must still be greater.

Deeply aware that, if it could be possible to prevail upon those in tolerably easy circumstances to examine into the state of the poor in their vicinity, much might be done to alleviate the present distress, the committee have made it a principal object to promote the establishment of local institutions, and are happy to say they have succeeded far beyond their expectations; and their funds, so inadequate in themselves for the purposes of general relief, have been made to act powerfully in promoting this desirable object.

Grants of money have been made on the condition that such local institutions should be formed; and the committee have had the satisfaction of finding that a gift of 30l. has stimulated the inhabitants of a place to form a local committee and raise 300l. among themselves: in other districts the grant of 100l. has been the means of raising 1000l. and many such instances occur in the correspondence.

The benevolence of the country has thus been excited in local efforts, and the relief already afforded by these means is incalculable.

In one extremely populous and suffering district, the committee thus formed has been the means of raising up six others in its neighbourhood, by offering to add one-fourth to whatever the inhabitants of each place might raise by subscription.

It is scarcely necessary to remark that local institutions possess many great advantages; the members of them have an opportunity of acquainting themselves with the wants and characters of the poor; and thus see that the funds are applied to the greatest advantage; while it has a soothing effect upon the unhappy sufferers, to observe that their case excites at least attention and sympathy.

The reports of the manner in which the poor have received the assistance afforded are gratifying in no ordinary degree, and abundantly prove even the political expediency of such an association as the present[....]

In all cases of real scarcity of that kind of food on which the poor principally subsist, whatever tends to increase the consumption of it must prove injurious to the community at large, by turning a dearth into a famine. The committee have therefore strongly dissuaded the selling of flour or oatmeal at reduced prices, wherever it was possible to procure other cheap articles of food. And again, as oatmeal is so extensively used by the poor in the northern counties, it becomes a great national object to lessen the consumption of oats for every other purpose than that of human food. The horses employed in this country consume a large proportion of grain; and as these animals can be maintained on food which would not subsist a human being, the Committee earnestly beg leave to recommend a reduction in the quantity usually given to them, as one means of producing a considerable degree of relief to the poor. Expedients for diminishing the consumption of articles of the first necessity will appear to be of still greater importance, when it is considered that not only whatever is thus saved from being consumed by cattle is something added to the stock of human sustenance; but when it is also taken into account that every such addition operates far more powerfully than inexact proportion to its own amount in reducing the price of the whole stock of the article, and not of that only, but of every other article of subsistence[....]

The success which has hitherto attended the exertions of this institution is only the earnest of what may be expected, if means are afforded for perfecting the plans now in progress.

It must, however, be remarked, that, owing to some untoward causes of political nature, arising out of the peculiar time and circumstances in which the Association was originally formed, and which have long ceased to exist, the support received by the Association was by no means such as might reasonably have been expected from the ordinary liberality of the public on similar occasions of inferior emergency. Nevertheless, in the space of seven months, with funds which even they themselves could not but conceive at first to be altogether disproportionate to their object, much distress has received direct relief: a spirit of active benevolence has been excited, a correspondence has been established through the kingdom, local institutions have been formed in many places where they did not exist, and measures have been taken to obviate the effect of a temporary pressure, by economizing the food on hand, and providing for an increased supply of a kind which at the same time is calculated to increase naval strength and prosperity of the country.

With a view to the prosecution of these objects on a scale still more extended, the committee solicit the pecuniary support of the public; and in such a cause they cannot but feel confident that they shall not solicit in vain. They cannot but hope that the relief which so honourably to our national character has been afforded to our foreign allies, will be extended no less liberally to our own industrious manufacturers.

33

ANON., 'DISTRESSES OF THE IRON MANUFACTURERS IN STAFFORDSHIRE'

Caledonian Mercury, 1 (August 1816), p. 4

Letters to the editor were a common means of representing the citizenry's concerns about the distress of the nation. In the following two letters, altruistic middle-class citizens intimate that, though well-intentioned, individual acts of charity could not possibly provide an effectual response to the overwhelming claims of poverty and distress occurring in the nation. An introduction to the letters and the letters themselves is included.

DOI: 10.4324/9780429198052-37

33. Anon., 'Distresses of the Iron Manufacturers in Staffordshire', *Caledonian Mercury* (1816)

We have been favoured with the perusal of two letters, one from the neighbourhood of Bilston, and the other from that of Birmingham, addressed to a respectable iron merchant in London, on the subject of the distresses under which the people employed in the iron works and collieries of these districts now labour. The following extracts from those most affecting compositions exhibit a picture of misery we really believe unprecedented in this country, and of which very few of our readers could have had any conception:—

"Coseley, near Bilton, Staffordshire, July 24, 1816.

When some of our principal iron works first failed, the whole extent of the consequent distress was not immediately apparent. The poor manufacturers had many of them made a little money: this, with the greatest frugality, did not last long: when expended, they ran in debt wherever they could gain credit; and when they could not be trusted any longer, they pawned or sold their furniture, article after article, till they had none to sell. When their goods were gone, they were obliged to have recourse to their parishes and to begging. The parishes were overwhelmed by the numbers applying for their aid, and could afford but little comparative support. The community in general (for commercial districts are usually generous) made great efforts to relieve their necessities. For my own part, I determined that I would fare harder, and that my children and household should do so likewise, in order to administer to their wants; and it was my desire that none worthy of relief should go away from my house unrelieved. It is true the succour was but small: they asked for nothing but a piece of bread, and bread for some time great numbers of them received; but I soon found that my very limited income, arising chiefly from uncertain sources, would not even furnish this scanty supply; and I was reduced to the necessity—to me a most painful one—of confining my charity within much smaller boundaries. Companies of five, or eight, or twelve poor manufacturers, able and willing to work, have been many times in the course of a day at my door, soliciting bread, and, what has often cut me to the heart, necessarily soliciting in vain.

Multitudes went through the country, offering to work at any thing merely for a little food, not even expecting wages, and thus gained little temporary employment and subsistence; but still their wives and children were at home in the greatest possible distress.

Within a small distance of my house is a large iron work; the machinery extends nearly half a mile; it was a noble manufactory. I passed by it one morning, after its operations were suspended, and was exceedingly affected with the sight; a little before, it was all animation and industry, affording the honourable means of livelihood to many thousands of fellow-creatures; the *silence* that now pervaded it spoke more eloquently and impressively to my heart than any language could possibly do—it was the silence of unmingled desolation! I visited a row of houses occupied by the workmen; the doors were used to be open, inviting the eye of the stranger to glance as he went along at their neatness, cleanliness, and felicity; little groups of healthful children accustomed to appear about the cottages, full of merriment and joy, and the inhabitants, strong and healthy, saluted you as you went by. But the scene was lamentably changed: it produced a melancholy on my spirits that I did not lose for a considerable period; the cottages were closed—the inhabitants could not bear to have it known that they were stripped of their little ornaments—no children played around the doors—the very plants trained up in their windows had pined and died—one man only appeared, emaciated and ghastly, a living spectre, as if the peaceful sepulchre had sent forth its inhabitants to fill with terror the abodes of the living.

When I have told these poor creatures that the parish must find them food or labour, they have replied, 'Sir, they cannot do either;' and some who have fared the best when our manufactories were flourishing around us, have said, 'We would rather die, Sir, than be dependent on the parish.'

It is unanswerable proof of the excellent disposition of these poor manufacturers [labourers in the factories], that although there are many thousands of them in the most distressed condition imaginable, there is very little depredation in the country.

If it will aid you in your benevolent designs, I will go through any part of our neighbourhood, from house to house, and give you a particular statement of the circumstances of each family; the labour will be to me a delightful remuneration; doing good I have long found to be its own reward. I would devote any portion of my time to procure you information.

Some, I believe, have really died of starvation; and in many cases, if not the *immediate* it was the *primary cause*. An insufficiency of wholesome nourishment, where they had been accustomed to great abundance, produced disease which terminated in dissolution.

Even *charity*, Sir, has left some of our districts. She has given all she had to give; the stream of her benevolence is dried up, and nothing remains but the grateful recollection of the channel through which it flowed, or emotions of despair lest it should never again be replenished.

I could send you many individual cases that come under my own personal knowledge. Not far from my house, a respectable individual, possessed of extensive information in the iron trade, who had been a confidential foreman in a large concern, and lived in much credit, has been for some time, with a wife and eight children, destitute of a sufficiency of bread. Many poor families, distinguished for their sobriety and industry, with five, six, seven, or eight children, are in the same disastrous circumstances; I have myself repeatedly saved a man, his wife, and six children, from absolute starvation, who were reduced to eat the cabbage stalks, and the refuse of their little cottage-garden, as the only food they could obtain.

Had I the pleasure, Sir, of being present at the meeting of your honourable society, I think I could plead the cause of these poor manufacturers till my strength would fail me, and I could plead no longer; their great distresses have taken deep hold of my heart. Shall the injured African readily find a multitude of the most able and eloquent of our nation to defend his cause, and to secure his rights; and shall there be none to commiserate our perishing *fellow-countrymen*, whose ingenuity and industry have spread the glory of Britain throughout the whole habitable globe? Shall no friendly hand be extended to wipe *away their tears*, and to prevent them sinking for ever under the insupportable pressure of accumulated woes? Forbid it honour, decency, humanity, religion!'

The other letter, with which we have been favoured, is dated

'Tibbington house, near Birmingham, July 25, 1816.

I have not lost a moment in distributing your donation of £.5 amongst some of the most distressing cases in my neighbourhood; and although the amount to each family was small, after dividing it amongst upwards of thirty, yet it was so very acceptable, that streams of gratitude flowed from the eyes of those who partook of it. Words cannot picture the distress that prevails in this neighbourhood; and what is still worse, it is likely to increase rapidly. Many of the ironworks, ironstone-works, and collieries that have been hitherto kept at work, are on the eve of being stopped. Indeed, hundreds of men have had notice within the last fortnight to seek fresh employment; and there are already some thousands who have been out of work many months, living upon charity and the household furniture which their late prosperity enabled them to provide.—The liberal and humane persons who have hitherto been a great support to such wretched objects, find the cases so numerous, that their funds of charity are thereby completely exhausted; and the only resort the poor creatures have left is to go to the fields, and from thence procure the best food they can for themselves and their children. The taste of bread is almost forgotten to many of them. I hope you will excuse my going into any further detail on the subject of such distress; for I assure you, the suffering my mind to retrace what I have before witnessed, without the ability to relieve, is too much for my feelings.'

34

ANON., 'DISTRESS OF THE NATION'

Morning Chronicle (29 August 1816), p. 3

Newspapers and magazines often cribbed from their counterparts; here *The Morning Chronicle* cribs an article from *The Montrose Review*. The article clearly finds fault with venues preaching that all was well in the country. This writer argues that the country was dealing with the greatest distress it had ever faced. The 'continental system' refers to Napoleon's use of a blockade of commerce between mainland Europe and England. Though criticising the Prince Regent for his paltry response to the distress, the article only calls for private charity to relieve mass hunger.

DOI: 10.4324/9780429198052-38

34. Anon., 'Distress of the Nation', *Morning Chronicle* (1816)

That Courtly Journal, the London *Courier*, in a late article on the state of the country represented trade in this quarter as in 'the most flourishing condition.' The falsehood of such a statement requires no contradiction at our hands; and we shall only hint to the Editor of that print, that we apprehend such base attempts to mislead the people are now too late to effect the desired purpose. Here numerous sequestrations are taking place amongst our farmers—many of whom, lately possessed of capital, must sink into poverty and wretchedness. Money has almost disappeared; and the properties of many respectable tradesmen are gradually shrinking from the repeated grasps of the tax gatherer, or lawyer. Indeed, every day brings fresh accounts of new distresses from different parts of these devoted kingdoms, and of the actual increase of the calamity where it has been felt before. In Dublin, hundreds of families are perishing for want; and above eight thousand are daily supplied with soup gratis. At no period in the history of Great Britain has so frightful and general a distress been known to prevail. In former times (the years 1796–7–8–9), when provisions were scarce and dear, those who suffered by this circumstance were few, comparatively speaking, and their sufferings of short duration; besides, labour was then abundant, and idleness a matter of choice, and not necessity; nor were the middle and upper orders of society at all prevented from supplying the wants of the lower. The evils of 1812, which resulted from the war with America, and the decrees of Bonaparte, were confined in the extent of their influence, and were immediately relieved by the wise revocation of the Orders in Council, and the destruction of the continental system. But our circumstances are now widely different from those of any former period. The distresses of the present period are felt universally; and though they are less poignant here, yet we are far, very far, from being freed from the general evil—an evil which extends to our manufacturers as well as to the owner and occupier of land—to the home trader, as well as to the merchant; and, consequently, our labourers are involved in universal distress, and many of their helpless offspring in a state of starvation. The return of peace, to which we all looked forward with so much pleasure as the consummation of all our wishes, has operated no relief to our burdens, but has increased their weight, and confirmed our ruin. To discover the cause of these evils is not an unimportant, though perhaps an ungracious, investigation. But we never will shrink from our duty, and shall certainly take an early opportunity of addressing *a Series of Letters*, on this very subject, to his Royal Highness the Prince Regent. In the mean time, nothing can be more foolish than to ascribe our distresses to the change effected by the peace. Our enormous taxation *alone* is the sole cause of frightful sufferings. If this burden was once removed, our trade would increase, and better times would shortly smile on us. In short, retrenchment of our national expenditure, is the only remedy for our distress that can at all be availing. But even the effect of this remedy will be slow; and, as the evil is great, something should be done for its mitigation immediately. For this purpose we know of no method likely to succeed better than the benevolence of individuals. This has, in many cases, been applied; and we are happy to find the sum collected by the Society in London exceeds 34,000*l*.—no thanks, however, to the Regent, and numerous sinecurists, whose paltry subscriptions are insulting to suffering humanity. We heartily recommend an imitation of this benevolent subscription to all who can spare anything from the wants of their own families. Compassion is the noblest virtue of man, and, with reverence be it spoken, it is the most prominent feature in the character of our Saviour, who was touched by its influence, and wept with Mary and Martha at the tomb of their brother, and restored to the disconsolate widow her only son. There is something powerfully attractive in this cause. This is not the complaint of noisy discontent, or willing indolence. We hear the sighs of honesty in indigence. We see the tears of ingenious industry in distress crying for want of bread! Let these sighs and these tears prevail; we are sure they must with all those who have hearts—hearts of flesh and blood! And we entreat them to put on 'bowels of mercy and compassion,' and relieve the misery of their fellow-men. And, as for those who have hearts of stone—who can squander thousands at royal fetes—strut away in the glare of a drawing-room, or the splendour of a feast,—and can hear with indifference the cries of their suffering fellow-creatures,—let them remember, if they dread nothing else, that a curse hath been pronounced by the pen of inspiration on him, who, having this world's goods, refuseth the participation of them to 'his brother who hath need.'

35

MR. HOLT, 'TO THE RIGHT HON. THE EARL OF DERBY, LORD LIEUTENANT OF THE COUNTY OF LANCASTER'

The Times (28 August 1819), p. 2

In this rather enlightened public appeal from a self-styled 'respectable manufacturer of Manchester', written just days after Peterloo, Mr. Holt asks the local presiding aristocrat, the Earl of Derby, to listen to the workers' distress so that other elements, such as so-called agitators, would not lead the workers astray; Holt suggests that all the labourers needed was food and employment to stop them from undertaking more radical actions.

DOI: 10.4324/9780429198052-39

35. Mr. Holt, 'To the Right Hon. The Earl of Derby, Lord Lieutenant of the County of Lancaster', *Times* (1819)

"As I have no object in view but the good of my country, I trust, noble Earl, thou wilt pardon the freedom I use, in thus addressing thee: I hold it to be the duty of every man, in times of imminent danger and difficulty, if he possess either influence or information, to use it, if possible, to arrest in their progress the growing evils of the day, which may have originated in the distress occasioned by the general pressure of the times, and are laid hold of by wicked and designing men, to create through the United Kingdom a general political ferment, dangerous to the peace and happiness of the country.

I have for many years had much to do with the labouring orders of people, and at the present time employ several hundreds: amongst these, occasionally, I have had to contend with much discontent and insubordination, arising, I am disposed to think, from the prevailing associations for the support of what they call the poor man's rights; and which have not unfrequently been carried to such an extreme, as to interfere most materially with the comfortable conduct of our manufacturers, as well as with the best interests of the workmen themselves. This being the case, the inconvenience could only be temporary, as the evil cured itself, without its being needful to resort to any strong or unconstitutional means for its suppression.

The alarm which has pervaded the country for some time back, particularly the manufacturing districts, seems to have been pressed upon the notice of every man: and though it has been generally admitted that the labouring orders have long been suffering severe privations, for want of employment, yet they have unfortunately been allowed to reiterate their complaints unnoticed; have been driven with their families to seek parochial relief; and from this state of wretchedness have easily been persuaded to throw themselves into the arms of modern Reformers, who, with this accession of power, promise to better their condition, by a more equal distribution of the good things with which the country abounds. That thousands—nay, tens of thousands, should flock to the standard of these men, is not to be wondered at, while men of rank and fortune fail to do their duty. Many who, by their successful prosecution of business, have, by the very labour which is now palsied and rests as a dead weight on the market, acquired princely fortunes—I say, while these men, who are alone competent to arrest the growing evils, look supinely on, indifferent as it were to those consequences which are inevitable, what can be hoped for unless relief is in some way administered?

It is in vain to look for a more prosperous state of things from the probable improvement of trade, as it regards a great proportion of our labouring poor; the means of production, aided by our numerous mechanical contrivances, are almost incalculable, and these press so upon all the markets to which thus far we have found access as to render our manufacturers of little value, leaving the industry of the country without hope of remuneration.

It is not from foreign competition alone that these evils proceed: it is from the mistaken policy of our manufacturers, who ought to be the natural guardians of the labour of the country, but who are ever bent upon reducing the price of that labour whenever the demand becomes languid; and thus producing a twofold evil, destroying the comforts of the operatives, and, in proportion as the prices are reduced, compelling them, by long hours and excessive exertion, to the production of an increased quantity of the very articles which are already too abundant.

I have too good an opinion of 9-tenths of the population of this country, for a moment to believe that the present ebullition deserves any such character as that given to it; but I am at the same time confirmed in my judgment, that great distress pervades a large body of well-disposed and well-affected men in the country, who would sit down contented with living in great moderation and plainness by their own industrious exertions. Give them but food and clothing, as the reward of their labour, and all the cant of universal suffrage, and annual Parliaments, with the rest of the catalogue of their demands, would disappear, or be found only with the itinerant politicians of the day. But when want stares them in the face, and the men of weight, of consequence, and of information, refuse to listen to their complaints, to whom, then, are they to look?

I am no party man myself, nor do I recollect ever, in the course of my life, attending a political meeting, or in any way interfering with the political contests of the day. But, surrounded as we are with alarm and difficulty, I could not excuse myself, if I did not state what appears to me to be calculated to tranquillize the public mind, and to restore order and comfort amongst us.

Permit me, with all due deference and respect for thy character and high rank in life, to suggest that, as Lord-Lieutenant of the county, if thou were to call a meeting of the nobility, gentry, landholders, and principal manufacturers, *for the purpose of taking into consideration the present distressed state of the labouring orders of people with a view to the devising of such measures as would give instant activity to the surplus labour in the several manufacturing districts*, I am of opinion that many expedients might be resorted to to effect this; and, probably, the manufacturers themselves might bring about a co-operation through the kingdom, for the purpose of raising the price of labour, and making its moderate exercise sufficient to procure the ordinary means of existence, without the degradation of parochial aid to eke out the scanty provision.

Could the poor but see the rich thus interesting themselves, to restore to them what the pressure of the times has gradually taken away; to what privations, during these efforts to serve them, would they not submit, with patient resignation?

I love my country, and greatly value its inhabitants. I cannot, therefore, contemplate the proposed emigration to the Cape of Good Hope as at all calculated to relieve our present distresses. Who, having the feelings of an Englishman, does not look with affection on the land of his nativity?

Let us then cherish that attachment, by a timely attention to the difficulties and distresses with which our suffering brethren are struggling. And this will, I'll answer for it, call them back to their duty and allegiance, and a time may come when they might prove themselves the country's best safeguard. The Crown and waste lands in the United Kingdom might, in my humble opinion, be parcelled out, under the direction and superintendence of Boards of Agriculture, composed of gentlemen who would most cheerfully give their services amongst the unemployed labourers and their families, to be held for a term of years free from rent and taxes.

Thus would profitable activity be given to the labour of thousands of families, and the districts where they are now hardly existing on pauperism, be relieved from a weight of expense which produces general distress and difficulty. This measure would give an increased value to the labour that remains; and it would be sought for at a price that would sustain life in comfort.

Should this plan be resorted to (and it has the sanction of a noble Earl, who is also the Lord Lieutenant of a northern district), no man, whose opinion is worth regarding, would dare to say, that it is a concession prompted by fear; because the precautions taken by Government, and all the constituted authorities through the nation, are of that formidable kind that cannot but convince the most desperate, that in the event of a general conflict nothing but destruction awaits them. The present poor-rates of the country amount annually, perhaps, to 1,000,000*l*. or 12,000,000*l*.: if what I would most respectfully recommend were taken up on a broad scale by Government, a fourth or fifth part of this amount might be fairly called for and easily furnished, as the means by which to carry into effect the proposed measure, because the operation of it would take the poor out of the several districts where they are the most burdensome; and, as a necessary consequence, would give a proportionately additional value to every man's property so relieved.

To ascertain the *degree* of distress prevailing through this country, (and of which some people affect to doubt), a commission of respectable, independent, and humane men, ought to be appointed, correctly to obtain the number of families out of employment who are willing to work, their general characters, usual occupations, *and how long this state of things has existed among them.*

Should this imperfect sketch, noble Earl, be found to contain any thing worthy thy notice and attention, I shall indeed greatly rejoice; and I do trust, that the motive which I am actuated will be admitted as a sufficient apology for the freedom I have exercised; and that thou wilt believe me to be, with all due deference and respect,

Thy obliged, and sincere friend,

8mo.10 [August 10] David Holt"

36

MR. BENNET, 'STATE OF THE MANUFACTURING DISTRICTS'

The Times (10 December 1819), pp. 2–3

MP Mr. Bennet (1777–1836) called for investigations into the plight of the workers who marched to Peterloo. Like so many others, he believed heavy taxation, left over from the Napoleonic Wars, burdened the country and had unequal and devastating effects on the lower classes. He also repeats a commitment to and belief in the need for the lower-class workers to live a comfortable existence, rather than enduring one constant trajectory towards subsistence levels.

Lord Robert Stewart Castlereagh's response to Bennet in the same sitting of Parliament illustrates the tension and arguments around Peterloo:

> It was a duty which the house owed to the unfortunate classes of society on whose behalf the inquiry was undertaken, not to cause expectation far beyond the means of parliamentary relief [....] Upon what principle could government act, if in seasons of difficulty they were to recognize the policy of taking from one class merely for the purpose of giving to another? Such a practice was equally inconsistent with all the rules of sound policy, and with the very nature of property in general.[85]

Note the translation for *Neque populi, aut plebis, ulla vox, sed attoniti vultus, et conversae ad omnia aures. Non tumultus, non quies, quale magni metus, et magnae irae silentium est* is 'Not a voice was heard from the people or even from the rabble. Everywhere were terror-stricken countenances, and ears turned to catch every sound. It was a scene neither of agitation nor of repose, but there reigned the silence of profound alarm and profound indignation'. Notice that Bennet names the date of Peterloo, a political gesture it would appear.

DOI: 10.4324/9780429198052-40

36. Mr. Bennet, 'State of the Manufacturing Districts', *Times* (1819)

[....] It was his [Bennet] decided opinion, that taxation was the great and decisive cause of our distress, and he could not conceive any grounds of doubt upon the subject, when the decline of trade and the depreciation of almost all commodities raised the rate of taxes from 15 to 25 per cent. (Hear, hear.) His object was to inquire into the peculiar distress, and the peculiar causes of that distress, in the few manufacturing districts, which had alternately excited the commiseration and the alarm of the community: he meant those districts in which disturbances had unhappily appeared. In Lancashire, the west riding of Yorkshire, and part of Scotland, the places to which he alluded, there were 'not fewer than 1,000,000 of persons,' which included the influx from Ireland of persons who, flying from great distress at home, betook themselves to Scotland in hopes of what they could not there find—a better state of existence. This increased, this great population, deprived of the trade and employment which they had some time enjoyed, were now reduced from a state of affluence and comfort, to a state of want and distress. The great staple of that part of the country having been the trade in cotton, the failure of that trade produced general ruin. One class, the opulent class, was involved in difficulty and embarrassment. The working classes, who were as three to one, were in a state of privation and distress, of which the house could form no conception. In the neighbourhood of Glasgow, in 1810, the weavers had 25s. a week; in 1812 their wages fell to 13s. a week; and in 1816 to 10s. At present they had not more than 5s. and 5s. 6d. (Hear, hear.) [....] Yet their clothes they were obliged to pawn while that was in their power; but soon the pawnbrokers became unable to supply any assistance, and fell themselves into the same distress as those whom they had relieved. This was not merely want, it was not merely poverty, it was not merely distress, it was literally starvation. (Hear, hear.) In this state of the hard-working, the affectionate, but the resourceless heads of families, for bread—the harrowing sense of present want aggravated by the recollection of past comfort—he put it to the house, whether with men in such a condition it was not a question of life and death. (Hear, hear.) He was the last man that would approve of any violence; but surely when we saw men placed under privations and feelings never presented to our eyes, and scarcely ever presented to our minds, we ought to exercise some degree of charity and interest[....] thousands were clamouring for bread, and thousands who had suddenly fallen into distress were not to be relieved by voluntary benevolence. The political direction which distress gave to their minds was neither surprising, nor very unreasonable[....] In England, the question at issue in the 17th century was, whether taxes were imposed by parliament, or to be levied at the pleasure of the crown; in short, whether the English government should be a representative government. To that question and its vital importance all Europe, at least all civilized Europe, was now awakened[....] While distress was so severe, and while the state of the representation was so painfully defective, could it be wondered at that discontent and other effects should have appeared among those classes of men?[...] He came next to call the attention of the house to the manufacturing districts of England[....] The shopkeepers were oppressed with taxes, which were exacted without mercy. The landholders might feel mercy in demanding their rents, but the shopkeepers found no mercy in the collectors of public taxes and parish taxes. The consequence was that many were driven upon the poor rates for support, because they had been unable to contribute to them. It would be mere waste of the time and attention of the house to go on describing the distresses in Scotland, which were of the same character as those which he had attempted to represent. The discontent and the disaffection, as it was termed, which were manifested in those districts, were occasioned, if not wholly, at least in the greatest, by distress. The people acted not from inclination; like drowning men who catch at straws, they grasped any projects that happened to be presented to them. The agricultural classes urged, that unless prices continued as high as they were, or higher, they could not exist; the manufacturing classes urged that they could not support themselves if prices were not reduced[....] It was not his intention to create division or hostility. He required only examination into the absolute condition of part of the country. In the hundred of Salford and in Manchester there were not fewer than 400,000 inhabitants, employed solely in manufacture and trade. Their population had grown up to this enormous rate in the course of a few years. But with the inconvenience of this enormous growth of population was to be connected the dispersion of the gentlemen from off their estates. The great population of the place consequently fell under a policy which had no natural influence in point of property or rank. Manufacturers, whose judgments as well as passions were directed by the nature of the trade they carried on, became the leading characters in that society; and clergymen, acting as magistrates, and indulging the influence of party-feelings, lost that influence and that authority over others which naturally belonged to the pure, exclusive, and humane exercise of their profession. The result was, that there existed not that mutual union between the higher and lower classes which ought always to exist[....] By the progress of education and knowledge, to the extent to which it had now reached, the people became attached to liberality of opinion and social liberty. The improvement of the people in the knowledge and manners which education produced naturally disposed them to feel impatient of the arbitrary and oppressive disposition of their magistrates. The result was, the unhappiest opposition and collision of the sentiment in the two classes. Here he would mention, that if among one class there was a union, which was called radical, there was in the other class a union of strange societies, or some other name equally invidious and offensive[....] He would now state the rate of weavers' wages in Manchester, Salford, Royton, Oldham, Middleton, and other places in that district. The best had from 6s. to 9s. and 10s. a week, for working 15 hours every day; another class had 8s. for 13 hours; a third 6s. for 13 hours; a fourth 7s. for 14 hours; and a fifth 7s.6d. for 14 hours. The very highest wages were from 11s. to 12s. 6d. He found the persons to whom he had alluded with no other bedding than sackcloth, and utterly destitute of wearing apparel. What they once possessed had been sold, in order to procure the more immediate necessaries of life. This was but a sample of the condition of things that prevailed generally throughout those districts; and he would ask, whether it was not natural, whether it was not an unavoidable result, that the people should look to Parliament for assistance? Could they be expected to endure miseries of this description without applying for relief to some quarter? If no relief was obtained, discontent must be consequence, and discontent would finally produce despair. He readily admitted that these feelings had been inflamed by the practices of designing men; but for the greater part they originated in, and were kept alive by, what approached to a state of famine. Give them but food and work, and the house would soon cease to hear of their distresses, or their discontents. Seeing, then, that this was the general disposition amongst these classes, and that their poverty and sufferings were undisputed, it might be worth while to advert a little to the view which was taken by them of the late transactions. It was a firm persuasion amongst them, that long before the meeting on the 16th of August, the municipal authorities at Manchester were their enemies[....] The house, too, in subsequently refusing to go into an inquiry upon [the magistrate's proceedings at Peterloo] had done more to excite distrust and inflame animosity, than by any proceeding for a long series of years. The belief and opinion which he had just mentioned as universally entertained amongst many classes, he himself knew to be the full and firm conviction of a most respectable portion of society at Manchester[....] Two questions therefore presented themselves with reference to this important point—what the state of feeling was prior to, and what it had been since, the 16th of August. His own belief was, that the fatal events of that day had led to a determination on the part of many to provide themselves with arms. Still they placed some dependence on the proceedings of Parliament. In the mean time, the utmost anxiety was shown for labour, in order not only to procure subsistence, but to provide means of defence. Ever since the 16th of August, an awful and portending silence had marked their ordinary intercourse. It bore too strong a resemblance to that state of public feeling so powerfully described by the historian, as having at one famous period of national misfortune characterised the Roman people:—'Neque populi, aut plebis, ulla vox, sed attoniti vultus, et conversae ad omnia aures. Non tumultus, non quies, quale magni metus, et magnae irae silentium est.' Many circumstances had long before occurred to produce resentment, but the latter had filled up the measure of what they conceived their sufferings and their wrongs[....] Most of the information of his Majesty's ministers on the subject of these discontents was obtained on the reports of spies and others, who he would not say were immediately connected with Government, but were employed by persons who were prone to be much too busy in their avocation[....] He could not exclude from consideration of the state and condition of the manufacturing classes, the causes of their present discontents. It might be found impossible to frame any plan of general or immediate relief, but he had no doubt that many measures might be adopted to correct and mitigate the evil. It had been just remarked, that, in this view, the people had done every thing, and the government nothing. Even small purchases of an article that was depressed in value had often been found extremely beneficial. The occasion, too, was a proper one for undertaking works of a public nature, he did not mean palaces, but works of solid utility, roads and canals by which all the operations of commercial and agricultural industry might be promoted. Even all this might be found insufficient, he admitted, to afford employment to the hundreds of thousands who stood in need of it; but if only thousands could be relieved, was not that an object of national importance?[...] His motion had for its object the restoration of peace to a distracted country—to unite and tranquillize where disunion alone unhappily reigned. He should indeed glory if he could be rendered the humble instrument of soothing misery and allaying discontent—of raising a temple of harmony on the spot which was now a scene of agitation, of suffering, and of strife. The hon. member concluded by moving for a committee to inquire into the state of the manufacturing districts, and particularly in Lancashire. (Hear, hear.)

37

ANON., 'MEETING OF THE COTTON-SPINNERS'

Morning Chronicle (6 July 1825), p. 4

This newspaper summary of a meeting held by activist cotton spinners illustrates the bubbling violence caused by the distress labourers were facing. The oath referred to is one that violent elements turned to out of desperation. This group is anxious to prove they did not take such an oath, though they do assert that they understood why a fellow labourer might join a group prone to violence. The piece reads in part as follows. This piece also appeared in the *Glasgow Free Press*.

DOI: 10.4324/9780429198052-41

37. Anon., 'Meeting of the Cotton-Spinners', *Morning Chronicle* (1825)

[....] Mr. THOMAS PATERSON (having been called to the Chair) first rose and addressed the assembly[....] Without more of prelude, he proposed that the meeting first proceed to consider of the accusation as regarded the 'Oath' which had been unfairly attributed to them as a body[....] The oath was then read by the SECRETARY, and was as follows:—

> 'I, A. B., do voluntarily swear, in the awful presence of Almighty God, and before these witnesses, that I will execute with zeal and alacrity, as far as in me lies, every task or injunction which the majority of my brethren shall impose upon me in furtherance of our common welfare; as the chastisement of nobs, the assassination of oppressive and tyrannical masters, or the demolition of shops that shall be deemed incorrigible; and also, that I will cheerfully contribute to the support of such of my brethren as shall lose their work in consequence of their exertions against tyranny, or renounce it in resistance to a reduction of wages; and I do further swear that I will never divulge the above obligation, unless I shall have been duly authorized and appointed to administer the same to persons making application for admission, or to persons constrained to become members of our fraternity.'

[....] PETER M'DOUGAL begged the indulgence of the Meeting[....] He would now turn for a moment to the 'oath' that had been attributed to the cotton-spinners as a body; and he would ask, was there a single individual now confronted with him who ever had, or would, become bound by such an oath? [cries of 'No! no!' from all present] [....]

WM. M'LEA [....] would be the last to break through every tie of human nature and humanity, to lend his aid to the fulfilment of the crime of assassination and bloodshed. Too true it was, also, violence had taken place; but were we to be blamed, as a body, for madness and outrage, brought on by the hunger & destitution of individuals?[...] and he sincerely trusted that there was not one of them now present, though fevered by hunger or utter starvation, who would be led to commit that which was unjust or illegal [cheers].

38

ANON., 'BURY, AUGUST 30. THE LATE MEETING AT MANCHESTER'

The Bury and Norwich Post, or Suffolk and Norfolk Telegraph (30 August 1826), p. 784

The Bury and Norwich Post features this article on a public meeting against the Corn Laws. Some of the working orders looked askance at the middle-class movement to repeal the Corn Laws because it often seemed proponents did not consider the needs of the labourers; but it was clear to workers that these laws always raised the price of bread at a time when labouring wages were falling.

DOI: 10.4324/9780429198052-42

38. Anon., 'Bury, August 30. The late Meeting at Manchester', *Bury and Norwich Post, or Suffolk and Norfolk Telegraph* (1826)

The late meeting at Manchester is too important an occurrence to be passed over in silence, and as placed in, and in some measure representing, a great agricultural district, we should neglect our duty if we did not enquire into, and where necessary, controvert the arguments which the commercial advocates have employed. The picture of distress which was drawn by the several speakers requires our deepest sympathy, and would supply an ample apology for any warmth into which they were betrayed, if apology could be needed for commenting with severity upon such injustice as they appear to think has been committed by the Corn Laws. 'The great mass of the working classes,' said the Chairman, 'are actually without the necessaries of life.' 'In no very distant circuit round Pendle-hill, another manufacturer asserted, '80,000 individuals are living, who rise every morning without food to eat, and without knowing how they are to get through the day.' The resolutions declare—'That this town, and the great manufacturing districts, of which it is the centre and the mart, are suffering, at the present moment, under the pressure of distress which is wholly unexampled in its extent and duration[...] which has deprived of all employment many thousands of skilful and industrious families of the labouring classes, degrading them into miserable dependents on the scanty pittance furnished by the poor rates, and by charitable relief; which is continually adding to the number of those who are so dependent; which, at the same time, gradually forcing down into the ranks of the necessitous many of the persons by whom those rates have been paid, and that relief has been given; and which is thus threatening to involve, in all the horrors of starvation, this most thickly peopled portion of the Three Kingdoms.'

39

ANON., 'ALARMING STATE OF THE PEOPLE'

The Examiner, 971 (1826), pp. 577–578

Leigh Hunt's radical journal pleaded the cause of the poor and had no patience with half measures, insisting that it was the State's responsibility to produce robust legislation to deal with the 'extreme sufferings' of the lower classes. The bottom line, the article asserts, is that under the auspices of Elizabeth 43, the starving who were willing to work had a 'right' to be fed and a right to a job.

 DOI: 10.4324/9780429198052-43

39. Anon., 'Alarming State of the People', *Examiner* (1826)

The accounts of the extreme sufferings of large multitudes of the labouring classes, in various parts of the country, from absolute want of food, and the horrible diseases resulting from that privation, have become so frightful, that it is impossible to think with patience of the sympathy shown by Government during the progress of mischief. It is difficult, no doubt, for men who are surrounded with everything that can tempt the appetite or contribute to the gratification of the senses, to whom a slight sensation of hunger is so great an enjoyment that artificial means are often employed to procure it,—it is difficult, we know, for the [comfortable] to sympathize with wretches suffering from the gnawings of the stomach, the languor and despair produced—not by repletion, but by a deficiency of food[....] yet in times like the present, when all classes are alarmed at the probable consequences of the condition of the labourers, when the journals teem every day with sickening details of the misery endured by tens of thousands in various parts of the kingdom, those men must be accounted deficient in common humanity, who, holding the highest powers in the State, neglect or even delay to administer relief[....]

The starving people have a *right* to be fed by those who possess the means. The law of England says, that every man willing to work shall be entitled to sustenance; and the poor-rates are the express means of providing it. But sufficient poor-rates cannot be collected in the populous manufacturing districts to keep the unemployed poor from starving. Recourse must therefore be had to the funds of the State, which should be enabled to bear this additional pressure by a tax on the rich exclusively. The labourers in this country have a double claim to such aid. They [labourers] produce more aggregate wealth than any two nations in the world together, although unhappily their own share of it is smaller than that of other labourers;—*and their present misery is caused by misgovernment*[....]

[....] We are justified therefore in saying that, be the effect of the subordinate causes more or less, the present want of employment among the manufacturers, and the general stagnation of trade, producing the starvation and misery of myriads of industrious people, is caused by the profligate expenditure, corruption, and the political ignorance, of Government.

Ministers tell us, that the distress is only temporary. Why hesitate then to apply temporary relief?[...] Had not a corrupt House of Commons allowed an interested party to defeat the Manchester and Liverpool Rail-Road Bill, how many thousands of poor spinners, now pining in idleness and hunger, might have been usefully employed on that great and profitable undertaking![...] and we must look forward to the horrible condition into which the addition of *cold* to *hunger* and *nakedness* will plunge whole multitudes of our countrymen and women.

40

ANON., 'CAUSES AND CURES OF THE PRESENT DISTRESS'

The Manchester Times (9 May 1829), p. 238

The relentless distress experienced across the first half of the nineteenth century amongst so much of the working classes is illustrated by articles on that distress in a range of conservative, moderate and radical venues. The continued call for 'inquiry' seems repetitive and indicative of the government's utter inability to and lack of motivation for facing its people's suffering. Terrified that starvation and unemployment would cause the poor to revolt, this writer implies that parliamentary reform meant implementing the six points of the Charter and modernising the civil service so that it could handle such disasters. With its pragmatic bent, this article also demands that the government rid itself of inefficiencies and sinecures in order to eliminate the 'cancer' that was affecting the body politic. The demand made for 'CHEAP GOVERNMENT' referenced a stipulation to repeal said sinecures. Whig MP Earl Grey (1764–1845) supported the Reform Bill and was Prime Minister from 1830–1834.

DOI: 10.4324/9780429198052-44

40. Anon., 'Causes and Cures of the Present Distress', *Manchester Times* (1830)

[....] The continued depression of trade, and the intense distress, which is experienced by the people in consequence of that depression, render an inquiry into its cause a subject, not merely of importance, but of the most pressing necessity. It is now obvious to every one, that if there be a remedy, that remedy must be applied soon, or our merchants and manufacturers will be reduced to hopeless INSOLVENCY, and those whom they have employed, to absolute STARVATION. It is therefore the bounden duty of all to take into consideration the causes of the depression, with the view of devising the means of averting the calamities which its continuance will occasion; and it is the duty of the Press, more especially, to diffuse correct opinion upon the subject, in order that public energy, instead of being wasted in fruitless efforts upon wrong points, may be concentrated, and directed with irresistible force upon the real causes of the evil.—Powerfully feeling the duty of exercising such influence as we may possess to avert a threatened danger, and hopeful of rousing the apathetic, and of directing the mistaken, we shall attempt to point out the causes of the national suffering, and to show the absolute necessity, for the salvation of the kingdom from calamities unparalleled in its history, of a general, united, and energetic effort to have those causes removed[....]

If[...] the manufacturer, who may for a time subsist on his capital, even if it yield him no income, how much more oppressive must it be to the mechanic or weaver, whose supply of daily bread is dependent on his daily earnings. What must be the despair of the unfortunate man who may be for weeks without employment; who when employed, earns only the half or two-thirds of what no longer than a year ago he could have earned; who sees this uncertainty of obtaining employment daily increasing, and the reward for his labour daily diminishing; what must be his despair when, instead of that reduction in the price of food which he anticipated, he looks forward even to an advance in its price; when instead of cheapness and abundance, he has the prospect before him of famine, occasioned by a scanty harvest, and the exclusion from our ports of the produce of other soils!

But it is not merely in preventing corn from falling to a rate at which it may be attainable by the impoverished manufacturer and the starving weaver, that the CORN LAWS aggravate the existing distress. This effect is, no doubt, highly oppressive to both classes, and more especially to the latter; but these laws operate in another and scarcely less hurtful manner, insomuch as they deprive us of customers who would willingly give us the grain which we need, and they do not need, in exchange for the manufactures which we are anxious to dispose of, and they are anxious to obtain. It is a species of political suicide to refuse to receive from other lands that food which God has intended for distribution amongst all his creatures; and it is still more preposterously, absurdly, aye, and WICKEDLY SELF-DESTRUCTIVE TO REFUSE TO RECEIVE IT, WHEN IT IS OFFERED IN EXCHANGE FOR THE VERY ARTICLES WHICH GLUT

OUR MARKETS, and which, while they remain on our hands, discourage the production of more, and consequently keep our people idle[....]

Can then our manufacturers and those whom they employ look on in sullen apathy while those execrable laws are at once raising the price of food, and limiting the number of their customers, and encouraging the growth of rival manufactures in other lands?[...] It is ridiculous to suppose that while means exist of giving a stimulus to their trade, and checking the growth of infant manufacturers in other lands, and obtaining food at reasonable prices, they will submit to ruin and starvation. Hunger, even when not unjustly caused, will break through stone walls; then how much more energetic will it be when it is occasioned by laws which are at variance with every principle of policy and justice, and every feeling of humanity!

What then is to be done? Why, what we have in good times and in bad times urged upon our townsmen, but which unfortunately they have always left undone till the danger is pressing and imminent. The Legislature is to be petitioned: it is to be told the monopoly of the corn-growers forces us to pay starvation prices out of our diminished means[:...] it is to be told that our population is STARVING AND IN DESPAIR; that hunger is not to be reasoned with, and that we anticipate the worst consequences, if such relief as equitable laws can give be not afforded[....]

[....] Great, indeed, worthy of our utmost efforts, would be our deliverance could we get these most important limbs of the body politic, the manufacturing interests, relieved from the dreadful paralysis, whose effects we have been describing; but, yet, were his relief effected, the whole body would still continue to suffer, in all its parts, from the cancer-like workings of the PRESENT SYSTEM OF TAXATION[....] Let things stop where they are, in the manufacturing districts, with regard to prices of the materials upon which our industry works; let things stop where they are, with regard to the scale of wages, and the rate of profit; and let there be such an alteration in the Corn Laws as would give us bread at the prices of 1822, such an alteration as would give us Wheat at two-thirds of its present value; let so much change in our favour be effected; and, still, as far even as the manufacturers are concerned, there could not, it is quite obvious, be any thing like a restoration of that sufficiency of the necessaries, and that moderate portion of the comforts of life, to which none, we hope of our readers will deny that the labouring classes are entitled[....]

[....] what we have to insist upon is, that even the people of the manufacturing counties, must, besides the alteration of the Corn Laws, have relief from the burden of Government Taxation[....] Let us not persuade ourselves that, if we get the palsy out of our limbs, we shall be well, though the cancer still remain in our vitals; but let us observe its ramifications and mark how it reaches every fibre even of the paralysed parts[....]

[....] What, then, is to be done? Is the revenue to be diminished to relieve the distress of the people? Is that annual account of the proceeds of taxation, which has, ever since PITT's days, been exhibited as the barometer of the nation's welfare, to show a constant falling off? Is it to show, quarter after quarter, the same downward progress as the mercury does in a frost? Yes; this is what we want to see; but not in such a way as the accounts have lately shown it, and not exactly from the same cause. The revenue falls off *now*, by so much as the wretched people's consumption of taxable articles is lessened by their want of means[;...] We want an adjustment between the people and those who have lived on the sweat of the people as consumers of the taxes. We want to have sinecures swept away; we want to have useless offices abolished; we want to have the salaries of the public functionaries brought down to a scale bearing some proportion to the services rendered[,...] we want the 'dead weight' rendered less intolerably heavy; we want the standing army to form a less frightful per-centage upon the whole adult male population of the kingdom; we want to see rigid economy, such economy as honest trustees would introduce into the affairs of an embarrassed tradesman, made to pervade every part of the affairs of this embarrassed and miserable country. We want to get rid of the monstrous anomaly of having the richest government, and most wretched people, that ever existed upon the face of the earth. This is what we want[....] we are glad to shelter ourselves from the shafts of folly and of malice, under the shield of EARL GREY, who most admirably expressed, in April 1826, in the House of Lords, what we believe to be the sentiments of all honest and sensible men upon this subject[....] 'Government must *take up the whole subject* with a sincere desire *to probe to the bottom all the evils that afflict us, and to propose those salutary reforms* which alone can restore us to health and prosperity. If only temporary palliations are resorted to, *distress will follow distress in succession, assuming a more aggravated form*, until, at last, it hurries on to A FEARFUL CONVULSION, from which I hope the country will have the strength to recover.'

Such, then, are the views which this noble lord took of our situation, at a period when the country was suffering exactly as it now suffers, and from the same causes. Those 'aggravated distresses,' those 'painful sufferings,' of which he speaks, do we not all feel?—and is there not, in the fearful anticipations with which every heart is filled, and every tongue is employed; in the prospects of starvation for the labouring classes, we ask, to be seen, the not obscure tokens of that terrible convulsion at which the firm-nerved Lord Grey could not glance, without something like expressions of horror? Go where you will, enter into what promiscuous company you may, you are every where met with the all-employing enquiries, *what is to be done? How long are things to go on at this rate?*[...] are [we] to see [ourselves] surrounded with an immense population, from whom nothing but cheap bread and low taxes can avert all the thousand horrors and crimes which wait upon starvation, and not make an effort to turn the current which is hurrying this mighty mass that destruction which will involve the great and small, the rich and poor together?[...] and while demanding CHEAP BREAD, let us demand what is equally essential to our welfare, a CHEAP GOVERNMENT. And to guard against the recurrence of misery which the people are now enduring, let us demand PARLIAMENTARY REFORM.

41

'J. R.', 'ART. IX. DOMESTIC ARRANGEMENTS OF THE WORKING CLASSES'

The London and Westminster Review, 3 (1836), pp. 450–466, on pp. 451, 459–460, 462–466

Putting forward a cooperative plan to save labourers from the high cost of food, this piece argues that the poor should pool their resources and live, essentially, in a commune. In a kind of modern understanding of the body's need for 'ease', the writer moves discussion about labourer's lives beyond subsistence and comfort to a higher form of peace of mind based on food security.

DOI: 10.4324/9780429198052-45

41. 'J. R.', 'Art. IX. Domestic Arrangements of the Working Classes', *London and Westminster Review* (1836)

[....] Poverty, in its widest sense, must be understood to mean, the privation of anything tending to physical, moral, or intellectual advancement; but our present purpose is to consider poverty principally in a physical point of view—the form in which it is most feared by those who suffer under its effects [...] we know that the progress from poverty to comfort is slower than is necessary, and that the change might be made rapid by proper guidance: in short, that Poverty is only another name for Ignorance; while Intelligence may be regarded as the synonyme of Comfort.

There are various conditions of physical poverty amongst nations which are called uncivilized; but the most demoralizing and deteriorating of all poverty is that which exists amongst civilized nations, and more especially in large towns[....] The crowded lanes, courts, and alleys of a large town, whose every house is one unseemly den of squalid hunger, strife, envy, hatred, malice, and all uncharitableness—these are the abodes in which poverty appears in her most fearful garb, surrounded by vice and every variety of misery[....]

[....] many poor people [...] exist in a condition of misery, produced by constant dread of starvation, or in an unimproving condition, caused by apathy arising from hopelessness. This is precisely the condition of many amongst the poorer classes in England and Ireland at the present day.

The remedy for this is not in reducing the rich, but in raising the poor[....]

[....] Every thing the working people consume, instead of coming to them direct from the producer, who would be content with a moderate profit, passes through so many hands, each of which adds something to the cost, that it reaches the poor consumer at a double price.

[....] In effecting a revolution for the better in the general condition of the working classes, it is evident that, before all things, it is necessary that they should enjoy physical ease; in other words, that they should be free from painful bodily sensations. To accomplish this, they require an abundant supply of food, clothing, warmth, and shelter. We have before shown, that there exist a considerable number of working men earning wages sufficient for their comfortable maintenance, but who nevertheless do not reap the full benefit of their earning, as these are dissipated in the payment of heavy rents for wretched lodgings, and exorbitant profits on retail purchases from day to day; and beyond this, there is a still larger waste of fuel and time, from which last loss no one can possible reap benefit—either consumer or distributor. Now what we propose is, to enable these producers to reap the whole benefit of their own earnings, instead of contributing a large portion of them to maintain a host of retail shopkeepers, and to pay the high rents of builder, ignorant of the superior economy of a more social life[....] It is better that the producers should be permanently bettered in their condition than that an artificial class should be kept up in perpetuity, on the earnings of others[....]

[....] We propose, therefore, to erect a quadrangle, with fifty dwellings on each side[;...] The tenants might have them, taxes included, for 10*l*. In the centre of the quadrangle we propose to erect a building consisting of a basement, a ground-floor, and a story: the basement to contain a steam-engine, an apparatus for pumping cold and hot water into pipes circulating through the whole of the dwellings. The open space between the dwellings and the central buildings might contain cellars for coals and durable provisions. The basement story is to be a kitchen, fitted with apparatus for cooking plain provisions of all kinds adapted to the supply of the two hundred families. The room above that would be adapted for a dining-room for such of the community as might choose to dine together[;...]The gas could be placed in lanterns in the walls of the dwellings—thus lighting the inside and outside at once, and preventing any offensive odour from entering the apartments. In addition to the other conveniences, there should be provided a sufficient number of warm and cold baths, and also a laundry and wash-house[....]

The liberation of the wives and daughters of these working men from drudgery in cooking, scrubbing, cleaning, water-carrying, and numerous other things, would give them a large amount of leisure for cultivation of their own intelligence and taste, and the training of the children. The men also, after the labour of the day was over, would come to cleanly homes and cheerful conversation: the gin-shop and the public house would be alike abandoned. The means of cleanliness would be easy and abundant as regarded their persons, and their health would be improved. So much as regards physical comfort; but in respect to facilities for the cultivation of the mind, the advantages would be very great indeed[....]

[....] And as such institutions increased in number, there would arise amongst them a generous emulation in improvement: they would be like fields separated by hedges, in which the relative excellence of the crops could be ascertained, and experiments usefully tried. They would form a general bond of union amongst the working classes, based on their true interests, and would teach them how to co-operate usefully for commercial and productive as we; as social purposes.

Earnestly do we wish that capitalists may see this plan in the same light as we do, and in making their own interest go hand in hand with the working-men's welfare, teach them to REGARD CAPITAL AND MACHINERY AS THE MOST EFFICIENT PROMOTERS OF THE INDEPENDENCE OF THE WORKING CLASSES.

Part 5

DIETARY, REAL AND IMAGINED

This section features particular references to the diets of the poor; it also includes satires on the order of Swift's 'A Modest Proposal', as well as at least one article that all but defies description in its obsessive efforts to produce bread from wood.

DOI: 10.4324/9780429198052-46

42

'M', 'ON MAKING BREAD FROM WOOD'

Edinburgh Magazine and Literary Miscellany (1817), pp. 313–316

Science meets absurd obsessions in this bid to feed the starving with the detritus of wood. At first one imagines this is farcical, but apparently Professor Autenrieth (1772–1835) was a real scientist working in Tübingen. Though Johann Heinrich Ferdinand von Autenrieth was a real person, it is unclear if he was involved in this experiment. To the nineteenth-century question of how to manage hunger and starvation, there are many peculiar responses, some so peculiar they breach generic expectations and push against the ability to understand irony. 'On Making Bread From Wood' by the anonymous 'M' is just such a generic oddity. In any case, the article puts into question a culture's willingness to resort to such extremely and literally distasteful methods to feed the poor, when, in reality, food itself was more than available and providing it would have been a more efficacious and practicable solution than the extraordinarily laborious procedures for creating bread out of wood described here.

DOI: 10.4324/9780429198052-47

42. 'M', 'On Making Bread From Wood', *Edinburgh Magazine* (1817)

We may admit it as an axiom in political economy, that the population of a state will adapt itself to the means of subsistence. But, as the amount of these varies from the operation of a variety of circumstances, we should often be exposed to all the miseries of famine, if there were not causes compensating the natural effects of the constantly fluctuating supply of food. In years of plenty, the excessive increase of population, which should naturally follow, is checked by the waste, which arises from cheapness, and by the speculation of merchants who export the surplus, or store it to meet contingent demands. In years of scarcity, starvation is prevented by the economy in the use of food, which is the effect of its dearness, and by the same speculative spirit of merchants who now dispose of their stored surplus, and import grain and provisions from other countries. By these means the balance between the population and supply of food is preserved, in most years, without great inconvenience. But in extraordinary cases, where the quantity of food is altogether insufficient for the wants of the people, extraordinary means of supply must be resorted to, and of these the most obvious and most efficient is the using as food of articles which are at other times rejected, such as the flesh of animals not commonly eaten, the horse, rat, frog, &c. or the parts not commonly used as food, the liver, lungs, and brain of larger animals and the whole blood and fat; also vegetables, and parts of vegetable not in common use[....] but beside those articles which we reject from mere prejudice, some are not eaten [...] because they are disgusting and disagreeable when eaten in a quantity, such as the whale, and other coarse fishes, and strong oils and fats; or because the compactness of their aggregation prevents them from being dissolved or digested in the stomach. Of this last description are most kinds of wood and bark, and woody fibre in general; and, as these are produced in great abundance in some countries, where food is always scarce, and in sufficient quantity in almost every country; when threatened with famine, it becomes a problem of great importance to discover the means of rendering them alimentary, at least so far as to assist in supporting the people until the danger of famine is at an end.

This has been attempted by Professor Autenrieth of Tubingen in regard to wood, and with considerable success. He considered that two circumstances rendered wood unfit for food, the foreign matters always mixed with the woody fibre, and the compact aggregation of the fibre itself. The former was to be overcome by rejecting those woods which naturally contain most foreign matter, such as the fir, on account of its resin, and the oak on account of its astringency; and by removing every thing that water can dissolve. He, therefore, preferred for his experiments those woods which have little taste or smell[....]

To render wood alimentary. It is necessary to reduce it to a state of extremely minute division[....] It also requires the repeated action of the heat of an oven, by which means it is not only better fitted for being ground, but probably also undergoes some internal change which renders it more digestible, as is evidently the case in regard to coffee. Wood prepared in this way acquired the smell and taste of corn flour. It, however, is never white, but always yellowish. It also agrees with corn flour in this, that it does not ferment without the addition of some leaven, and in this case sour leaven of corn flour is the best. With this it makes a perfectly uniform and spongy bread, like common brown bread, and when it is thoroughly baked, and has much crust, it has a much better taste of bread than what in times of scarcity is prepared of bran and husks of corn.

To make wood flour in perfection, the wood, after being thoroughly stripped of its bark, is to be sawed transversely into disks of about an inch in diameter. The saw-dust is to be preserved, and the disks to be beaten to fibres in a pounding-mill. The fibres and saw-dust, mixed together, are next to be deprived of every thing harsh and bitter which is soluble in water, by boiling them in a large quantity of water[....] The whole is now to be completely dried, either in the sun or by fire, and repeatedly ground in a flour-mill, till it pass through boulting cloth.

The ground wood is next to be baked into small flat cakes, with water rendered slightly mucilaginous, by the addition of some decoction of linseed, mallow stalks and leaves, lime-tree bark, or any other substance[....] These cakes are to be baked until they are quite dry, and become of a brownish yellow colour on the surface. After this they are to be broken in pieces, and again ground repeatedly[....]

[....] If wood flour, tied up in fine linen, be long kneaded in a vessel of water, the water is rendered milky, and deposits slowly a quantity of starch, which, with boiling water, forms a thick, tough, trembling, tenacious jelly, like that of wheat starch; and it is only necessary to see this starch to be satisfied that the wood flour is soluble and nutritious[....]

Professor Autenrieth next tried the nutritious effects of wood flour on animals; and for this purpose, after confining a young dog a whole day with only water, a gruel of indifferently-prepared wood flour, salt, and water, was set before him. At first he ate very little of it, and in the evening was very weak, having nearly fasted for twenty-four hours. During the night he had ate a good deal of his gruel, and was in the morning lively. He now got as much gruel as he could eat four times a-day; and in a few days he seemed to be quite reconciled to his new diet, and at the end of seven days was perfectly well, and even seemed to have grown. He was then hanged, one hour and a half after a full meal, to ascertain the fact of digestion by dissection[....]

Professor Autenrieth and his family next tried it themselves, in the form of gruels or soup, dumplings and pancakes, all made with as little of any other ingredients as possible; and, although they ate these preparations in satiety, they found them palatable, and suffered no inconvenience from them[....]

[....] Professor Autenrieth found fifteen pounds of birchwood flour, with three pounds of sour wheat leaven, and two pounds of wheat flour, mixed up with eight measures of new milk, yielded thirty-six pounds of very good bread[....]

Professor Autenrieth made the following experiment with this bread:—He at a quarter of a pound of it with weak coffee to breakfast. The bread he ate the rougher it became, and somewhat constringed the throat, but was not bitter. The last bit, which, on that account, he chewed little, was unpleasant, and afterwards his stomach was oppressed, and he was convinced that the continued use of wood bread alone would have injured him. But, at mid-day, his appetite had returned, and he ate of several kinds of soup made with this flour, with some other preparations of it, without any inconvenience. In the evening he ate another quarter of a pound of the bread, with some milk, without any dislike or oppression at his stomach. He slept well, and was next morning in his usual health.

From these experiments, it is obvious, that in cases of necessity wood may be made to furnish a considerable quantity of nourishment, but it is no less obvious, that the process is so troublesome and expensive, that it never can become an article of food, except when there is an absolute scarcity of provision.

43

ANON., 'REAL RELIEF FOR THE SUFFERINGS OF THE POOR'

Moral reformer, and protestor against the vices, abuses, and corruptions of the age, 1 (1831), pp. 138–145

Praising bread as the poor man's source of life, this article reviles the Corn Laws as well as any other laws, economic or political, that put food out of reach of the poor.

DOI: 10.4324/9780429198052-48

43. Anon., 'Real Relief for the Sufferings of the Poor', *Moral reformer, and protestor against the vices, abuses, and corruptions of the age* (1831)

AMONGST the social duties of life, none is more important than that of taking care of the poor. Under the best guarded system of policy, there will be instances of distress, and which, no doubt, are wisely permitted, to call into exercise the benevolent feelings of our nature. Every child in misery, every son of affliction, is a call upon our sympathy; and, in a world where trouble is the common lot, it ought to be cherished to the greatest extent. To relieve the poor is every where commanded; and, if done from proper motives, has the sanctions of religion, and the promise of its best rewards. I have before divided the poor into *three* classes—those who are impoverished by their own vices,—the able-bodied poor, whose wages are so much below the price of living,—and the naturally poor, including the widow, the fatherless, the infirm, and the aged. For the first there is no remedy but *personal* reformation; in favour of the second and third classes I beg again to put in my plea.

While we hear of whole counties in Ireland in a state of famine and starvation; whilst nearly the whole of our labourers and weavers are reduced to the degraded rank of paupers; whilst cases of appalling misery are daily occurring—in the midst of a land abounding with wealth, and favoured with almost unlimited powers of production,—if efforts are not made, and made immediately, to afford a general and permanent relief, who would regret what consequences came upon a nation so deadly insensible to the obligations of justice, and to the duties of humanity?[...] the poor of England want CHEAP BREAD[....] *bread* is what the cravings of the stomach demand every day. Oh! how I grieve to think of the sparing divisions which the mother is obliged to make in every meal, among her hungry children; and especially when she has to delay the breakfast an hour or two, in order to meet the impossibility of providing for the usual number of meals! Think of this ye bloated, overgrown epicures, ye hard hearted tyrants, who not only reap the labour of others, but impose every obstacle in the way of rational relief[....] Shall we make laws to allow foreign competition to bring down the wages of artizans, and at the same time, laws to keep up the price of bread?[...] *A removal of all useless burdens from the land, and a repeal of the Corn Laws*, I repeat, is the only remaining hope[....]

[....] let corn be reduced to the price of calicoes; let the woman's dinner be as cheap as her bed gown, and then, I assert, we shall see the return of the rosy bloom of health, and the smile of satisfaction into many a poor man's cot. If we bear in mind that *food* is on request at least three times a day, that a moderate sized family should spend about fifteen shillings every week in food, and that the same family perhaps does not spend one shilling in a month in any of the cheapened articles of manufacture, we may easily see, whilst the middling and higher classes, including all the land owners, are benefitting by cheap goods, there is little or no advantage to the poor. Bread, they must have, and until that is cheap, either by improved methods of cultivation, or by foreign importation, we might as well think of moving the heavens, as persuading the people to be content[....]

[....] The advocates of the poor laws may take credit to themselves, if they please, for exclusive knowledge of 'moral and political economy,' but all arguments for the English poor laws, are arguments for *perpetuating* misery[....] The aim of many 'vestries' is not to understand the whole truth of the case, and to give them *sufficient* relief, but to *get clear* of them with as *little* as possible[....] Starvation and mendicity are the result of the present laws[;...]

[....] While I have, under this head, particularly dwelt on the *abolition of the corn/ laws*, I by no means wish to overlook *the abolition of every expensive monopoly*—the *remission* of the *oppressive taxes*—the *correction of absentee-ism*—and the discovery of fresh *sources of employment*[....] May the time soon arrive when crime, poverty, and misery shall no longer disgrace our land!

44

ANON., 'THE GENERAL FAST'

Figaro in London, 14 (1832), pp. 53–54

During the Victorian period, it was common for the government to call for State-sponsored prayers and fasts in response to famine, war and other historical events. This piece draws a comparison between what the poor and rich might eat during such a fast to show the hypocrisy of these political rituals. The graphic that accompanies the article illustrates the stark differences, with the rich man featured feasting at the groaning board, as it were, in contrast to two poor starving men sitting on a stoop in tattered clothing. The writer savages the underlying reason for the State fast: it is intended to take the public's attention off the government's refusal to care for the lower classes in a time of calamity.

DOI: 10.4324/9780429198052-49

44. Anon., 'The General Fast', *Figaro in London* (1832)

We present to our readers this week a contrast in the shape of a pair of pictures, illustrative of the approaching General Fast, and the manner in which it will be likely to be observed by two different degrees of society. The well-fed aristocrat will luxuriate for a day in a change of diet: the poor man will take his customary meal of never-varying scantiness. If eating fish be indispensably necessary to keeping the Fast, how is he to obey the proclamation who depends for his daily sustenance on charity? He may, perchance, be enabled to purchase a ha'p'oth of dried sprats, which may be as efficacious for the purposes of piety, as the most sumptuous of fish dinners. A General Fast in the higher ranks will, we imagine, turn out to be a day of general epicurism. Already has the ingenuity of the professed cooks been, as we find from the papers, put into requisition to devise methods of dressing fish, in order to tempt the appetites of the rich on a day when the viands under which their tables usually groan, must be shunned as impious. Were we but acquainted with the technicalities of cookery, we could enumerate a catalogue of dishes to be formed by culinary skill from fish alone, which will be eaten in the houses of the wealthy, on the 21st of March, with the assumption of spiritual humility, but with all the real relish of the grossest animal gluttony. We cannot sufficiently reprobate the weakness and want of sense evinced by the ministry in acceding to the canting proposition of the would-be-saintly Perceval. We put it to them as men of common understanding, do they suppose that the Fast they have ordered will be likely to prove acceptable in the eyes of heaven? Putting out of the question the hypocrisy to which it must give rise, do they imagine that even a sincere Fast would in any way tend to make the country more worthy than it is of divine protection? Is a man's holiness to be estimated by the quality or quantity of his food? If so, what hope is there for one who dines regularly every day on a joint? But how irrevocably damned is he who impiously ventures to eat a mutton chop to his breakfast? On the other hand, he who partakes but sparely of animal food may, according to this strange doctrine, hope for salvation; and one who can manage to live on tea and bread and butter may confidently expect a snug corner in Abraham's bosom. We suspect the lower classes of England, with all their ignorance, are too well informed to believe that eating meat must in time send a man to the devil, or that a regimen of salt fish and egg sauce is sufficient to put on in training for a cherubim. It may be very convenient for those who have too much of the good things of this life, to inculcate such a belief as would reconcile to their lot that large portion of the community who have too little; but starvation is not the road that one would naturally choose, in taking a journey to heaven. It is certainly a short cut out of this world, but we cannot suppose it will help us on very far in the next, more especially as it is a path, which those holy personages, the Bishops, never by any chance think of adopting. The pretext for the General Fast, is one which we have already in a preceding number of *Figaro* shown to be ridiculous, it being ordered according to the King's proclamation, to avert the ravages of the cholera, which a want of proper food is known to encourage. It is, however, we suspect, proposed from a deeper reason than that which the ministers have assigned:—it is intended to draw away the public attention from oppressive injustice, productive of want—the parent of disease, and lay the calamity with which England is afflicted to the charge of divine providence. Let the Bishop of London before he presumes to blaspheme against his maker, and charge him with disseminating a pest—let his holiness try the effect of a little charity, and by giving some of his superfluity for the benefit of the poor, endeavour to find out whether the monopoly of such persons as himself is not, instead of providence, the true cause of cholera. We take leave of the subject of the fast with contempt. If it is essential to religion, the poor are already sufficiently virtuous, and as to the rich a fast will never effect any improvement in them, unless they will consent to observe it for a twelvemonth, and give away in charity the surplus of their enormous incomes, of which an abstinence from meats during that period would leave them in possession.

45

'DIETARY TABLES ISSUED BY THE POOR LAW COMMISSIONERS FOR CIRENCESTER UNION, DECEMBER 1836'

Hansard, HC (1836), Volume 40, Image 3

These dietary tables illustrate assumptions made about what the State owed its lower-class citizens when they faced calamity. One can see from the stinting and rather cold-hearted approach why so many of the poor refused to go into the workhouses, even if they were facing starvation.

DOI: 10.4324/9780429198052-50

45. 'Dietary Tables Issued by Poor Law Commissions for Cirencester Union, December 1836' (1836)

DIETARY FOR ABLE-BODIED PAUPERS.

		Breakfast.		Dinner.				Supper.	
		Bread.	Gruel.	Bacon.	Potatoes.	Beef Soup.	Pudding	Bread.	Cheese.
		oz.	pints.	oz.	lbs.	pints.	oz.	oz.	oz.
Sunday	Men	7	1½	2½	1	- -	- -	7	1
	Women	6	1½	2½	1	- -	- -	6	1
Monday	Men	7	1½	- -	1½	- -	- -	7	1
	Women	6	1½	- -	1½	- -	- -	6	1
Tuesday	Men	7	1½	- -	½	- -	14	7	1
	Women	6	1½	- -	½	- -	12	6	1
Wednesday	Men	7	1½	2½	1	- -	- -	7	1
	Women	6	1½	2½	1	- -	- -	6	1
Thursday	Men	7	1½	- -	1	1½	- -	7	1
	Women	6	1½	- -	1	1½	- -	6	1
Friday	Men	7	1½	- -	½	- -	14	7	1
	Women	6	1½	- -	½	- -	12	6	1
Saturday	Men	7	1½	- -	1½	1½	- -	7	1
	Women	6	1½	- -	1	1½	- -	6	1

Refractory to be allowed sixteen ounces of bread, with water, per diem.

46

ANON., 'STARVATION WHOLESOME'

The Champion and Weekly Herald (25 December 1836), p. 119

The date of Christmas is key for reading this short entry that sarcastically trades in the idea that starvation is 'wholesome'. The cutting snippet appears in the radical journal *The Champion.* Tuifnell (1806–1886) was a civil servant.

DOI: 10.4324/9780429198052-51

46. Anon., 'Starvation Wholesome', *Champion and Weekly Herald* (1836)

Mr. Tufnell, one of the Assistant Poor-law Commissioners, has addressed a letter to the Guardians of the Bromley Union, in which he labours to prove, from statistical sources, that the diet table of their workhouse, instead of being too scanty, is by far too profuse, and that in fact, the less poor people have to eat the longer they live. We wonder whether this well-paid gentleman has ever tried his own theory upon himself.

47

TESTIMONY FROM MR. THOMAS BOURNE, *SELECT COMMITTEE ON POOR LAW AMENDMENT ACT: THIRD REPORT*

Hansard, HC (1837), Volume 40, Images 32–33, 35, 37–39, 47–49

This is a report of a parliamentary interrogation of Mr. Thomas Bourne that took place on 14 April 1837, three years after the New Poor Laws were established; Bourne was the Master at the Fareham Workhouse. He disciplined three children for having 'dirty habits' (question 4332), which included bedwetting and soiling their underclothing during regular bouts of diarrhoea. Bourne's persistent fealty to harsh discipline (including putting the children in the stocks and reducing their food intake) was shocking to the Lords investigating these particular incidents, in part because of how the withholding of food was used as part of the punishment. Ultimately, Bourne decided to have the children removed from the workhouse.

DOI: 10.4324/9780429198052-52

47. Testimony from Mr. Thomas Bourne, *Select Committee on Poor Law Amendment Act: Third Report', 19th Century House of Commons Sessional Papers* (1837)

4337. Did you direct that there should be withheld from those children a part of their food, in consequence of their habits?—The schoolmistress had a general direction from me, and those children were treated as other children were.
4338. You diminished their food with a view to prevent those [dirty] habits?—Yes.
4339. Was the medical man acquainted with the diminution of the food?—I am not aware that he was.
4340. Did you or not consider it your duty when you were treating those children for what might be considered a complaint [diarrhea], either by a diminuntion of food or any other particular mode of treatment [he had them put in the stocks], to make the medical man acquainted with that circumstance?—The medical man was ultimately acquainted with it, when they became more dirty in their habits[....]
4344. How far did you carry this diminution of food?—My directions were only to stop for a day generally.
4345. The whole food?—No.
4346. What quantity?—The half of the food in a day[....]
4347. And you did that with a view of correcting those dirty habits?—Yes[....]
4353. Were those children submitted to this punishment of the stocks at the same time that their food was diminished?—I believe they were[....]
4358. Were you told by the schoolmistress, or anyone else, that their health began to decline?—She made that observation to me when she remarked that the punishment did not appear to have any effect.
4359. How soon after they were in the house did the schoolmistress observe to you that their health appeared to decline?—It might have been, I suppose, a month.
4360. What did you do when their health appeared to decline?—I desired her to discontinue their punishment.
4361. Including the diminution of their food?—Yes.
4362. Did you, when you were told that their health began to decline, communicate it to the medical officer?—Yes, he saw them.
4363. What did he direct to be done when he saw them?—He did not direct anything; they were chiefly in their beds, when they got so filthy that they could not be kept up for any time together; they were no sooner up than they were dirty, and were obliged to be put to bed.
4364. Were they in bed in consequence of their dirty habits, or in consequence of their declining in health?—In consequence of their dirty habits[....]

[Bourne decided to have the children removed from the workhouse.]

4377. Did he [the medical officer] express any doubt as to the propriety of their being removed?—No; one of the children, Warren, had been very ill, a fortnight before, of fever, and he had expressed himself that he did not think it was possible that he could live[....] [They were removed to Bishop's Waltham]

4387. Did you ever hear it represented that the children had arrived in Bishop's Waltham in a state of great exhaustion and debility, and were very ill?—I afterwards heard that[....]

4419. Have you any knowledge of those children having been beaten also; have you heard of such a thing, or have you done it yourself?—I have done it myself once or twice, with a small birch rod, the same as I would beat a child of my own[....]

4482. Did you ever punish them for any thing else?—Not without the knowledge of the board of guardians.

4483. For having taken any leeks out of the garden?—Yes, two were ordered to be punished for that offense by the board.

4484. Do you know whether they ate the leeks?—They were detected with them, they did not eat them.

4485. How were they punished?—They were flogged by the birch over the breech by the board's order, with 12 stripes[....]

4518. Have you any children of your own?—Yes.

4519. Are they ever ill?—I have only one child living.

4520. Would you consider, if a child was ill and relaxed in its bowels, and therefore dirty in its habits, that that was a proper mode of treating your child, to put it in the stocks?—I should consider that they deserved punishment of some kind for this repeated fault; the habits of these children were so, without relaxation of the bowels.

4521. Do not you consider that a child, doing that, does it from weakness?—No, I do not.

4522. You think that he does it on purpose?—I consider that he does it from sloth; because I have had experience of that; and the mode of punishment that I have adopted has had the effect of curing many.

4523. That mode of punishment being by putting them in the stocks, and reducing the quantity of their food?—That has had a good effect upon many[....]

4775. You state that in January those children were removed into this out-building [with no heat nor windows], and you state that the reason for that was for fear that they should infect the other children?—Yes.

4827. How long was the short allowance [of food] continued?—For about a month after they came there, I should think[....]

4831. Did it not appear to you that as you were wreaking the powers of the body by continuing the short allowance, that you were thereby increasing the cause of the evil?—As soon as I found that it had no avail, I ordered it to be discontinued.

48

ANON., 'SUPPRESSED PAPERS OF THE BRITISH ASSOCIATION, LEFT IN NEWCASTLE UPON TYNE IN AUGUST LAST'

Northern Liberator (8 December 1838), p. 3

'Suppressed Papers of the British Association' handily spoofs the assumptions of the Poor Law, and suggests sarcastically that the poor should learn to live on air; set next to the article on how to make bread from wood, this piece illustrates how many in the middle and upper classes simply could not imagine that any of the poor deserved to have food, raiment and shelter. Lord Brougham's plan to urge the poor to emigrate was a common suggestion amongst many in the upper classes who thought that it was easily accomplished. They obviously were not considering the emotional and economic stresses such plans would wreak on the labouring classes. Lord Howick is Earl Grey and John Bowring was an economist (1792–1872). Francis Beaumont (1584–1616) and John Fletcher (1579–1625) were prolific playwrights of the seventeenth century known for their comedy. Sir Humphry Davy (1778–1829) was an inventor and chemist. Francois Magendie (1783–1855) was a French physiologist.

DOI: 10.4324/9780429198052-53

48. Anon., 'Suppressed Papers of the British Association, 'Left in Newcastle Upon Tyne in August Last', *Northern Liberator* (1838)

When the British Association, for the Advancement of Science, was at Newcastle in August last, we became acquainted with a fact connected with its general management, which we are now anxious should be made public[....]The fact is, that certain papers had been sent to the statistical section to be read to the members; but these were suppressed; they were all returned, and placed in our hands, with the words written on each, '*not admissible.*'

This will seem rather a strange affair when we tell our readers that these papers were from the pens of some of our most intelligent and profound citizens who are nightly burning the midnight oil to benefit mankind in general; we need hardly mention the names of Lord Brougham, Mr. Jos. Hume, M.P., Dr. Bowring, Lord Howick, &c. It does seem extraordinary these papers should have been passed over, but so the fact is[....] Now we believe that the fact is true as here stated, but the cause of it arose from the extreme modesty of the writers. They did not like to obtrude themselves on such an august body of men as the British Association[...] Indeed, every one knows the close and inviolable connexion between bashfulness and mental superiority, therefore, we think the Committee ought not to have rejected the papers in question[....]

The first paper was one from Mr. Joseph Hume, Member for Kilkenny. It was entitled '*The best means of finding when hens are with egg, and how to turn this useful discovery to the public good.*' The paper, with the exception of spelling and grammar, was concise and lucid enough. It set forth that you must go to the hen roost pretty early in the morning, and catch the hen before she breaks her fast. You then place her gently on the left arm, give her two or three chucks under the chin in a playful mode, and then delicately place your two fore fingers and thumb where naturalists place the *Ventris Extremum*; give a gentle jerk upwards, and you will find the rudiments of what you are seeking after. The writer then went on to state that he had for a long period applied his mind to this subject. He had disinterestedly kept three clerks to make calculations how the public weal might be promoted by the government keeping an extensive *hen roost. Ten millions* of hens might be kept in some convenient spot in England, under the guidance of a few Commissioners and Clerks.—Means might be taken, though he professed himself ignorant of the physiological rationale of the matter, to make these hens lay every day in the year. This would produce *three thousand six hundred and fifty millions* of eggs a year, which might be sold at two for a penny, for nearly *seven millions* per annum, which would make a sinking fund sufficient to redeem the whole of the national debt in three or four years[....]

The next paper was an extremely interesting one from Dr. Bowring, and somewhat akin to the preceding one. He had been sent to Egypt by the present government on divers interesting missions, and had there obtained knowledge highly useful to the people of this country. It is well known that Egypt was deeply skilled in what is now termed 'political economy' more than four thousand years ago.

This was undoubtedly an excellent field for the Doctor's skill and erudition. The subject which principally engrossed his attention in this country was the manner of hatching chickens with artificial heat. A brilliant idea struck his fancy, as he witnessed this ingenious process in Cairo, Alexandria, and other towns, that the plan might be profitably introduced into this country, and might relieve the nation of a great portion of its 'redundant labour.' Instead, however, of having kilns or stones for bringing the chickens to life in the eggs, he purposes to have a large national establishment of men, women, and children to sit upon the eggs, with feather breaches, till they hatch, and <?> up the tender offspring till they fatten, and are fit to eat. Such an institution might be placed by the government under the direction of half a score of commissioners, with a requisite number of assistants, clerks, book-keepers, runners, and who would pay the greatest attention to the separation of the sexes during the season of incubation. This would be a most profitable, easy, and comfortable mode for two or three millions of working people employing themselves; for all they would have to do would simply be to sit quiet, keep themselves in a cozy heat, and feed themselves with the produce of their own peaceful labours[....]

The next paper was from my Lord Brougham[....] [who deduced that the] plain simple fact was, that clothing of all kinds might be advantageously dispensed with, in case of the poor especially, who were a grievous burden to the country, and if not curtailed in their extravagant habits and notions would ultimately make himself, and every nobleman in the land, complete beggars in a short time. All that would be necessary to keep the cold and moisture out from the human body would be a certain kind of *varnish*, which might be rubbed over the whole outer man, varied in colour in the different sexes, black for the man, and blue for the females, to preserve the blessings of moral restraint[....] He felt confident a great national saving would be effected in the workhouse especially; and it would tend to raise the character of the English peasantry out of that dependent, lazy, and profligate condition in which they had so long been immersed[....]

The next paper that comes under our notice was by the Right Honourable Lord Howick, and was entitled a, 'Proposal to accustom the poorer classes to live upon air.' This is a very curious paper, and shews the great chemical as well as politico-economical lore of his lordship. One would suppose that it had been written, Beaumont and Fletcher like, by Malthus and Sir Humphrey Davy in conjunction. By an elaborate chemical analysis his lordship shews that the nutritive part of all food whatsoever may be resolved into the gas called nitrogen. Beef and mutton, broth and potatoes, black puddings and hodge-podge, he shews are only clumsy vehicles for conveying nitrogen into the stomach by tempting the palate to swallow it. This clumsy expedient of Dame Nature, which is only akin to giving children medicine in sugar or treacle, his lordship proposes gradually to set aside. He shews that the stomachs of the poor might be gradually accustomed to the reception of nitrogen in its uncombined and unadulterated state, and proves by experiments, of Magendie of Paris, that the only danger would be that this aerial food would be too rich even for hard-working people. Magendie, Lord Howick observes, proved by experiment, that an exclusive diet upon substances which contain this nutritive gas in the most condensed state are very prejudicial[....]This once effected, here is a cheap dietary for the bastiles; as nitrogen can be obtained from various substances at a trifling expense in copious volume. His lordship calculates that one hundred cubic feet of nitrogen would support fifty adult paupers for seventeen days, and the expense would only be a fraction of a farthing per diem per head!

49

JOHN EAGLES, 'NEW SCHEME FOR MAINTAINING THE POOR'

Blackwood's Edinburgh Magazine 43 (1838), pp. 489–493

This piece, like the previous one, is very much in keeping with Swift's famous 'A Modest Proposal', to which the article directly refers. In this case, the tongue-in-cheek writer, John Eagles, would do away with the aged and youthful poor but not before using their skin to advantage for the needs of the Poor Law Commissioners. Again, Lord Brougham is mentioned as a kind of bogey-man, having evil designs on the poor. References to Indian cannibalism project (and elide) homefront anxieties onto Indian culture, yet still focus squarely on the British government's culpability. There seems to be a reference to the article on making bread from wood, as well. 'Vivite sylvae!' means 'live forests', and Lacedemonians is a name for Spartans.

DOI: 10.4324/9780429198052-54

49. John Eagles, 'New Scheme for Maintaining the Poor', *Blackwood's Edinburgh Magazine* (1838)

One would think that Swift's serious proposal of killing, selling, and eating the children of the Irish poor must have found favour in the eyes of Liberals, Utilitarians, and Political Economists[....] great progress having been already made in our civilisation, much more may be expected; vulgar prejudices on the necessity of much feeding may be obliterated, and the poor be made readily to acquiesce in a system of maintaining each other, upon the principle of the lamps that are made to consume their own smoke.

To attain so desirable an object is well worth the deepest study of all philosophers whatever; and the right of disposing of the poor for the benefit of the poor can no longer be disputed. Nature, say the philosophers, furnishes an ample table for a certain number of guests; all who come after the seats are filled are not to be thought of; there must be no crowding, and but that the feast is amply provided for the select number, all aftercomers might be fairly made minced meat of to supply any lack of provisions. I, as every one must, subscribe to this, but only on the plea of necessity. All I say is, that there might be a more humane method of feeding. I propose a plan, and I do hope that, when in an age not very distant it shall be in full play, I shall be considered at last as great a benefactor to mankind as Lord Brougham. He would teach them algebra—I would keep them alive. He would do his part at other's people's cost—I mine at no cost at all.

I am fully aware that science has long been at work, and some admirable inventions are advancing to an astonishing maturity. I have recently attended the lectures of a great political economist, who performed the wonderful operation of making loaves of bread out of saw-dust—wherein it was fully shown that the poor may be made to 'lick the dust' with great advantage to themselves and the rest of mankind; 'Vivite sylvae!'—and the saw-mill for the tread-mill—and there will never be a lack of grist. I had scarcely recovered from my wonderment at this wonder of wonders, when it was declared, to the infinite satisfaction of a number of Poor-Guardians present, that very good bread had been made out of granite—so that it is to be hoped the sciences may yet come, when, without shame, the poor shall ask for bread and you shall 'give them a stone!!!' But however ingenious these inventions are, I fear the process will require more scientific knowledge than our common bakers are likely for some time to come to possess; at least until the New Schools for Universal and Useful Knowledge shall have been in play half a century. Considering, therefore, the already too expensive machinery set in work by the new Poor-laws—it is to be feared the little saving in the material, should saw-dust and granite supersede wheat, would be eaten up, and perhaps in a more palatable way, by new commissionerships and appointments of scientific bakers, which an earlier adoption of these inventions would absolutely require. It is with great pleasure, therefore, that I lay before the public my more simple, and perfectly practicable scheme; and I more particularly recommend it to the notice of the Poor Law Commissioners, because they will see at once that to enforce it, their full authority will be required, and consequently their importance and their salaries will be secured forever. It must be assumed that luxuries are not to be admitted into a poor-house. That the maintaining the poor at all is an evil not to be endured but through necessity; and rather to preserve ourselves than them. This is evidently the admitted maxim, the very principle running through the late Poor-laws. And I certainly heard one of the itinerant assistant Commissioners, when developing the laws and promoting the unions, boast that the new poor-houses would not be 'too comfortable,' that they would be so hard to the inmates, that none, not even the most idle, would stay in them longer than they could help, nor when they might, in any degree short of starvation, maintain themselves, that is keep body and soul together.

Three-fourths of the inmates in a union poor-house may be put down as aged and infirm—the other fourth as children and idiots—so that the large majority being composed of the aged and infirm it follows that there must be rapid succession—that in the course of Nature they must die faster than any other portion of the population, and the course of Art under the new medical poor regulations may vie with that of Nature in accelerating the much-wished-for consummation. I would have, then, those that drop off support those that live on; and I think after the scheme had been in operation a little while, the supply would be regular and certain. There are but two prejudices to get over—the foolish and unphilosophical repugnance to any kind of flesh, and the very useless and wasteful one of burying the dead[....]

[....] The man who bequeaths his own body, as some do, to fertilize the earth, and looks forward to vegetate a full-grown cabbage, proud in death of his philosophy, is undoubtedly a great benefactor to his fellow creatures. All will not thus bequeath themselves—but as those who consume other people's property become themselves substantially other people's property, it is but fair they should be at other people's disposal. There is no getting over that sound principle—so those who consume should by that law be themselves consumed[....]

I would have set up in every union poor-house a patent digester upon a new scale, and upon the most improved principles, such as the toughness of some of the materials may require. I would have every man, woman, and child, that shall die in these union houses, boiled down, and made into soup, which will be, I am persuaded, sufficient in quantity to support all the living inmates, if the fast-days are as religiously observed as they ought to be; and in quality quite equal to the celebrated 'Black Broth,' the public meal of that great people and notable economists, the Lacedemonians.

Still, after the flesh has been all boiled off the bones, it is manifest there will be an overplus—the bones themselves, which must likewise come within the 'appropriation clause' of my scheme. These bones may be partly manufactured into forks and spoons and ladles for the use of the poor. The rest I would have regularly *ground*, made into bread, and distributed to the poor on Sundays. Tread-mills may here be of great use, and thus will be accomplished the great scheme, so long the desideratum of all philosophers—of GRINDING

THE POOR FOR THEIR OWN BENEFIT. I am here only taking into account the infirm and aged. Sickly and delicate constitutions will occasionally require something approaching to luxury[....] I think the sickly poor may be brought to relish the more tender food of infants and children, who must of course occasionally die in the houses; a regular certificate from the surgeon and registrar of deaths being just put up in some conspicuous place in the kitchen and eating-rooms that they have not died of measles, no meats, under such circumstances, being considered wholesome. I have been told by a retired sausage-vender that children under twelve years of age, particularly females, are as good and as tender as chicken; of which, indeed, I have heard a confirmation, from the fact, that a converted Indian woman, in a dying state, upon being asked by a missionary, 'What he could do for her?' said, she thought she could pick the small bones of a little child's hand, but that now none of her people would kill her one. This was the speech, and more than half-request of one well acquainted with the delicacy, and who had a return of appetite, as the 'ruling passion strong in death.' It must have been very shocking to hear. But let it not for a moment be supposed that our guardians would, any more than the missionaries themselves, sanction the killing. If, under any emergency, they may seem to do so, it would be under the mildest form of 'killing no murder,' when it would be an absolute cruelty to prolong the life of the believer.

But my scheme does not end here. I would have no loss whatever, but all profit. A cow does not die, but she is honoured in her skin; a sheep-skin has dignity conferred upon it, conveys lands and houses to the latest posterity, and is treasured up in iron chests, and why should not the skin of an old woman-pauper, already half-tanned, have its posterior use, and be made serviceable as it might be many ways. I have preferred to mention the skins of old women, because they are believed to be more durable, are better preserved and wrapped in flannels during life, have less wear and tear, and have been less exposed to weather and whipping. Well, I would have these thoroughly tanned. I would have them made into coverings for the Commissioners' chairs, and the great tables used to cushion the Guardians' pews[....]

[....] I would then have the said skins hereafter, in all cases, to be used for covering and binding of such books and registers as the clergy are desired to keep[....] And it should be considered a great privilege and honour to the poor to bear on their backs after they are dead, generations yet to come while they are living. Thus they will be themselves their own veritable genealogical trees, which I cannot but think a source of commendable pride to them who have so little to be proud of[...] I really think the poor will take much more care of their own skins than they have hitherto done[....]

The skins of very young children I would have sold for ladies' albums; for which purpose, embossed with cherubim heads, they will fetch a great price; and the proceeds may greatly help towards paying the salaries of the Poor-Law Commissioners, and the significant innocency of the one source of this income make their office appear more respectable.

I would likewise have the skins of all bastards, and idiots especially, set apart to register those miscalled marriages which have not the sanction of the Church.; and I would have them for this purpose stamped, that there may be no mistake[....]

I have here fully developed my scheme. Until it shall be taken up by the Government, many evils of the new Poor-Laws must go on;[...]

50

TESTIMONY FROM REV. D. WILLIAMS (CURATE OF SHALBOURNE), 11 MAY 1838, AND FROM JOHN BOWEN (GUARDIAN OF BRIDGWATER UNION), 5 JULY 1838, *SELECT COMMITTEE OF HOUSE OF LORDS ON OPERATION OF POOR LAW AMENDMENT ACT*

Hansard, HC (1837–1838), Volume 41, Images 107–108, 889–890

In this questioning of a curate named Reverend Williams and of Bridgwater Union Guardian Mr. John Bowen Parliament recovers, second-hand, how a poor child might feel if made to choose between food and one's parents.

DOI: 10.4324/9780429198052-55

50. Testimony from Rev. D. Williams (Curate of Shalbourne) and from John Bowen (Guardian of Bridgwater Union), *Select Committee of House of Lords on Operation of Poor Law Amendment Act* (1838)

Testimony of Rev. D. Williams, 11 May 1838

Do you imagine that [Isaac] Watts [a poor man with many children] would[....] have sent his Children into the Workhouse?

I do not know that he would. I do not know that poor People would avail themselves of the Privilege; their Feeling is very strong against the Workhouse, insomuch that I questioned the Wife of Watts on Tuesday last[....]

What did Mrs. Watts say?

[....] She came, and she said, 'No; I do not wish my Children to go to the Workhouse; I would much rather that they should suffer at Home than that they should go to the Workhouse'.

[....] Have you ascertained with respect to any other Persons—Townsend or Knight [other poor men with lots of children] [...] whether they would like to have their Children taken away?

Knight was from Home at the Time I called, and his Wife said she would rather have her Children suffer at Home. When I saw this Girl of Watt's (she is a sharp little Girl) I questioned her upon the Subject; I said, 'You have been in the Workhouse; mind you tell me the Truth; would you like to go to the Workhouse rather than be at Home?' 'No;' she said, 'I would much rather be at Home.' 'Why?' I said; 'Because I had not Victuals enough at the Workhouse.' 'What did you get at the Workhouse?' I asked; 'what was your Breakfast?' 'Why, I had Bread and Gruel.' 'What was your Dinner?' 'Why, I had Meat for Dinner Three Times a Week, Beef or Bacon;' and after I had questioned her as to all this, I asked,' What do you get at Home?' She said, 'I get Bread for Breakfast.' 'Tea, do you get?' 'No Tea; but Mother gets a little weak Tea sometimes.' 'And Mother gives you a little, I suppose?' 'No, she does not,' she said. 'Do you get Bread and Butter?' 'No, not always; sometimes I do.' 'What is your Breakfast?' I said. 'Bread,' she said. 'Nothing but Bread?' I asked, and she said, 'Nothing but Bread;' and I said, 'Bread and Gruel in the Workhouse is better than Bread at Home?' 'No; but there was not enough to satisfy Nature;' that was her Answer. I suppose she meant the Cravings of Hunger.

Testimony of John Bowen 5 July 1838

[....] Do you think the Wages are sufficient to support a Man and his Family?

They are not; not in Comfort.

If they get on with them, how do they get on?

I do not know how a Man on 7*s*. a Week lives.

Do you think the Remedy for the State of Things be a Payment out of the Poor Rates?

I think not; but until some other Remedy is provided the poor Man has nothing to provide for a rainy Day; he is actually brought down to the Brink of Starvation; and if you stop that Source of Supply, though it may be a vicious one, without providing him with any other, you either drive him to dishonest Courses or you put him to Death.

51

CHARLES HORACE WALL, 'HOW DO POOR MEN LIVE?'

Tait's Edinburgh Magazine, 6 (1839), pp. 13–22, on pp. 13–16, 19–20

Including a list of the necessities of the poor needed to survive, this text shows how the labourer's wages could not possibly have covered these subsistence level requirements. By focusing on how the labourer only had 'property' in his labour, this writer shows how contemporary economists simply did not see the difference between what property meant for the rich and for the poor. Also, the article builds on the assumption that a great nation must take care of its poor or the body politic might erupt in violence. The attention paid to how the poor refused to follow 'beneficial' leaders illustrates a downright discomfort with the democratic dynamics of political association, while the mystifying of the poor becomes a sign of the alienation between classes. Richard Oastler (1789–1861) was a Tory and commission agent for years before becoming interested in the needs of the labourers. Sir Thomas Bernard (1769–1834) was an Irish MP. Bernard is supposed to have said: 'It is a melancholy truth—and the concealment of it will prevent the correction of the evil—that the poor of England are not properly fed'.[86]

DOI: 10.4324/9780429198052-56

51. Charles Horace Wall, 'How Do Poor Men Live?', *Tait's Edinburgh Magazine* (1839)

[....] How the poor of our fellow-creatures live, is an inquiry pressing on all men pretending to be Christians and philanthropists; but it is the special duty of legislators and rulers not only to know how the great mass of the People live, but to see that they subsist in a condition that may prevent any reasonable cause of discontent[....]

Some perilous crisis, if not anarchical revolution, can only be averted by the timely adoption of real reforms—[....]

[....] As matters now stand, it may be said that the promise of God has failed the British isles, and that men are no longer able, by the sweat of their brow, to earn their bread; that it is a necessary law of society, that the rewards of industry should diminish, in proportion as its capabilities and exertions are increased.

One alarming symptom of the present popular discontents, is, that the mass of the poor have no accredited leaders in whose wisdom and integrity they may with safety confide. They despise the Whigs, and they abhor the Tories; that is, where they indulge political feelings at all; for, while they clamour after such men as Mr. Oastler, it does not appear that any leader has much wholesome influence among them, or any that is likely to be either beneficial or permanent. But such considerations lead to a wider range of speculation than we propose to take. We do not mean to enter into political discussion; but to adhere to the mystery involved in the narrow text, '*How do poor men live.*'

We apprehend this mystery was as clearly solved as the case admits, by the poor woman, who, when the question was put to her, probably by a poor-law assistant-commissioner, replied—'Lord bless you! We do not *live*, we only *bides!'* Many of the poor of England cannot, indeed, be said to live—they merely exist.

[....] The chief lesson which the operatives require, is not how to accumulate, but how they are to gain such an amount of wages as, without starvation, admits of saving[....]

[....] The mass of the people of this country have, at this moment, the conviction riveted into their minds, that the interests of the higher orders, is diametrically opposed to their interests; that they must be ground to dust, in order that the capitalists and farmers may become wealthy, that the rich may live in luxury, and the great maintain their magnificence[....]

In the meanwhile, How poor men live—how they keep soul and body together—is the standing miracle which few regard. From the late reports of statists—though they are always more or less inaccurate, and moreover, generally disposed to err on the flattering side—the average wages of artisans in towns may be rated, at the very highest, at 1l. per week; and we believe that, if times of dull trade and want of employment were taken into account, 15s. would be much nearer the truth. We say this confidently, as there are many callings—such, for examples, as that of printers—where, although 30s. or £2 may be gained by hard work and night-work when work is plentiful, a settled yearly wage of 18s. or 20s. would be preferred by a prudent compositor[....] And in how many trades to the workmen, for a few years, increase their wages by spending their capital—namely, their health, vigour, and skill—untimely worn out? If a working man must spend his whole wages as he goes along in the necessary maintenance of his family—and, alas! how seldom does that little all suffice for its comfortable subsistence!—if he make no accumulation against the evil day, he is assuredly living upon and exhausting his capital; that which ought to be stored against the season, not merely of fluctuation in trade, and sickness, but of diminished strength and ability of labour, and finally against decrepitude, old age, and the workhouse[....]

[....] A work on domestic economy, published some years ago by Colburn, contains numerous household estimates—and the lowest income estimated is exactly one shilling more than our sum, or 21s. a-week. We are content to throw that shilling into the total, which thus makes net 3s. 6d. a-day for every working-day in the year, and now give the particulars of the weekly bill:—

Bread and flour for five persons	£0	3	6
Butter, cheese, and milk	0	1	9
Sugar and treacle	0	0	9
Rice, oatmeal, salt, &c	0	0	6
Butchers' meat or fish, say meat, 61b. at 4 ½ d.	0	2	3
Vegetables, including a ¼ cwt. of potatoes, 4lb.a-day,	0	1	2
Table-beer		1	6
[Coals and wood], 1d.	0	1	9
Candles—average ½ lb., at 7d.	0	0	3½
Soap, starch, blue, for washing	0	0	3½
Sundries, for cleaning, scouring, &c., 1d.;	0	0	
Total for household expences,	0	13	6
Rent,	0	2	6
Clothes and haberdashery,	0	3	6
Total expense,	0	19	3[....]

[....] we cannot imagine any man objecting to even one of those items, who values the health, morals, and happiness of the operative class. We have allowed of no indulgence or luxury whatever, save two family holidays; scantily provided for many necessaries; and left nothing for savings against old age, sickness, or misfortune; and yet there is a deficit of £1.18s.—and this is in a high income, as wages run throughout the country.

How then do poor men live? We fear Sir Thomas Bernard was in the right. The poor of England, and workmen of England are not properly fed; they are not properly clothed; they are not sufficiently lodged and warmed[....] half-starving—they will sometimes weather through, no one can say how[....]

He is convinced that there is, for his Order, no protection save by obtaining a direct influence in the legislature through extended suffrage. And who is entitled to the first right of a free citizen, if he is not?

Part 6

VIOLENCE, REVOLUTION, CRIME

16 August 1819 was an infamous day in Manchester, when up to 80,000 labourers marched peaceably to St. Peter's Field square to hear an oration by the radical speaker Henry Hunt. Learning from spies that the labourers were practising military marching in preparation for the event and fearing violence, the town magistrates called up the local yeomanry and militia, ostensibly to keep the peace; instead, they charged on horseback into the mass of peaceful marchers that included women and children. Attacking the group with sabres, the militia caused a panic as protestors were pressed against the narrow confines of the square. Eighteen people were killed and over 400 people were wounded. Afterwards, the square looked like a battle had occurred there, and the press likened it to Waterloo, hence the name 'Peterloo'. Whether they agreed with the labourer's goals, many in the country were horrified that English soldiers attacked freeborn Englishmen, women and children who were protesting peacefully. This event became immortalised in Chartist and other rhetoric as well as in regular memorials throughout the rest of the century. This event is believed to be one of the many stepping-stones the lower classes navigated towards obtaining universal suffrage.

An article entitled 'Politic and Social Experiments of 1819', which appeared in *The Morning Post* on Monday, 26 July 1819, illustrates the tensions going on just prior to Peterloo. The writer avers that,

> If we do not *now* make *some experiment* of relieving ourselves and the poor, by starvation, typhus, the gallows, or emigration, we *must* make the experiment of giving them employment *at home* and fair *wages* for their *labour;* or *food* without work—or land to dig—or something else.[87]

In light of Peterloo, Parliament might have been more prescient if it had focused on the reasons for the protest: hunger and unemployment. Over the next few months after Peterloo, *The Times* featured numerous articles trying to make sense of what actually happened at Peterloo and of its import for society at large. Seeing itself as the mediating voice of reason, *The Times* could not fully rationalise this event. In 'London, Tuesday, August 24, 1819', Britain's premier newspaper ultimately

DOI: 10.4324/9780429198052-57

argued that bread and butter issues were what should have been focused on by Parliament in its response to the masses and their distress, saying:

> We are of the number of those who feel that the condition of the labouring class of cotton-manufacturers required to be amended for the good of the whole community; [...] and that some vicious and unwholesome principles which have crept into trade and into the laws which affect the labourer, are powerful causes of the heartbreaking misery which he suffers.[88]

Other responses are featured below.

52

ANON., 'LONDON, TUESDAY, AUGUST 24, 1819'

The Times (24 August 1819), p. 2

The Times saw itself as the arbiter of what it saw as the war taking place between 'rich and poor' in the aftermath of Peterloo. But, given its own argument internal to the article, it is clear that the rich should not have been the judges of the measures taken by the masses to ensure their voices were heard. Too often the well-to-do referred to the poor as 'wretches' and inarticulate clunky oafs, all but seeing them as alien beings. In keeping with rhetoric across this topic, England saw itself as needing to be above violence, which sniffed of what they saw as French extremism. Noting that it could only rely on its sources because it had no understanding of Manchester 'whatsoever', the writer asserts, then refutes, the 'entitle[ment]' of the lower class to make demands on the upper classes. The piece is responding, in part, to an article in the *Courier* a few days earlier, its provenance not given aside from the reference to the *Courier*.

DOI: 10.4324/9780429198052-58

52. Anon., 'London, Tuesday, August 24, 1819', *Times* (1819)

[....] a sentence in the *Courier*, importing that persons on the spot were the most competent judges of the state of affairs around them; and we urged as a strong objection, that magistrates were naturally imbued with sympathy for the masters, and indignation or resentment against the labouring classes, seeing that the magistrates were also masters, and likely to take part with themselves[....] We are of the number of those who feel that the condition of the labouring class of cotton-manufacturers requires to be amended for the good of the whole community, that their wages are too low, and ought to be raised to a level with the price of food and clothing, and religious instruction of their children; and that some vicious and unwholesome principles which have crept into trade and into the laws which affect the labourer, are powerful causes of the heart-breaking misery which he suffers. But when the poor of the manufacturing districts, squalid, crowded, desperate, and almost innumerable, make known their wants to those above them, it is not, perhaps, in the most persuasive or conciliatory accents. The clamours of an immense multitude for relief to their wants must ever be, under and circumstances, formidable to every man of property who hears them; and when the passions of these poor wretches are still further inflamed by mischievous representations of redress which they ought to seek, and of the manner in which they are entitled to demand it, there is little wonder if the dispute itself, should bear the complexion to the affluent and timid, of a general war of poverty against wealth; or, in other words, of a general scheme for the robbery of every man who has a house to hold him. All the accounts from the manufacturing country, and from Manchester, its great metropolis, unconsciously divide the loyal and disloyal by their grand classification of rich and poor. This it is which must make every man, who has lived long enough to see and reflect upon revolutions in other countries, and rebellions in our own, most anxious, not only that power should be exercised on moderate and patient principles, but that it should be wielded by thoroughly impartial and unsuspected hands. There is nothing at all disgraceful in a man of property at Manchester apprehending great mischief from the excesses of a mob—mischief to himself and to his fortunes. We merely say, that *any* such man of fortune, acting under the impression of such fears, must be more apt than others would be, to exert precipitately the power intrusted to him; for precipitation is incidental to a state of alarm[....]

We see with increasing dislike and concern, the advertisement of more meetings both in London and in the north. The capital is menaced with one for tomorrow at Smithfield. What can the wretches mean? Are they so little conversant with political or individual nature, as not to know that the abuse of a right in the one case, as of a faculty in the other, is too frequently followed by the loss of it. That these meetings, although it be more probably that the real purpose of those who hold them is the overthrow of the State, may still be kept within the letter of the constitution, is a fact we shall not question. But when the whole world are convinced of their profligate as well as frantic objects, and convinced also that such frequent assemblages of the people may have a tendency to promote those objects, what *can* be the consequence but this?—that the cords of law will sooner or later be drawn so tight, as to restrain the well-disposed part of the nation from ever meeting for any purpose whatever; and thus to stifle the public voice—the last, best hope of political society.

53

ANON., 'THE DEBATE UPON THE ADDRESS'

The Times (26 November 1819)

Condescending to the Peterloo marchers, this *Times* article also finds fault with the excessive military response, thus recognising the poor as citizens deserving protection from their country. *The Times* also essentially recognised that poverty was not a crime and that 43 Elizabeth invoked a contract with the labouring classes. Henry Addington, known as Lord Sidmouth (1757–1844), was the Home Secretary from 1812 to 1822, and in that position had enforced the unpopular Six Acts of Repression that responded to the labourers' efforts to obtain suffrage and other progressive measures. James Stuart Wortley (1776–1845) was a military man and politician.

DOI: 10.4324/9780429198052-59

53. Anon., 'The debate upon the Address', *Times* (1819)

[....] The most important feature with respect to the assembly at Manchester, is, whether it was legal or not? And it was asserted by Ministers, that no lawyer would stake his reputation upon an opinion that the meeting was legal. Why, the Magistrates themselves, in their first published communication with Ministers, did state their conviction that the meeting was legal; saying, 'As the law now stands, we cannot interfere with these meetings, notwithstanding our decided opinion of their mischief and danger.' Surely, then, in a case of so much difficulty, some indulgence should have been shown to the ignorant illiterate men assembled; who, goaded, as it is on all hands allowed, by distress, and inflamed by profligate demagogues, thought that they were met in order to produce some undefined good to themselves: and when the leaders were quietly taken prisoners, the followers should *not have been cut down, or ridden over* by the military[....]

The next subject of inquiry—that is to say, for we must be well understood here, if the lives and limbs of Englishmen are worth inquiring about at all—in that case the next subject of inquiry is, whether the Riot-Act was read or not[....] Monstrous, then, as the thing may see, this important fact [of whether it was read or not] rests in every stage of uncertainty[....] but neither in nor out of Parliament has any one man been adduced or spoken of by name who hear it read. The most essential purpose, therefore, of reading it was lost.

There is another subject to which we solicit attention. The first of the documents produced is a letter from the New Bailey Court-house, addressed to Lord SIDMOUTH by five Magistrates, SILVESTER, WRIGHT, MARRIOT, ETHELSTON, AND NORRIS, which speaks of 'The deep distresses of the manufacturing classes of this extensive population.' *It adds, that 'when* the people are *oppressed with hunger*, they (the signing Magistrates) do not wonder at their giving ear to any doctrines which they are told will redress their grievances.' Here, therefore, is the cause of the disaffection, or apparent disaffection, laid open, and the remedy suggested by these Magistrates. Distress, amounting even to 'hunger,' is the reason why the people listened to seditious demagogues. Did Ministers, then, adopt any measures to relieve the distress thus pointed out to them, and the consequences of which, they were assured, would be so fatal to the public peace? This letter is signed on the 1st of July, six weeks before the meeting. Sufficient *time, therefore*, was allowed for preventing any such meeting; and that, not by the Yeomanry's sabres or constables staves, or the reading of the Riot Acts, but by such means as humanity prescribes, and just policy would adopt. What, then, we ask, did Ministers in consequence of this intelligence? Did they take any measures to prevent men 'in deep distress and suffering from hunger' from joining the disaffected? All these, it is obvious, are subjects of broad and general inquiry, and might well be scrutinized by Parliament. They cannot form the gist of any action at law, or criminal prosecution, and can only come before the Courts collaterally. Their investigation, therefore, by the *grand inquest of the nation*, is natural, and we hope will take place.

54

ANON., 'PARLIAMENTARY INTELLIGENCE. HOUSE OF LORDS AND HOUSE OF COMMONS, TUESDAY, NOVEMBER 30'

The Times (1 December 1819), pp. 1–2, 4

In a recap of discussions in the House of Lords, this article notes the Lords' discussion of 'distress', crisis and peril, and hones in on the debates about whether to focus on forcibly maintaining the peace in the face of purported radical insurrections after Peterloo or on the underlying cause of the insurrection—distress. Whig MP, the Marquis of Lansdowne (1780–1863), served as Home Secretary and Chancellor of the Exchequer over his long political career. While Lansdowne favoured strong measures for putting an end to violence and sedition, he also saw the importance of getting at the root cause for such disruptions by the lower classes. Indeed, in this speech, he acknowledges that there must have been something wrong since so many members of the lower classes were listening to the agitators and protesting their condition. His speech also highlights the 'sacred' trust so many MPs believed in, the laissez-faire principle of leaving the markets alone to right themselves—his willingness to interfere in the market suggests just how perilous the situation had become.

MP Lord Grenville (1759–1834) served a long career in government, including in the House of Commons and as Home Secretary and Foreign Secretary. Grenville also shows willingness to depart from 'sacred' duties to market principles in order to save the people from such overwhelming distress. Earl Grey shows disgust for the 'complacency' of MPs who claimed there was no distress or that there was no need to respond to it.

In the House of Commons a similar conversation was going on. Lord Charles Milton's (1786–1857) shocking depiction of Peterloo indicates a traditional sense of the social contract between the classes and how to maintain it. Like Milton, George Tierney (1761–1830) believed that the deep causes of distress had to be examined and rooted out.

DOI: 10.4324/9780429198052-60

54. Anon., 'Parliamentary Intelligence. House of Lords and House of Commons', Tuesday, Nov, 30', *Times* (1819)

STATE OF THE COUNTRY

The Marquis of LANDSDOWNE: [....] sedition of every kind was to be put down by the law. But when the violence was repressed, and the sedition subdued, was not the evil which had led to that state of things to be explored?[...] It was not sufficient for them to know, that itinerant demagogues had travelled over the country, addressing seditious harangues to multitudes of people; they were bound to make themselves acquainted with the causes which had produced these extraordinary effects, and to ascertain why so many tongues were thus employed, and why they found so many ears disposed to listen to them[....] he was again compelled to point to those who were suffering under the greatest degree of distress. Among the cotton-manufacturers, whose situation was worse than that of any other class, the spirit of radicalism had been carried to the greatest extent. It was important that their lordships should feel the truth of this view of the subject, in order that their attention might be fully directed to the state of the manufacturing districts[....] It became their lordships to turn their attention to this distress, and to investigate its causes[....]

[....] Having exhausted all their means in a struggle between life and misery, was it surprising if nothing was done to remove the cause, that they should proceed from poverty to crime, till society, grown weary of the load, wished to shake off the incumbrance?[...]

If, indeed, he could bring himself to the opinion that the evil was temporary, that it depended in a great measure on the distress of other countries, and that the means suggested would give effectual relief to the distressed population, then he might be induced to depart from those principles of political economy which, under other circumstance, he should be disposed to hold sacred. If he could be persuaded that a parliamentary grant would carry the people of the distressed districts over their difficulty, he would not hesitate to give it his concurrence[....]

Lord GRENVILLE: [....] he was satisfied that the root of the evil lay deeper, he believed, nevertheless, that it would not have been possible to work a portion of the population into the state of ferment in which the papers presented proved them to be, but for the concurrence of other circumstances originating in present and pressing distress. He was therefore convinced that if it were possible by any measure of Parliament could adopt—*even departing* on the urgency of the occasion from those principles relating to commerce and manufactures, which, in ordinary times, ought to be held sacred and inviolable[....] to alleviate the existing distresses[....]

Earl Grey: [....] th*at distress* [...] was the main and operative cause of the disturbed state of the public mind[....] His noble friends [Parliament], indeed, had allowed, and had expressed themselves with great complacency—a complacency natural to so consoling a topic—that the people were not generally disaffected.

How Is this to be explained?[...] Was it, therefore, inconsistent with humanity and justice to say, that when the circumstances of this dangerous influence on the public mind were under consideration, their lordships should in the first instance look to the cause, and *endeavour to check the evil in its source*?[...] He was grieved, therefore, to hear that Latin quotation of the noble marquis, which implied that the whole people were filled with fury and detestable malice against the government, and all indiscriminately combined against the institutions of their country[....] There was, indeed, no real defence in any country, especially in a country under such a constitution as that of England, but a system of liberty which should conciliate the affection and esteem of the people[....]

Lord Milton (House of Commons): [....] *It was not* by riding through a body of men, or mowing them down by soldiery [Peterloo], while they were assembled at a meeting of this character, that the people of England were to be subdued, but by means and measures of a more lenient and conciliatory character[....]

Mr. George Tierney (House of Commons): [....] if severe laws were to be passed, and if a resolution was to be adopted to restrict still further the liberty of the country, it was their bounden duty to take into consideration the distress, and the causes of the distress, which now prevailed. The noble lord, indeed, had asked them, whether they would wait and postpone the passing of his measures, until, they had inquired into the necessity of enacting them. 'With as great reason might the poor man turn round and say to the noble lord, 'will you postpone to relieve me, when I am starving, until you have inquired into the means of removing my distress?'

55

WILLIAM JOHNSTON, 'THE PRESENT CRISIS'

Blackwood's Edinburgh Magazine, 28 (1830), pp. 690–694

This article by Irish journalist William Johnston suggests that the nation was facing violent revolution if it refused to listen to the poor and provide them with the simple necessity for which they were asking—food. In this regard, he warns that if the new Parliament did not respond to the people's distress the possibility of revolution was very real. Nevertheless, his pride in the 'sober' slowness of English institutions in responding to crisis ignores the fact that the hungry could not wait— for obviously if their starving condition was ignored too long it would lead to death. The Irish Famine and famines in India, China and elsewhere would prove the British State's glacial slowness in responding to calamities was ultimately inhumane and inefficient. Johnston makes his argument, in part, by referring to England's own non-violent Glorious Revolution (1688–89, which he distinguishes favourably from the violent French Revolution), when James II, a strict Catholic, was removed as king and William III (along with James's Protestant daughter Mary II) replaced him.

DOI: 10.4324/9780429198052-61

55. William Johnston, 'The Present Crisis', *Blackwood's Edinburgh Magazine* (1830)

There is a tide in the affairs of nations, as well as of individuals, and the present tide is that which sweeps on towards the uncertain shore of revolution. The madness, or conviction, or sentiment, or whatever be its right name, is as general as that of the Crusades and from the Mediterranean to the Baltic, the people are in a ferment[....] Nations, like the people before the flood, become 'corrupt before God;' but a more merciful dispensation, instead of drowning the world, gives us wars and revolutions; and they operate as a purge, exhausting for the moment, but sanative; and the kingdoms grow strong again, till a recurrence of the disease shall require a repetition of the remedy. All this is not very new perhaps but it is worth while to dwell a little upon these reflections, in order to dissipate those of a more gloomy nature, which the present angry aspect of the political world is so apt to occasion.

The present crisis is one which no man, who reflects at all, can look upon without very lively interest; for, in no period of modern times, has the settled order of things appeared to be so extensively under the influence of desire for change[.....]

[....] Our Parliamentary debates, if very unargumentative talking may deserve that name, and our newspapers and magazines, notwithstanding the adverse of a Whig Attorney-general [James Scarlett, whom we've seen before in the discussion about the Poor Laws], are quite sufficient safety-valves, to let off the ill-humour of the people; and our institutions, however slow and expensive in their working, and although clogged with abuses in their details, are yet of certain efficacy to secure us from such perversion of authority as would call for the forcible intermeddling of the common people; or would justify an *ostentatious* applause of such intermeddling. The common people here, as everywhere else, will catch up what appears on the surface, without seeking to go deeper, and if they find the forcible interference of their brethren on the continent the theme of public and inflated panegyric, they will draw their conclusions at once, and without stopping to make nice enquiries as to the circumstances of the case, in which this much-lauded interference took place.

It is not like Englishmen, it is not consistent with common sense, to rush headlong into this public admiration of that about which we know so little, except that from the rapidity of the change, (we refer to the affairs of France) it is almost impossible that the new system of government, struck off at the first heat, can be permanent[....] That which is to endure, must be done soberly, and thoughtfully, and deliberately; but that which is done with the rapidity of the shifting of a scene, is likely as soon to give place to another. The French did us the honour very frequently in their late brief proceedings, to refer to our Revolution as a model, as well as an example; it would have been well if they not only recollected what we did, but the way in which it was done[....] In the peculiar circumstances of this country, impoverished by a mistaken system of commercial policy, embarrassed by the contraction of the circulating medium, and the consequent increase of the pressure of taxation,—dissatisfied with a cabinet which has but slender reputation for ability, and none at all for political integrity,—and harassed by the distress of an unemployed population[....]

[...] Let it be shewn by all those who have property, and have a mind to keep it, that they are not unmindful of the condition of those who have none; and let them rather endeavour to stop with food, than with unnourishing argument, the mouths of those who complain, that they are willing to work, but can get no bread[....] But let the dinner be provided, and the argument loses nearly all its point. Abstinence is said to quicken the reasoning powers, and the observation applies as well to those who reason themselves from defective premises into wrong conclusions, as to others[....] but if it be true, as it seems to be almost universally admitted, that a sour and sullen spirit of insubordination is gaining fearful ground among the people, the first thing needful, in order to bring them to a better spirit, and to secure a considerate hearing for whatever may be addressed to them, in the way of good advice, will be to relieve their abject penury or at the least, to shew an honest and anxious desire to do so.

Parliament will very soon meet, under circumstances of a very peculiar and trying nature; and it will require no slight effort on its part to command the respect and confidence of the people. Never was a British Parliament more narrowly watched than it will be. It is not merely that it is a new Parliament, under a new sovereign, and that the affairs of government generally over the world are in an unusual state of disturbance; the Parliament has a character to make with the people. The contempt which the people entertained for the last Parliament was freely spoken of within the walls of the Houses. It was felt that Parliament was deficient in sympathy with the people, or, at all events, destitute of the energy and ability necessary to give effect to that sympathy, if it did exist; and the eagerness with which the public look for redeeming proceedings on the part of the new Parliament is unparalleled in its intensity and universality. It is, indeed, come to this: that, with the present temper and in the present circumstances of the people of this country, the very existence of the Parliament as at present constituted, and the permanence of the power interwoven with its present constitution, depends upon a revival of its energy, and a display of such qualities as may satisfy a thinking and examining people that it is worthy to have the management of their affairs. We earnestly hope, therefore, that no attempt will be made, as at the commencement of the last session, to escape from the question of the common people's condition; that Parliament will not hesitate to grapple with the truth and discuss it manfully and fearlessly; and thus shew itself worthy of the people's confidence. The best way to prevent revolution, is to shew the people that they have nothing to gain by it; and that those whom they permit to govern them, take as good care of them as any other whom they could choose[....] Much as has been said of the wasting away of respect for Parliament, in consequence of its not having kept pace with the intellectual improvement of the people at large, we are inclined to think that [Parliament] has lost much more of its influence, and of the sympathy which the people used to feel with it, through an affectation of political, which indulging itself in cold generalities and abstract propositions, seems to forget the present necessities of the people, and turn an unwilling, if not a contemptuous ear to their complaints[....] It is impossible for the sufferer not to feel a desire to bring down his kind advisor to the level of his own distress, that he might then see how his philosophy would console him in hopeless hunger[....] Now, without being in the least disposed to underrate the immense value of the power derived from machinery, and fully satisfied that to the aid derived from this power are we indebted for the high rank which we hold among the nations of the world, we would yet warn members of Parliament, and others, against supposing that the complaints of those who suffer from the use of machinery are unenlightened and absurd, and worthy only of derision[....] If instead of going backward in the view of the use of machinery, we carry it forward, and assume that all the work now done by manual labour may be done by machinery, this, according to the absolute principle of its utility, would be a great advantage. But what would then become of all those who live by the remuneration of labour, and who have no property? Would those who have property, and who avail themselves of the cheapness of machinery, share it with the people whose labour was no longer of any value as an equivalent? They would not;—but starvation would grow desperate, the rights of property would be violated, and a social chaos would ensue. The use of machinery, therefore, concurrently with the present system of the right of property, may be carried to such an excess, as would lead to the destruction of the latter[....] but while property continues in the hands of a few, and the mass of the people have nothing but their labour to offer in exchange for so much of it as their daily wants require, it is easy to see how the depression of the value of that labour may be carried so far as to compel them to resort to the law of nature, and violate the regulations of a society whose advantages they have no means of sharing in.

We have ventured to say so much upon this subject, because in the present period, when revolutions and new governments occupy a portion of almost every one's thoughts, the first principle of the social compact must necessarily come into frequent discussion, and the new powers of mankind be taken as an element in such considerations. When we consider how wonderfully the powers of production have been altered and improved, and how generally throughout the world we find suffering following from abundance, and perceive a want of demand equal to the powers of supply, it seems to be almost time that some serious alteration in the system of society should take place, so as to give mankind at large a fairer share of the advantages which our great improvements are capable of affording.

But whatever is done, we trust that in England it will be courageously, and soberly, and discreetly, after the manner of our fathers. Above all things, we hate a melodramatic air in politics; and a 'coup d'etat' is our special aversion. England cannot stop the progress of events; and if the world is changing, she must change with it; yet still, we venture to predict, maintaining her ancient character for boldness, regulated by calm and reflecting prudence.

56

WILLIAM COBBETT, 'FEELOSOFICAL QUACKERY'

Cobbett's Weekly Political Register, 74 (1831), pp. 551–558

William Cobbett (1763–1835) was certainly an irascible character, and that is why his writing is so fascinating to read. He saw the Industrial Revolution as a kind of insult to the rural and communal nature of life before the rise of the machine and capitalist economics. In this article, Cobbett shames those supposed altruists who viewed the poor as 'ignorant' and who saw education as their primary need. He suggests that the violence on the part of the working classes was occurring because the traditional home ties between the classes were now gone. Thus, rather than educating the so-called ignorant poor, Cobbett says the upper classes and their philosophers needed to be [r]educated themselves, as it were—in other words, they needed to learn, again, that the only answer to the violence was to help the labourers to live well and not starve. Referring to political economists as 'feelosofers' and 'quacks', Cobbett points out that it is necessary to feed a person before one can teach them—hence the need to 'establish well-loaded bacon racks in the villages instead of libraries'.

He begins by pointing out the faults of an article of 'quackery' in *The Morning Chronicle* of 23 November 1831, in which it was said:

> Why should there be a single district or corner of the country devoid of such excellent institutions as infant and industry schools, schools for mutual instruction [...]? Why are the poor unassisted by Governments in their endeavours to frame such establishments, and left to struggle for their attainment through destitution and difficulties, without any certain and definite aid? The aid is withheld, and the people are induced to consider the governing classes as the enemies [....] We may remember what a vast proportion of *the incendiaries* and rioters in the south last winter were *unable to* read—had not attained the first step to-wards *mental improvement* [....] *how can such ignorant beings* comprehend and feel the *advantages* resulting from the *guardianship of property,* even to him whose sole property consists in his daily labour?

Cobbett acidly analyses the article to amplify his own agenda for the poor.

DOI: 10.4324/9780429198052-62

56. William Cobbett, "Feelosofical Quackery', *Cobbett's Weekly Political Register* (1831)

There are but too many in this country who indulge in the delusion, that one part of society may set an example of heartless injustice, engrossing selfishness and rapacity without bound or limit, while the rest of society will contentedly respect and obey the laws[....] they say, or would say to the inquiring or disaffected poor, 'Thou art accustomed to comment on measures and interests that are beyond thy limited reason, and thou knowest that thy opinions have already drawn displeasure on thee. The ignorant and the low are to the state as children whose duty it is to obey, and not to cavil.' The day for this language to produce its effect in this country *is gone for ever*. Let us look around in every direction, and we shall see disaffected paupers, unwilling slaves, alienated from the institutions of a society which they think has treated them with injustice. The torch of the incendiary throughout all the agricultural counties of England ought to warn us of the danger of being surrounded by fellow-creatures between whom and ourselves there are no ties of sympathy, over whose minds we cease to possess influence[....]

[....] The *feelosofers* lay it down as an *axiom*, that *riots* and *fires* proceed from the *ignorance* of the perpetrators; and that *ignorance* consists in an inability to *write*, and to *read newspapers* and Brougham's stupid stuff called '*Useful Knowledge*.' This they lay down as an *axiom*. For want of being able to read thus, they hold that the poor creatures cannot comprehend the 'blessings of *accumulation*' they cannot 'comprehend and feel the '*advantage* resulting from the *guardianship* of *property*.' No, poor things, they cannot comprehend the advantage that results to them from barns and stacks being kept safe for the use of those who deny them all but potatoes, and hardly a stomach full of them. *The poor 'ignorant beings'* cannot comprehend and feel this advantage without the aid of 'apartments to read' Brougham's *Useful Knowledge*: much less can they comprehend and *feel the advantages* resulting from their being (men, old men, boys, and women) compelled to *starve*, or to draw carts and waggons like beasts of burden. it really does need a 'Labourers' Institute' to 'convince that it is advantageous to young women to have their long hair cut from their heads by a brutal hired overseer, and to have their bodies covered with serge with a badge on it; or to be compelled to be *prostitutes*, or to *starve*.' Poh! You miserable Scotch quacks! It is the employers that want to be *educated*: the landlords, parsons, and big farmers, want to be taught that it is their *true* interest in the end, to cause the working people to live well, and to possess the means of being well dressed[....]

But the *roguery* at the bottom is this! Those who put forth this quackery want the present *funding* and *taxing system* to go on: because, if it stop *they must go to work*. They rail against the *tithes*, indeed; but they want *all the rest to* go on. Now, it cannot go on without starving the labourers. These tax-eaters do not dare to say, in direct terms, that they wish the labourers to starve; and, therefore, they will *never allow* that the riots and the fires are *caused by the pinchings of hunger*. Hence they beat about for causes and, just at this time, their favourite cause is want of *'labourer's institutes,'* in which the labourers are made to see clearly, that it is *reasonable* and *just* that they who make to come all the meat and bread and beer and wool and leather, to live upon potatoes and water and go half-naked in their bodies and barefooted. Poh! You quacks; you Scotch quacks; establish well-loaded bacon racks in the villages instead of libraries; teach the landlords and farmers to feed and clothe the working-people well; and then they may sleep in safety: otherwise they never will again, though the world be inundated by your miserable roguish quackery.

57

ANON., 'THE INTERPRETER: WHERE MAY ONE STARVE?'

Figaro in London, 2 (1833), pp. 169–170

This piece hilariously and caustically points out how nothing stops hunger and if the State did not ensure a comfortable level of living to labourers, it had to expect crime to increase, in some cases because prison at least provided decent meals, in contrast to the workhouse.

DOI: 10.4324/9780429198052-63

57. Anon., 'The Interpreter: Where may one Starve?', *Figaro in London* (1833)

Dialogue Between a Magistrate and a Beggar

—A miserable-looking young man, named *William Walworth*, having been proved guilty of soliciting charity near the reservoir in the Green Park, the following dialogue took place between him and Mr. White, the Magistrate:—

Magistrate. —Well, master, what have you to say to the charge?—

Prisoner —I thought it better to beg than steal, your Worship.

Magistrate —I think so too, but you must know that both are offences against the law; and it is told us that, as soon as we are able to read and write, we ought to get our living in the sweat of our brow.

Prisoner —Very true, Sir, but it appears that I am doomed to get my living by the sweat of my brow at the tread-mill.

Magistrate —Pray where do you come from master?

Prisoner —I come from Finching, in Wilts, your Worship.

Magistrate —Why did you not stop there, master? What did you come here for, eh?

Prisoner —Why I thought I might as well starve here as there. I thought I could better my condition here.

Magistrate —In the course of my experience I have found many such as you, who would rather starve from home than at home; but it is my duty to send you to the House of Correction for fourteen days.

Prisoner —Thank you, master, I am much obliged to you.

Prisoner was then removed to the lock-up.—*Daily Papers*[....]

[....] In the instance above recited, White with humanity so peculiar to the magisterial bench, sends a man to prison for fourteen days, because he has ventured upon the horrible offence of attempting to avoid starvation by asking charity. The conclusion come to is nothing new, but the dialogue which led to it is worthy of remark, from the novelty of some of the opinions broached by the magistrate. White is courteous enough to admit that begging is better than stealing though he sees enormity in both, and wisely suggests that 'men should look to the sweat of their brows for a livelihood.' Now does White presume to declare that a man may live upon mere sweat, a suggestion which savours equally of filth and cruelty. The beggar shrewdly enough observes, that 'it seems he must get his living by the sweat of his brow at the tread-mill.' The mendicant was right—sweat he must somehow, if he expects to live, even when his perspiration does no good to any one. White then enquires why the poor devil did not stay to starve in his native place, and actually commits him to prison for daring to have any choice as to the place where he should undergo the process of starvation. It is a refinement indeed on oppression when a man is not only left to the most utter destitution, but is positively thrust into a dungeon because he has presumed to use his own discretion as to the place for starving in. If a man must die of want, surely he has a right to die in town, without being packed off to the tread-mill, for being found among the arrivals in the metropolis. An empty pocket and a vacant stomach are never very welcome visitors anywhere, but in London where people regard one another just in proportion as they hope to make something out of one another, poverty and hunger are things almost certain to find their way in a week to the tread-mill.

58

ANON., '*THE TOWN*, A MINISTERIAL PAPER'

Leicester, or Commercial Agricultural Chronicle (1 June 1833), p. 4

This humourous piece goes far in deconstructing the radical cause through transmogrification of its rhetoric. As such, 'The Town' gives a 'skeleton' or snapshot of a radical's speech by using what we might now refer to as all the 'dog whistles' one might expect from radical ideologies of the time. Those dog whistles are racist; in particular to Africa and Native Americans. But though this spoof undermines radical righteous anger, it ultimately recognises the distress fueling such rhetoric. Indeed, starvation quietly stands at the centre of the litany, indicating that, at the very least, the writer understands that lower-class hunger *was* the point and that starvation would always viscerally parlay its demands in one form or another.

The tattoo is a musical performance by a military group. Many of the names mentioned are fictional; but Richard Carlile (1790–1843) was a notable radical of the time and Henry Hetheringon (1792–1849) was a radical bookseller; MP John Josiah Guest (1785–1852) was a Welsh ironworker; I have been unable to find an MP from this time period with the last name of George. The reference to the standing army was an acknowledgement that there had been no standing armies before the Napoleonic Wars and that the State was now using them to round up and intimidate the labourers who protested. Labourers felt a standing army was essentially a means of undermining democracy. The poor reviled taxes on windows, a crude means for the government to make money; 'aquafortis' is another name for 'nitric acid'.

DOI: 10.4324/9780429198052-64

58. Anon., '*The Town*, a Ministerial Paper', *Leicester, or Commercial Agricultural Chronicle* (1833)

The Town, a ministerial paper, gives the following as a text-book of 'Radical Rhetoric:—A meeting was held on Wednesday, in the borough, at which Mr. Bailey acted as Chairman, and made the following energetic speech:—Police—bloody brutal Whigs—murder—bludgeons—massacre—scalps war-whoop, Cherokees—African lions, tigers, hell-hounds—tyranny, bloody, savage ambition—people must fight—rights, liberties, constitution, violation, despoliation, damnation—brickbats, pokers, spits, scythes, toasting forks, broom sticks, cabbage stumps, rotten eggs—caps of liberty, flags, banners, death's dead and cross bones, union. Messrs. George and Guest seconded a resolution to the following effect:—Whigs, villains, monsters, hippopotami, salamanders, murderers, manglers and Muscovites—no faith, defiance, hatred, detestation abhorrence, revenge, courage, union, order, peace, love, justice, justifiable homicide, manslaughter for ever! Mr. Lee, who ran off with orator Mee, spoke in the following energetic manner:—England, glory, price power, debt, misery, starvation—bayonets, standing army, tithes, bishops, blood, callous hardened Pharoahs, Genghis Khan, Tamerlane, Barbarossa, Nero, Caligula, Marius, Sylla, Brutus, liberty, freedom, equality, destruction, reformation, excitation, agitation, reservation, light of nature, window taxes, taxes of candles, God of nature, wheat a shilling a bushel, Christianity, takes of newspapers, Carlile, Hetherington, bloody *Times* glass bottles, flint stones, smashification, battering rams, blunderbusses, raw head and bloody bones, Terrific Register, daggers, poinards, bomb shells, red host balls, two edged swords, double-headed shot, fire, horror, death or liberty—patience, petition, tattooing, carbines, gunpowder, vitriol, aquafortis, millstones, peace, fury, safety, blood, obedience, revenge, pity, slaughter, love, murder, hellfire, brimstone, sulphur, happiness, torment, chaos, order, smoke. We have given these skeleton speeches, and shall be happy to supply them to all the radical orators of the day, as they embody the leading articles of all the topic necessary for a red-hot speech, or boiling lava kind of address, so necessary at the present crisis.

59

PETER QUIZ, 'RADICAL SHOOTING. LETTER TO EDITOR OF THE *BRIGHTON PATRIOT*'

Brighton Patriot and Lewes Free Press (7 April 1835), p. 4

This is another example of brilliant witty writing from the voice of a radical defying British suppression of the lower-class voices in the order of Swift's 'A Modest Proposal'. It also portends the modern short story 'The Most Dangerous Game' by Richard Connell, in which hunting and killing human beings is represented as the ultimate game. Apparently Captain Shelley (dates unknown) had made a rousing speech at a dinner at Town Hall in Brighton and is reported to have said that he 'was quite sure that the army was ready to shoot every radical', to which Peter Quiz found good grounds for his satirical response.[89]

DOI: 10.4324/9780429198052-65

59. Peter Quiz, 'Radical Shooting. Letter to Editor of the *Brighton Patriot*', *Brighton Patriot and Lewes Free* Press (1835)

RADICAL SHOOTING.

To the Editor of the Brighton Patriot.

SIR,—In your zeal for the radical cause, you appear to have overlooked the motives which actuated Captain Adolphus Shelley, when he expressed his belief that 'the Army was ready to shoot all the Radicals.' It is the misfortune of contracted minds that they only look to the surface of things; and permit me to say that I am surprised you should not have sufficient discrimination to discover the grand and comprehensive designs which pervaded the brains of Captain S. when he made that noble and patriotic speech. Brains did I say! Perhaps I am in error. If so, I humbly beg pardon:—I have no wish to accuse any man of possessing that which does not belong to him. Be this as it may, Captain S. deserves the thanks of the country; and who is there, even amongst the Rads themselves, whose heart does not beat with grateful joy at the bare thought of being shot by a lord or a lordling! Only think of the honor of receiving an ounce of warm lead from the exalted hands of an Earl or Duke! Think of the ecstatic delight attending the dying under such circumstances! But I must not dwell too long on this theme, lest it create so violent a competition to be shot, among the radicals, as to be attended with inconvenience.

My object is to convince you (who it seems have no taste for imaginative pleasures and such as these), by reason and argument, of the national blessings and benefits which this radical shooting is certain to produce. In the first place you confess that many of the radicals are in want of the common necessaries of life;—why then would you deny them the privilege of a short and pleasant death? Cruel, heartless man! Would you wish them to linger in starvation. You acknowledge a dearth of employment. Short sighted mortal! Is it not evident that, thinning the Rads in this way would lessen the demand for it, and consequently produce an abundance of work and high wages for those left behind? You complain of the game laws—would not this neutralize them? Who would care about a trumpery partridge, if we were permitted to bag several good fat radicals in the course of a day; and with what pleasure would one of our aristocratic sprigs read an invitation worded thus:—

> 'Captain Sir Adolphus Shootrad presents his compliments to Lord Henry Augustus Bring-emdown, and would feel honoured with his company at Popaway Hall, on Tuesday next, for a day's radical shooting.

P. S. Excellent sport is expected, as a public meeting will take place the same day[....]

After so many years of profound peace, the inefficiency of the army will be readily admitted. Here then is an opportunity for excellent practice. Instead of firing at targets or such like children's toys, they would be able to exercise their courage and skill on *real* men, and to acquire a knowledge of military tactics without the danger of being hurt[....]

If asked what should be done with the dead game, I answer that on this point I pride myself, establishing as it will a new era in political economy. Let it be pickled; part of it should be sent to the starving Irish in return for their exports, part used for home consumption, part reserved for contingencies:—to victual our fleet, for instance, in the event of a sudden equipment, and the remainder placed at the disposal of the Poor Law Commissioners. This may appear monstrous to persons of squeamish sensibilities; but in this age of innovation we must not suffer ancient prejudices to stand in the way of useful improvements. It will have the effect of reducing the price of provisions, so necessary to the poor man's comfort; and I have no doubt that when the practice becomes general, the radical tub in the labourer's cottage will be as common as the pork tub was formerly. In conclusion Sir, if this project should be deemed impracticable, allow me to suggest that in order to exterminate the radicals, they should be obliged to eat each other, and that, following the example of the surviving hostile cat, means should be devised to make the last one eat himself.

I am, Sir, your obedient Servant,
PETER QUIZ.

60

TESTIMONY FROM REV. GEORGE STRINGER BULL, 14 AUGUST 1838, *SELECT COMMITTEE OF HOUSE OF LORDS ON OPERATION OF POOR LAW AMENDMENT ACT*

Hansard, HC (1837–1838), Volume 41, Images 232–234, 255–256

In this exchange George Stringer Bull (1799–1865), the cleric and reformer who despised the premises of the Poor Laws, strongly condemns the State for committing 'murder' when it ignored the needs of the poor. Thus, he turns the tables on the reasoning that poverty itself was a crime.

 DOI: 10.4324/9780429198052-66

60. Testimony from Rev. George Stringer Bull, 14 Aug 1838, *Select Committee of House of Lords on Operation of Poor Law Amendment Act. Report, Minutes of Evidence, Index* (1838)

Are not the Union Workhouses generally called and considered Prisons or Bastiles?

That Name is frequently used as a Term to characterize them; and I apprehend it could be proved that not Six Persons out of a Hundred applying for Relief that are offered Relief in the Workhouses accept the Offer.'

[....] 'Have you ever used the Word 'Prison'?

I have called them Workhouse Prisons.

How do you define a Prison?

Because Persons are there subject in a very great measure, as I am informed, to Prison Discipline, frequently to Prison Dress and Prison Confinement, and I must say frequently to worse than Prison Fare.

[The Question is repeated.]

A Place of Confinement and Coercion.

With or without the Consent of the Person confined?

In the Case of a Prison, without the Consent of the Person confined.

And out of which he cannot get whenever he chooses?

Certainly.

Is that the Case with any of the Union Workhouses?

In the Case of the Workhouse the Consent of the Person is obtained upon, I conceive, unreasonable and illegal Conditions. Hunger drives him there, and he must submit to the Confinement of the Prison, and must consent to submit to it, before he can satisfy his Hunger.

He can come out of it when he likes?

Yes, but he must submit to Starvation as the attendant Condition of Liberty.

Has this Boy [a child he helped] submitted to Starvation as the Alternative of his not going to this Prison?

No, he has not; he has found a Friend.

If all these Horrors existed in the Poorhouse at Towcester [a 'Black Hole' for those not following rules, which is next to the 'Dead House,' mandatory cutting of hair, physical discipline, illegally separating husband from wife] how came it that you have not stated them either to the Board of Guardians or to the Poor Law Commissioners, in order that they might be removed?

I have thought best to appeal to Parliament, who have the Power of removing the Root of the Evil.

It would take some Time to remove the Root of the Evil; but would it not be a more ready Way to apply to those Persons that could have immediately removed the Evil?

I think not; I think the best Way is to lay the Axe to the Root of the Tree[....]

Do not you think that the Workhouse being only provided for Persons who are unable to support themselves, and can show that they are unable to support themselves, that it is necessary that it should in some Degree be a rigorous System?

I consider that there ought to be no Rigour whatever in granting Relief to the Poor.

Do you think that Persons in the Workhouse ought to be better off, and have as little Restraint as they would have in their own Houses?

No; but I think they ought not to be worse, because Poverty is not a Crime.

In that Case, how would you prevent all the Inhabitants who happened not to be in very good Circumstances from going into the Workhouse?

I conceive that, according to the Suggestion in the Question, Prevention is better than Cure, and that if the Legislature, whose Duty it is to attend to these Matters, had endeavoured to prevent Poverty, rather than to adopt a rigorous System for punishing it, it would have been far better.

How are they to prevent Poverty?

There might be many Regulations adopted for the Purpose of encouraging Industry and preventing Poverty; but it is not for me to suggest to your Lordships, whose special Duty this is, what should be done in such Cases[....]

[....] What Class of Persons do you call Oppressors of the Poor?

Any Persons who by harsh Measures drive the Poor to commit such Acts [suicide] as were there alleged.

[....] Do you mean that the Three Estates of the Realm [monarchy; nobles; and the lower and middle classes], who passed the Act of Parliament, are the Oppressors of the Poor?

[....] I think that the Act has that Effect[....] If any Person knowing that to be the Effect of an Act enforces it to the Destruction of the Poor, or to drive them to Self-destruction, I conceive that they are morally guilty of Murder.

[....] Therefore if the Board of Guardians under the Orders of the Commissioners who are entitled to give such Orders by that Act of Parliament [the Poor laws], refuse Relief to a Pauper, and he hangs himself, they are guilty of Murder; is that what you mean to say?

I do mean to say that; I mean to say in effect that whatever harsh and severe Regulations are pressed upon a Pauper leading or driving him to Self-destruction, the Persons so exercising those Regulations are morally guilty of Murder, in my Opinion.

61

ANON., 'STEALING FROM STARVATION'

The Champion and Weekly Herald (2 December 1838), p. 4

This is a spoof on the Poor Laws and their complexity and obscurity. But it also shows their irrational effects, that is, that it quickly becomes apparent to the poor and hungry that it is better to commit a crime in order to be fed in prison than to remain a good citizen and starve.

DOI: 10.4324/9780429198052-67

61. Anon., 'Stealing from Starvation', *Champion and Weekly Herald* (1838)

[....] The COMMON SERGEANT: Well, sir, how is it that you make your second appearance here so soon?

Prisoner: Why, my lord, the fact is, I came out of the House of Correction in August last without a penny and with my character blasted; and I assure you, my lord, I have since that time travelled 800 miles in search of work; but, unfortunately, without success. Our trade has, in many parts, been entirely broken up; and the opening of the Birmingham and other railways has thrown more than 2000 shoeing smiths out of employ.

The COMMON SERGEANT: But notwithstanding you are poor, you should not resort to thieving.

Prisoner: Oh, my lord, hunger and starvation will drive a man to commit acts which he would otherwise scorn.

The COMMON SERGEANT: Then you should apply to your parish, and they will relieve you.

The prisoner shook his head.

The COMMON SERGEANT: Where do you belong to?

Prisoner: [....] Really, my lord, there are so many clauses in the Poor-law Amendment Act which clash one against the other, that no person seems able to understand them. (Laughter.) It's all very well laughing, but I declare I had no food for two days, nor a bed for three nights, before I committed this offence, and I will candidly admit I did it on purpose to be taken into custody; what else could I do[....] I would certainly rather leave the country than be compelled to starve in it.

62

A COMMISSIONER, 'INTERCEPTED REPORT OF A POOR LAW COMMISSIONER'

Figaro in London, 21 (1839), p. 18

This is another satire, illustrating the view that the rich were using the Poor Laws to rid the country of the poor through 'exterminat[ion]' by starvation. Here the famous Prime Minister John Russell becomes the butt of the joke.

DOI: 10.4324/9780429198052-68

62. A Commissioner, 'Intercepted Report of a Poor Law Commissioner', *Figaro in London* (1839)

TO LORD JOHN RUSSELLL.

My Lord.—I am happy to have to inform your Lordship that the job in which we are mutually interested, namely, the continuance of the Amended Poor Law Commissions, has every prospect of being continued; for though nothing can be more unpopular than ourselves as a body, still by our unbridled power, we have contrived to obtain such a sway, that nothing short of the devil himself could shake us, and as, my Lord, the devil happens to be all on our side (not to say our immediate patron), there is no fear of any hostility in that quarter.

Your Lordship is, I believe that our unpopularity is chiefly among the poor, and therefore, my Lord, it has appeared prudent to us to exterminate the poor as speedily as possible.

I am happy to have to inform your Lordship that we are getting rid of the poor rapidly in every quarter of the kingdom, and I am delighted to add, that we have been aided in our views by several fatal diseases, which have decimated the work-houses, and of course, therefore, greatly diminished the evil of poverty. We shall continue to adhere rigidly to the principles of starvation, upon which we have to the present so successfully acted, and I remain, my Lord, your Lordship's obedient servant.

A COMMISSIONER.

Notes

1. A. Sen, *Poverty and Famines: An Essay on Entitlement and Deprivation* (Oxford: Clarendon Press, 1981).
2. S. Devereux, *Theories of Famine* (New York: Harvester Wheatsheaf, 1993); M. Davis, *Late Victorian Holocausts; El Niño Famines and the Making of the Third World* (London: Verso, 2001), p. 39.
3. P. Mandler, *The Uses of Charity: The Poor on Relief in the Nineteenth-Century Metropolis* (Philadelphia: University of Pennsylvania Press, 2016), p. 1.
4. L Schlossberg, '"The Low, Vague Hum of Numbers": Malthusian Economies of *Jane Eyre*', *Victorian Literature and Culture*, 29 (2002), pp. 489–506, on p. 494.
5. A. Brundage, *The English Poor Laws, 1700–1930* (Basingstoke: Palgrave, 2002), pp. 29, 36, 40, 25.
6. E. P. Thompson, 'The Moral Economy of the English Crowd in the Eighteenth Century', *Past and Present*, 50 (1971), pp. 76–136; see A. Bentley, 'Reading Food Riots: Scarcity, Abundance and National Identity', in Peter Scholliers (ed.), *Food, Drink, and Identity: Cooking, Eating, and Drinking in Europe Since the Middle Ages* (Oxford: Berg Press, 2001), pp. 179–193, on p. 182.
7. D. Reisman, *Thomas Robert Malthus* (New York: Palgrave Macmillan, 2018), p. 22.
8. J. L. Hammond and B. Hammond, *Village Labourer, 1760–1832: A Study in the Government of England before the Reform Bill* (London: Longmans, Green, 1920); qtd in S. A. Shave, *Pauper Policies: Poor Law Practice in England, 1780–1850* (Manchester: Manchester University Press, 2017), p. 2.
9. '*Spectator*', 'Economical Suffering and Political Discontent', *Bradford Observer*, 21 June 1838, p. [1].
10. A. Kidd, *State, Society and the Poor in Nineteenth-Century England* (Basingstoke: Macmillan, 1999), p. 5.
11. J. Burnett, *Plenty and Want: A Social History of Food in England from 1815 to the Present Day*, 3rd ed. (New York: Routledge,1989), p. 35; qtd in C. Boyce, 'Representing the "Hungry Forties" in Image and Verse: The Politics of Hunger in Early-Victorian Illustrated Periodicals', *Victorian Literature and Culture*, 40 (2012), pp. 421–449, on p. 423.
12. I. Gazeley and S. Horrell, 'Nutrition in the English agricultural labourer's household over the course of the long nineteenth century', *Economic History Review*, 66 (2013), pp. 757–84, on p. 770; S. Szreter, 'Economic Growth, Disruption, Deprivation, Disease, Death: On the Importance of the Politics of Public Health for Development', *Population and Development Review*, 23 (1997), pp. 693–728, on p. 694.
13. E. Griffin, 'Diets, Hunger and Living Standards During the British Industrial Revolution', *Past and Present*, no. 239 (2018), pp. 71–111, on pp. 76–77, 97, 103.

14. Gazeley and Horrell, pp. 769, 759; see also R. Floud, K. Wachter, and A. Gregory, *Height, Health and History: Nutritional Status in the United Kingdom, 1750–1980* (Cambridge: Cambridge University Press, 1990), pp. 134–154.
15. Gazeley and Horrell, pp. 767, 782.
16. See Griffin, pp. 83, 89, 76; D. Davies, *The Case of the Labourers in Husbandry Stated and Considered* (1795). F. M. Morton, *The State of the Poor: A History of the Labouring Classes in England* (London, 1928).
17. British Library (hereafter BL), Collections, Printed and Ms., Relating to the Repeal of the Laws against Combinations of Workmen, 1734–1826, vol. 8, Forming an Appendix to Add Mss 27798. 1734–1826. MS Radical Politics and the Working Man in England. Part One; Additional Manuscripts 27789-27830, 27806, p. 346. Nineteenth Century Collections Online (hereafter NCCO).
18. Qtd in A. Bashford and J. E. Chaplin, *The New Worlds of Thomas Robert Malthus: Rereading the Principle of Population* (Princeton: Princeton University Press, 2016), p. 2; Wrigley, 'Standing Between Two Worlds', in E. A. Wrigley and D. Souden, *Works of Thomas Robert Malthus* (London: Routledge, 1986).
19. D. Hume, *Political Discourses*, ed. William Bell Robertson (London: Walter Scott Publishing), p. 19; Project Gutenberg: https://www.gutenberg.org/files/59792/59792-h/59792-h.htm.
20. Schlossberg, p. 493.
21. W. R. Greg, *Enigmas of Life*, 4th ed. (London: Trübner, 1873), p. 59.
22. *An Essay on the Principle of Population* (London: J. Johnson, 1798), p. 1, https://www.gutenberg.org/files/4239/4239-h/4239-h.htm; qtd in Schlossberg, p. 494.
23. Boyce, p. 424.
24. https://www.gutenberg.org/files/4239/4239-h/4239-h.htm.
25. S. Bhattacharya, 'Victorian Hunger: Charles Dickens, Elizabeth Gaskell, Henry Mayhew' (PhD thesis, University of Southern California, Los Angeles, 2002), p. 1; qtd in T. Moore, 'Starvation in Victorian Christmas Fiction', *Victorian Literature and Culture*, 36 (2008), pp. 489–505, on p. 490; Schlossberg, p. 496.
26. Schlossberg, pp. 494–495; J. P. Huzel, *The Popularization of Malthus in Early Nineteenth-Century England: Martineau, Cobbett and the Pauper Press* (Farnham, Surrey: Ashgate, 2006), p. 3.
27. Anon., 'Art. V. Corn-Law Fallacies, with the Answers', *Eclectic review*, 5 (1839), pp. 79–98, on p. 97.
28. Anon., 'Mr. Godwin's Work on Population', *Morning Chronicle*, 26 December 1820, p. [4].
29. Schlossberg, p. 494.
30. Brundage, p. 11.
31. Anon., 'Seditious Meeting Bill', *Times* (hereafter TDA), 1 December 1819, p. 3.
32. Anon., 'Seditious Meeting Bill', *TDA*, 1 December 1819, p. 3.
33. See Thompson, 'Moral Economy', pp. 76–136; and Bentley, p. 182.
34. C. Fitzwilliam, *First, Second, and Third Addresses to the Landowners of England on the Corn Laws;* qtd in Moore, p. 492.
35. Anon., 'Progress of the Corn Law Question', *Examiner* (1842), p. 771.
36. [Alfred Mallalieu], 'The Corn Law Question', *Blackwood's Edinburgh Magazine*, 35 (1834), pp. 792–802, on p. 798.
37. T. de Quincey, 'Dilemmas on the Corn Law Question', *Blackwood's Edinburgh Magazine*, 45 (1839), pp. 170–176, on p. 170.
38. Qtd in J. R. Wordie, 'Perceptions and Reality: the Effects of the Corn Laws and their Repeal in England, 1815–1906', in Wordie (ed.), *Agriculture and Politics in England, 1815–1939* (London: Palgrave Macmillan, 2000), pp. 33–69, on pp. 35–36; see also Wordie, pp. 36, 45, 49, 50.

39. B. Harris, 'The New Poor Law and the Relief of Poverty, 1834–1914', in *The Origins of the British Welfare State: State and Social Welfare in England and Wales, 1800–1945* (Basingstoke: Palgrave Macmillan, 2004), pp. 40–58, on p. 45; M. D. Button and J. A. Sheetz-Nguyen, (eds), *Victorians and the Case for Charity: Essays on Responses to English Poverty by the State, the Church and the Literati* (Jefferson, North Carolina: McFarland, 2014), p. 21; see also D. Vincent, *Bread, Knowledge, Freedom: A Study of Nineteenth-Century Working Class Autobiography* (New York: Methuen, 1982).
40. Anon., 'On the Poor Laws', *Brighton Patriot and South of England Free Press*, 15 August 1837, p. [4].
41. Anon., 'Poor Law Murders', *Figaro in London*, 6 (1837), p. 83.
42. Anon., 'Art. V. Corn-Law Fallacies, with the Answers', *Eclectic Review*, 5 (1839), pp. 79–98, on p. 81; Anon., 'The Guttling and Guzzling System of the Whigs', *Morning Post*, 14 September 1836, p. [3].
43. Kidd, pp. 14, 25.
44. Kidd, p. 27.
45. Huzel, p. 1; K. Polyani, *The Great Transformation: The Political and Economic Origins of Our Time*, 2nd ed. (Boston: Beacon Press, 2001), p. 87; qtd in Huzel, p. 1.
46. 'Poor-Laws Bill', Commons Sitting, Hansard, HC © British Library Board vol. 8, cols 865–921 (19 February 1807).
47. Brundage, p. 11.
48. This information comes from Susan Brink, 'What Happens to the Body and Mind When Starvation Sets In?' National Public Radio, 20 January 2016: https://www.npr.org/sections/goatsandsoda/2016/01/20/463710330/what-happens-to-the-body-and-mind-when-starvation-sets-in; see also Ancel Keys and the University of Minnesota, Laboratory of physiological Hygiene, *The Biology of Human Starvation* (Minneapolis: University of Minnesota Press, 1950).
49. Boyce, p. 424; Mandler, p.1.
50. Anon., 'Investigation of the State of the Poor', *Literary Panorama*, 2 (1807), pp. 225–255, on p. 251.
51. Kidd, p. 30; Boyce, pp. 422, 444; Vernon, p. 17; qtd in Boyce, pp. 424–425.
52. Wordie, p. 39; E. Hobsbawm, 'The Machine Breakers' in *Labouring Men: Studies in the History of Labour* (London: Weidenfield and Nicolson, 1968), p. 59; qtd in Bentley, p. 183.
53. Anon., 'The Relative Condition of Rich and Poor Considered', *Poor Man's Guardian* (1833), pp. 25–26, on p. 26.
54. Anon., 'ART. I. –Further Observations on the State of the Nation', *Critical Review*, 5th series, 4 (1816), pp. 441–456, on p. 442.
55. Anon.,'Public Meeting at Glossop', *Northern Star*, 10 March 1838, p. 3.
56. Anon., 'Public Meeting at Glossop', *Northern Star*, 10 March 1838, p. 3; Anon., 'The Victimized Cotton Spinners', *Northern Star*, 24 March 1838, p. 3; Anon.,'The Damnable Act', *Northern Star*, 24 March 1838, p. [3]; Anon., 'Consolidation of the Productive Classes', *Poor Man's Guardian*, 30 August 1834, p. 237.
57. Anon., 'A Comparative View of the Vices and Virtues of the TWO Orders of Society, viz. the RICH and the POOR', *Black Dwarf*, 1 (1817), pp. 287–288, on p. 287.
58. Anon., 'Public Meeting of the Inhabitants of Glasgow, in the Bazaar', *Northern Liberator*, 13 January 1838, p. [1].
59. Anon., 'Public Meeting in Favour of the Glasgow Cotton Spinners', *Northern Liberator*, 18 November 1837, p. [4].
60. Anon., 'The Distress', *Sheffield Independent*, 8 June 1833, pp. 1–4, on p.1.
61. T. Sokoll, *Essex Pauper Letters, 1731–1837* (Oxford: Oxford University Press, 2001).
62. Anon., 'An Address from the Framework-Knitters to the Gentlemen Hosiers of the Town of Nottingham', *Nottingham* Review, 29 November 1811.

63. OED. https://www-oed-com.libproxy.unm.edu/view/Entry/55762?rskey=b5PZts&result=1&isAdvanced=false#eid.
64. J. L. Hammond and B. Hammond, p. 220.
65. Anon., 'Proposed Refusal to Support the Poor, and to Abolish the Poor Laws', *Black Dwarf*, 6 (1821), pp. 773–778, on pp. 773, 774.
66. Anon., 'Acts of the "Collective Wisdom" of the "Thunderers"', *Black Dwarf*, 8 (1822), pp. 345–355, on p. 348.
67. Anon., 'Interesting Statements Respecting the Manufacture of Nottingham and Its Neighbourhood', *Nottingham Review*, 29 November 1811.
68. Anon., 'State of Public Feeling in Scotland', *Blackwood's Edinburgh Magazine*, 31 (1832), pp. 65–76, on pp. 67–68.
69. Anon., 'Machine-Breakers and Stack-Burners Against the Boroughmongers', *Voice of the People*, 8 January 1831. Working Men-Machine Breaking—National Association for Wages, Etc. 1831–1839, MS Radical Politics and the Working Man in England, Part Two, Set 51, p. 143. NCCO.
70. Anon., 'Address of the Relief Committee of Stockport to the Public', Cotton and Silk, 1811–1832, MS Radical Politics and the Working Man in England: Part One, Set 16; Vol. 2. BL. NCCO.
71. E. Curran, 'Manchester Weavers Petition', to Mr. Joseph Hume (1827), Cotton and Silk, 1811–32, MS Radical Politics and the Working Man in England: Part One, Set 16; Vol. 2. BL. NCCO.
72. Anon., 'Meeting of the Cotton-Spinners', *Morning Chronicle*, 6 July 1825, p. [4].
73. Anon., 'The Infernal Enactment', *Northern Liberator*, 26 May 1838, p. [3].
74. 'Currency, Corn Laws, and Crime, To the Editor of The Morning Chronicle', *Morning Chronicle*, 6 December 1825, p. [3].
75. R. Moore, Secretary to Weaver's Committee to Unionize the Workers, 'Address to the Much-Injured Part of the Community, the Cotton Weavers, Petition', 1 March 1825. Collections, Printed and Ms., Relating to the Repeal of the Laws against Combinations of Workmen, 1734–1826, vol. III, App. To Add. Mss. 27798. NCCO.
76. Anon., 'The Reform Egg', *Figaro in London*, 2 (1833), pp. 169–170.
77. R. Taylor, Secretary, 'To the Manufacturers, Mechanics, Artisans, and Others, (Inhabitants of Manchester and Its Vicinity) Who Signed and Supported the Late Petition to the House of Commons'. Letters and Papers Supplementary, 1811, September to November 1811. MS Home Office (hereafter HO) Papers and Records, Part Five: HO 42, Box 117. NCCO.
78. 'Political Power and British Economic Life, 1650–1870', in R. Floud, J. Humphries, P. Johnson (eds), *The Cambridge Economic History of Modern Britain, Vol. I: 1700–1870* (Cambridge: Cambridge University Press, 2014), pp. 345–367, on p. 361.
79. *The Trial against Isaac Eaton, for publishing a supposed libel, intituled Politics for the people; or, hog's wash: at just hall in Old Bailey* (London: Daniel Isaac Eaton, 1794). NCCO.
80. 'Letter from a Briton', 27 May 1812. Letters and Papers 1812, May, MS HO Papers and Records: Part Five: HO 42, 1810–1812 Box 123, National Archives, Kew (hereafter NA). NCCO.
81. p. 40.
82. Anon., 'Bristol Election. An Account of Mr. Hunt's Public Reception in Bristol, May 18, 1812' (Bristol: W. Major, 1812), pp. 4, 5, 7. Letters and Papers. 1812. July 1812. MS HO Papers and Records: Part Five: HO 42, Box 125. NA. NCCO.
83. Anon., 'Folly and Villainy of the Ministry—Manchester Meeting', *Sherwin's Weekly Political Register*, 5 (1819), pp. 221–236, on pp. 221, 223.
84. pp. 4, 8, 36, 37.

85. 'State of the Manufacturing Districts', *TDA*, 10 December 1819, p. 2.
86. Quoted in this article on p. 14.
87. 'Politic and Social Experiments of 1819', *Morning Post*, 26 July 1819, p. [2].
88. 'London, Tuesday, August 24, 1819', p. 2.
89. See 'Local News', *Brighton Patriot*, 24 March 1845.

INDEX